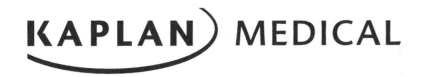

KAPLAN) MEDICAL

T0351872

CLINICAL MANAGEMENT REVIEW 2023–2024 VOLUME 2

FOR USMLE® STEP 3 AND COMLEX-USA® LEVEL 3

USMLE® (United States Medical Licensing Examination®) is a joint program of the National Board of Medical Examiners (NBME) and the Federation of State Medical Boards (FSMB). COMLEX-USA® is a registered trademark of the National Board of Osteopathic Medical Examiners, Inc. (NBOME). These organizations are not affiliated with Kaplan, and neither endorse nor contribute to the creation of this product.

USMLE® (United States Medical Licensing Examination®) is a joint program of the National Board of Medical Examiners (NBME) and the Federation of State Medical Boards (FSMB). COMLEX-USA® is a registered trademark of the National Board of Osteopathic Medical Examiners, Inc. (NBOME). These organizations are not affiliated with Kaplan, and neither endorse nor contribute to the creation of this product.

This publication is designed to provide accurate information in regard to the subject matter covered as of its publication date, with the understanding that knowledge and best practice constantly evolve. The publisher is not engaged in rendering medical, legal, accounting, or other professional service. If medical or legal advice or other expert assistance is required, the services of a competent professional should be sought. This publication is not intended for use in clinical practice or the delivery of medical care. To the fullest extent of the law, neither the Publisher nor the Editors assume any liability for any injury and/or damage to persons or property arising out of or related to any use of the material contained in this book.

© 2023 by Kaplan North America, LLC

Published by Kaplan Medical, a division of Kaplan North America, LLC.
1515 West Cypress Creek Road
Fort Lauderdale, Florida 33309

All rights reserved. The text of this publication, or any part thereof, may not be reproduced in any manner whatsoever without written permission from the publisher. This book may not be duplicated or resold, pursuant to the terms of your Kaplan Enrollment Agreement.

10   9   8   7   6   5   4   3   2   1

Course ISBN: 978-1-5062-8329-6
Course Kit ISBN: 978-1-5062-8333-3

Retail ISBN: 978-1-5062-8577-1
Retail Kit ISBN: 978-1-5062-8331-9

Kit items come as a set and should not be broken out and sold separately.

Kaplan Publishing print books are available at special quantity discounts to use for sales promotions, employee premiums, or educational purposes. For more information or to purchase books, please call the Simon & Schuster special sales department at 866-506-1949.

EDITORS

Pediatrics

Eduardo Pino, MD
Associate Professor, Department of Pediatrics
Marshall University School of Medicine
Medical Director, Pediatric ICU
Cabell Huntington Hospital
Huntington, WV

Gynecology and Obstetrics

Elmar Peter Sakala, MD, MA, MPH, FACOG
Professor of Gynecology and Obstetrics
Division of Maternal Fetal Medicine
Department of Gynecology and Obstetrics
Loma Linda University School of Medicine
Loma Linda, CA

Surgery

Mark Nolan Hill, MD, FACS
Professor of Surgery
Chicago Medical School
Chicago, IL

We want to hear what you think. What do you like or not like about the Notes? Please email us at **medfeedback@kaplan.com**.

Table of Contents

PART I

PEDIATRICS

CASE 1

Chief Complaint

"My eye is red."

History and Physical Examination

A 16-year-old girl comes to the office with a 2-day history of a watery, red left eye with a yellowish discharge. She reports crusting upon awakening. She denies eye pain and does not recall any trauma to the eye. Physical examination reveals diffuse conjunctival hyperemia of the left eye associated with a mucoid discharge and pupils that dilate normally with mild photophobia in the affected eye. There is no adenopathy. The funduscopic examination, eye movement, and visual acuity are all normal.

Differential Diagnosis

1. Bacterial conjunctivitis
2. Viral conjunctivitis
3. Acute glaucoma
4. Anterior uveitis
5. Trauma: corneal abrasion/foreign body
6. Allergic conjunctivitis
7. Chemical conjunctivitis
8. Periorbital/orbital cellulitis

Clues

- Unilateral
- No eye pain
- No trauma
- Mucoid discharge
- Normal pupillary dilatation
- Normal eye movement
- Normal visual acuity

CLINICAL PEARL

Always ask about a history of trauma or chemical contact.

CLINICAL PEARL

Because this is an adolescent, be sure to ask about sexual activity. Always consider *N. gonorrhoeae*, *C. trachomatis*, and herpes simplex (if vesicles are present). Unilateral versus bilateral erythema is a good first step in thinking about the differential diagnosis.

CCS NOTE

Always check vision, eye movement, pupillary size, and reactivity. Perform fundoscopic examination.

CLINICAL PEARL

Routine prophylactic antibiotic eye ointment at birth may delay the presentation of ophthalmia neonatorum from hrs to days.

Initial Management

Setting: outpatient workup and treatment

Diagnostic/Therapeutic Plan

- Snellen chart visual acuity

- Consider Gram stain and culture for *N. gonorrhoeae* and PCR or antigen test for *C. trachomatis*, depending on possible history of sexual activity or child abuse

Test Results

- Visual acuity: normal

- Gram stain/culture: negative

Assessment

- Unilateral red eye with mucoid, yellowish discharge and crusting upon awakening is the classic presentation of a bacterial conjunctivitis. Viral conjunctivitis is likely to be bilateral with a watery discharge.

- Allergic conjunctivitis should have itchiness, be bilateral and watery, and have a seasonal component and perhaps other history of allergic disease.

- With no history of pain or trauma caused by a foreign body, chemical conjunctivitis or corneal abrasion is highly unlikely.

- Normal vision and no ophthalmoplegia or proptosis, normal and symmetric pupillary size and reaction rule out anterior uveitis, orbital cellulitis, and glaucoma. Also, there is no description of periorbital or orbital erythema/edema and no fever or other systemic findings.

Further Management Plan/Results

Bacterial conjunctivitis will most often resolve spontaneously after several days. However, it is most commonly treated with a topical ophthalmic antibiotic.

- Trimethoprim-polymyxin drops

- Polymyxin-bacitracin ointment

- Fluoroquinolones (not to be given parenterally if age <18 yrs)

Do not use topical steroids if you are unsure of the diagnosis.

Discussion

Neonatal red eye

- **With eye drainage**: perform Gram stain and culture for *N. gonorrhoeae* and PCR or antigen test for *C. trachomatis* (ophthalmia neonatorum)

  - If positive for *N. gonorrhoeae*, treat for both: ceftriaxone IM × 1 with eye irrigation until clear for *N. gonorrhoeae* and erythromycin for 14 days with eye irrigation until clear for *C. trachomatis*

  - Otherwise, treat for positive *C. trachomatis*

- **With no eye drainage and suggestive of glaucoma**: megalocornea, tearing, photophobia, blepharospasm (refer to ophthalmologist)

- **With no eye drainage or evidence of glaucoma**: conjunctival hemorrhage, corneal abrasion (uncommon in neonate)

Infant, child, adolescent red eye

- **History of or suspicion of contact with a chemical**: irrigate and refer to ophthalmologist

- **History of foreign body**: examine eye and irrigate if nonpenetrating foreign body; otherwise, refer to ophthalmologist

- **Trauma, no foreign body**

  - Topical anesthetic (tetracaine) × 1 for thorough eye exam and vision testing

  - **Fluorescein with Wood lamp examination: corneal abrasion**

  - Topical ophthalmic antibiotic drops

  - Patching no longer recommended

- **Nonconjunctival inflammation**

  - Blepharitis: crusting, redness, itching of eyelids

  - Dacryocystitis: inflammation inferomedial to inner canthus

  - Dacryoadenitis: inflammation of upper, outer eyelid

  - Periorbital cellulitis: periorbital erythema, edema, warmth

  - Orbital cellulitis, **proptosis**, pain, visual changes, ophthalmoplegia; refer to ophthalmologist immediately

- **Signs and symptoms suggestive of glaucoma**: refer to ophthalmologist

- **Signs not suggestive of glaucoma:**

  - Keratitis: adenovirus, herpes simplex

  - Anterior uveitis: IBD, juvenile immune arthritis, Reiter's syndrome, sarcoidosis, Behçet's disease, early disseminated Lyme disease, early in Kawasaki's

- Itching, tearing, conjunctival edema, **seasonal**: allergic conjunctivitis

Remember, if it hurts, it is serious.

Final Diagnosis

Bacterial conjunctivitis

CLINICAL PEARL

For both periorbital and orbital cellulitis, cover for *S. aureus, S. pneumoniae*, and *H. influenza*, and consider possible resistance. Orbital cellulitis is an emergent condition and needs immediate referral to ophthalmology. MRI of the orbit and surrounding tissue should be performed to aid surgical drainage. Start IV antibiotics immediately.

CASE 2

Chief Complaint

Rash on legs

History and Physical Examination

A 6-year-old boy is brought to the office because of a rash that started as a superficial accumulation of several small vesicles on his legs below the knees. There is no fever or chills. He lives in the suburbs and often walks outside in the local woods in short pants. Vital signs are T 37.0° C (98.6° F), BP 110/70 mm Hg, pulse 84/min, and respirations 16/min. Physical examination shows honey-brown, crusted lesions with an erythematous base on both legs. There are other lesions as well, in various stages of crusting and openness. The examination is otherwise normal.

Differential Diagnosis

1. Impetigo
2. Cellulitis
3. Erysipelas
4. Varicella
5. Folliculitis (*S. aureus*)
6. Herpes simplex
7. Scabies
8. Contact dermatitis (e.g., poison ivy)
9. Dyshidrotic eczema

Clues

- Honey-brown, crusted lesions with an erythematous base
- Various stages of crusting and openness

Initial Management

Setting: outpatient workup and treatment

Diagnostic/Therapeutic Plan

- No cultures need to be done; this is a classic description and the diagnosis is clinically obvious

Expected Etiology

S. pyogenes (group A strep or *S. aureus* [can present as non-bullous])

Assessment

This is the **classic description** of a streptococcal impetigo (lower extremities, honey-brown lesions with an erythematous base, combination of ulcerated and crusted lesions). The presence of lesions on exposed legs (the patient wore short pants) and walking outside in the woods suggest some form of problem secondary to contact. The absence of fever and constitutional/systemic findings should lead you to assume a benign, localized disease.

Skin lesions due to staphylococcal infections are more likely to occur at the base of follicles and will range from papulovesicular to bullae. There is no evidence of any deeper or more widespread disease, such as cellulitis, erysipelas, or staphylococcal scalded skin syndrome. Patients with staphylococcal scalded skin appear much more toxic.

Management Plan/Results

Topical antibiotic treatment is warranted if disease is mild and localized: mupirocin is usually first-line. (Over-the-counter combinations of bacitracin-neomycin-polymyxin B are less effective.)

Otherwise, treatment is oral, with dicloxacillin/cloxacillin, cephalexin, or clindamycin. Oral treatment is warranted if there are widespread lesions or bullous lesions.

Discussion

A summary of vesicles and bullae is as follows.

Age birth to 2 mos

  Generalized

  - Disseminated herpes simplex

  - Disseminated candidiasis

  - Erythema toxicum: common, benign neonatal rash

  - **Epidermolysis bullosa**: inherited blistering disorder; usually begins in neonatal period; blistering in areas of trauma or pressure (extensor surfaces)

  - **Incontinentia pigmenti**: hereditary multisystem disorder (hair, eyes, CNS, teeth); mostly females; usually starts in first 2 wks of life with crops of bullae on trunk or extremities that become verrucous and then pigmented

  - Congenital varicella

  - Staphylococcal scalded skin syndrome

  Localized

  - Sucking blisters: dorsal surfaces of hands, fingers, forearms

  - Bullous impetigo

  - Localized herpes simplex

  - Localized candidiasis (perineal)

Age >2 mos

  With systemic illness

  - Varicella

CLINICAL PEARL

- With increasing resistance of S. pyogenes and S. aureus, macrolides should not be considered.

- If methicillin-resistant S. aureus (MRSA) is considered, then trimethoprim-sulfamethoxazole or clindamycin is a good choice.

- Vancomycin is not recommended for oral use but is highly effective intravenously, especially for MRSA.

- Hand-foot-mouth disease: coxsackie virus; painful, ulcerating vesicles on mouth, hands, and feet
- Staphylococcal scalded skin syndrome
- Stevens-Johnson's syndrome: most serious form of erythema multiforme; need skin and 2 mucous membranes
- Toxic epidermal necrolysis (Lyell's disease): widespread erythema and tenderness, followed by separation of skin between epidermis and dermis; also with bullae and positive Nikolsky's sign

Without systemic illness

- Generalized
  - Impetigo, bullous impetigo
  - Scabies: especially palms and soles; extremely pruritic; excoriates easily
  - Erythema multiforme: vesiculobullous, hypersensitivity eruption; target lesions
  - Epidermolysis bullosa
  - Pemphigus: usually seen in adolescents or adults; severe chronic blistering disorder
- Localized
  - Impetigo, bullous impetigo
  - Contact dermatitis
  - Insect bites
  - Burns
  - Herpes
  - Dyshidrotic eczema
  - Scabies
  - Epidermolysis bullosa
  - Pemphigus

CLINICAL PEARL

Nikolsky's sign is seen in staphylococcal scalded-skin syndrome (SSSS) or toxic epidermal necrolysis. With touch or pressure, skin will easily exfoliate.

Follow-up Management and Prevention

Typically, 7 days of therapy is sufficient for mild cases.

- Crusted lesions may be washed gently.
- Scratching can spread the organism.
- As with most infectious diseases, good handwashing can help prevent spread of disease.

Complications of impetigo include post-streptococcal glomerulonephritis. Treatment of skin infection does not seem to prevent this complication.

Final Diagnosis

Impetigo

CASE 3

Chief Complaint

Neonate with nasal flaring, cyanosis, and grunting

History and Physical Examination

A 17-year-old African American girl (G2P1) with unknown LMP and no prenatal care comes to the emergency department complaining of contractions every 5 minutes. Obstetric U/S is consistent with a gestational age of 28 weeks. Estimated fetal weight is 1,000 g and the baby is in breech presentation. The patient is started on $MgSO_4$ for tocolysis and betamethasone for fetal lung maturity. Contractions space out within 1 hour, and the patient is transferred to the antepartum service.

Forty-eight hours later, spontaneous rupture of membranes is confirmed, and the patient is transferred to the labor and delivery floor for further monitoring. There she develops late decelerations and is thus prepared for an emergent cesarean section, which is uneventful. She delivers a baby girl with Apgar scores of 7 at 1 min, 8 at 5 mins, and weighing 1,140 grams. The baby is transferred to the neonatology ICU. Within an hour, the baby develops tachypnea, nasal flaring, subcostal and intercostal retractions, cyanosis, and expiratory grunting.

Differential Diagnosis

1. Respiratory distress syndrome (RDS)
2. Pneumonia
3. Meconium aspiration syndrome
4. Transient tachypnea of the newborn (TTN)
5. Nonpulmonary causes, i.e., hypothermia, hypoglycemia, anemia, polycythemia, metabolic acidosis
6. Congenital heart disease
7. Diaphragmatic hernia/other congenital pulmonary anomalies
8. Primary pulmonary hypertension of the newborn

Clues

- Prematurity
- The physical findings are indicative of respiratory distress in general. "Grunting" is expiring against a partially closed glottis, and indicates that the baby is making attempts to increase alveolar end-expiratory pressure to preserve oxygenation.

CLINICAL PEARL

Apgar scores are done every 5 minutes as long as there are still resuscitative efforts.

CLINICAL PEARL

Pulmonary artery hypertension is more commonly secondary to hypoxia because of a primary underlying cardiopulmonary problem, compared with primary (idiopathic) pulmonary hypertension of the newborn.

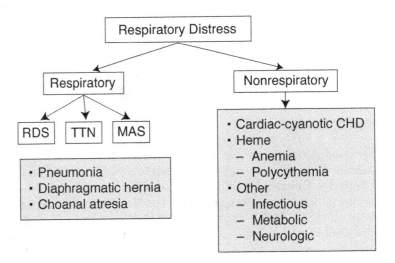

Respiratory Disorders: Overview

Initial Management

Setting: inpatient in delivery room

Diagnostic/Therapeutic Plan

Intervention	Results
• Place baby in open radiant warmer with skin electrodes attached	Done
• Place on cardiac and respiratory monitors	HR 160/min; RR 60/min
• Place in 100% oxygen (hood or nasal canula)	Done
• Place pulse oximeter on baby	Oxygen saturation 88% in room air; 99% in 100% oxygen
• Wean oxygen so that pulse oximetry is 93–96%	Pulse oximetry 95%
• Order chest x-ray and echocardiogram	Done
• Place umbilical venous catheter (UVC) for fluids/medications and umbilical arterial catheter (UAC) for blood draws/ABGs; begin 10% dextrose solution via UVC	Done
• Draw and send ABG, and send blood to lab for CBC and differential platelets, glucose, calcium, and blood culture	ABG: pH 7.29, pCO_2 50, pO_2 90 BE −1; other labs WNL
• Place baby on nasal CPAP of +4–5 cm H_2O with continued O_2	Baby has less grunting; O_2 sat 98%
• Perform sterile suprapubic bladder tap for U/A and C and S	Done
• Transfer to neonatal ICU	Done

Patient Safety Note

Don't forget about hyperoxia and the risk of retinopathy of prematurity.

Initial Assessment

A premature baby with respiratory distress and hypoxemia most likely has RDS (surfactant immaturity and deficiency). The most important first steps are to place the baby on a heat source (radiant warmer), place monitors, provide oxygen, and then re-evaluate.

Although the pulse oximeter shows good oxygen saturation, the continued grunting with the hypoxemia, hypercarbia, and acidosis indicates that the baby continues to have respiratory distress. Nasal CPAP (n-CPAP) would be the first step to open collapsed alveoli in an attempt to improve the respiratory problem. Re-evaluation is needed.

Always perform a sepsis workup (CBC, blood culture, sterile urine culture, $\pm$ CSF) and then begin empiric antibiotics in any sick newborn; infection is always a possibility. Also check for hypoglycemia and hypocalcemia.

Initial fluid in a newborn is a source of dextrose only (usually D10); electrolytes will not be needed until at least another 24 hrs; newborn may need calcium depending on serum level (transient hypoparathyroidism).

Further Diagnostic Plan/Results

1. Start antibiotics: ampicillin and gentamicin	Done
2. Obtain CXR results	Decreased lung volume; reticulogranular pattern with **air bronchograms**
3. Re-evaluate respiratory status	ABG in 70% O_2: pH 7.28, pCO_2 52 mm Hg, pO_2 50 mm Hg, BE -1
4. Intubate, place on ventilator, and give **surfactant** via the endotracheal tube	Done
5. Follow oxygen saturations and wean FIO_2 as needed; follow ABGs carefully and wean ventilator as needed	Being done
6. Obtain cardiac echocardiogram results	Large persistent ductus arteriosus; no cyanotic heart lesions
7. Begin **indomethacin** therapy for persistent ductus arteriosus	Done

CLINICAL PEARL

Don't forget to cover for group B streptococcal pneumonia, *Escherichia coli*, and *Listeria monocytogenes*. Ampicillin and gentamicin are appropriate if meningitis is not suspected. Otherwise, ampicillin + a third-generation cephalosporin (e.g., cefotaxime) are needed.

CLINICAL PEARL

Although this is the classic appearance of RDS, group B streptococcal pneumonia has a similar appearance.

CLINICAL PEARL

We know there will be a persistent ductus arteriosus. The echocardiogram is to rule out cyanotic heart disease. Never give indomethacin until this is known because it will adversely affect a ductal-dependent heart lesion.

Basic Science Correlate

- Surfactant is responsible for decreasing surface tension, thereby preventing alveolar collapse and atelectasis. It is produced in the type II alveolar cells, which start to form at about 24 wks' gestation.

  - Surfactant composition

    - Lipid-mostly phosphatidylcholine

    - Protein-surfactant proteins A, B, C, D

  - Preterm babies have decreased quantity and quality of surfactant

  - Incidence of RDS drops as gestational age increases; incidence significantly drops after 35–36 wks' gestation

Discussion

The best **initial diagnostic test** for sorting out the various etiologies of respiratory distress is **chest x-ray**. Look for the following:

- Ground glass appearance (reticulogranular pattern)

- Air bronchograms

- Atelectasis

The definitive test is amniotic fluid or tracheal aspirate for lecithin-sphingomyelin (L/S) ratio (part of the full lung profile).

- Done on amniotic fluid before delivery

- Ratio >2 indicates low risk for RDS

A major problem with RDS is hypoxemia due to alveolar collapse at end-expiration, and therefore, ventilation-perfusion mismatching. Hypercarbia and acidosis occur later with respiratory failure and the effects of a left-to-right shunt via a persistent ductus arteriosus.

Immediate intubation is not always necessary with RDS. One can either **start oxygen and n-CPAP before re-evaluating** or **perform intubation and give prophylactic surfactant**. Both methods are considered appropriate.

Oxygenation must be followed carefully to prevent hyperoxia and ventilation must be performed carefully to prevent barotrauma. The patient must be weaned constantly based on examination, pulse oximetry, blood gases (and pulmonary function measurements).

Final Diagnosis

Respiratory distress syndrome (RDS)

CASE 4

Chief Complaint

"My baby has been vomiting for 2 days."

History and Physical Examination

A 3-week-old boy is brought to the emergency room with a history of vomiting after each feeding. The symptoms started 2 days ago and have been worsening over the last 24 hours. The mother describes the vomiting as projectile and occurring within 30 minutes after he feeds. He has appeared to be a bit lethargic over the last 12 hours. There is no history of fever or diarrhea. The mother states that the infant wants to have the formula and is hungry. She just fed him 20 minutes ago, and urine was passed within the hour. There is no history of recent upper respiratory infection or exposure to any such cases. The infant was fed formula from birth, and for the first month had an intake of about 4 ounces every 4 hrs. There was the passage of 5–6 stools per day of a pasty consistency and yellow in color, along with the passage of urine about 7 times per day.

The mother is a 24-year-old white woman who had regular prenatal care and a normal spontaneous vaginal delivery. The newborn weighed 6 lb, 4 oz and had an uneventful postnatal course; the mother and newborn left the hospital within 3 days after delivery. The infant appears very irritable but consolable in his mother's arms. Physical examination shows no acute respiratory distress or evidence of an exanthem. His skin is warm to the touch with average skin turgor. Further examination shows:

HEENT: normocephalic, atraumatic; anicteric sclera, pink conjunctiva, positive red reflex bilaterally; anterior fontanelle open and soft; external auditory canals are WNL bilaterally; bilateral tympanic membranes with positive light reflex; nasal septum in midline, no evidence of polyps; oral cavity shows moist mucosa; no exudates or other abnormalities

Neck: supple, no adenopathy, no thyroid masses

Lung: good respiratory effort, clear to auscultation within the limits of examination

Cardiovascular: SI, S2 regular; no murmurs appreciated

Abdomen: positive bowel sounds, no organomegaly appreciated; during examination, infant had nonbilious projectile vomiting; on palpation after the vomiting, a palpable, hard, mobile, nontender mass was appreciated in the epigastrium to the right of midline

Genitalia: Tanner stage 1, testicles descended bilaterally; no inguinal masses found

Extremities: full ROM; no cyanosis or edema; no subluxation click found

Neurology: no focal deficits; normal infant with positive Moro reflex; good muscle tone in all extremities

CLINICAL PEARL

A major indicator to the severity of illness is that the neonate still wants the formula and remains hungry despite the vomiting.

- In any patient with vomiting, diarrhea, or decreased oral intake, always establish state of hydration through history and physical examination.

- Vomiting alone in a neonate should be considered GI obstruction until proven otherwise.

CLINICAL PEARL

This is the description of an "olive." The best time to feel for this mass is after an episode of vomiting.

Initial Management

Setting: initially outpatient, but inpatient admission will be necessary

Differential Diagnosis

1. Pyloric stenosis
2. Gastroesophageal reflux
3. Viral gastroenteritis
4. Malrotation with intermittent volvulus
5. Infection
6. Inborn error of metabolism

Clues

- Male, firstborn, Caucasian
- Age 3–4 wks
- Nonbilious projectile vomiting
- Remains hungry, wants to feed
- Palpable "olive"

Initial Diagnostic Plan/Results

1. CBC with differential	WBC 12,700/mm^3; neutrophils: 68%, bands: 6%, lymphocytes: 24%
2. SMA-7	Na 129, Cl 92, HCO3 28, K+ 3.1, BUN 24, glucose 92, creatinine 0.8
3. Urinalysis	Normal, except specific gravity 1.030
4. U/S	Hypertrophied pylorus

CLINICAL PEARL

In the evaluation of hydration status, it is always appropriate to check electrolytes, BUN/creatinine, glucose, and urinalysis.

If U/S is unavailable, perform an upper GI series. Results would show vigorous gastric peristalsis with little emptying of the contrast material. An elongated narrow pyloric canal is seen as a single tract (string sign).

Assessment

Classic lab findings are hypokalemic, hypochloremic metabolic alkalosis (loss of Cl and HCO$_3$ and shift of K). The child may have hyponatremia or isonatremia.

The **diagnostic procedure of choice** is the **U/S.** The "target lesion" is seen—a dark outer ring of hypertrophied pylorus with small, white central lumen.

Treatment

Treatment is surgical (pyloromyotomy). Start IV fluids to correct any dehydration and electrolyte abnormalities (Na, Cl, K). After surgery, slowly increase intake to full feeds over 48–72 hrs.

Initial Workup

- If evidence of infection: diarrhea (check stool for blood), known exposures, fever
- If evidence of partial or complete obstruction: plain radiographs, barium studies
    - Decreased or lack of passage of stools
    - Abdominal distension, decreased bowel sounds
    - Radiograph to check air/fluid level, lack of distal bowel gas
- When there is likelihood of pyloric stenosis, do an U/S of the pyloric region
- Evaluation of hydration status (history, examination, electrolytes, U/A) with fluid/electrolyte treatment (oral or IV)
- When evidence of acute abdomen, get surgical consult
- For possible gastroesophageal reflux

Treatment depends upon diagnosis and whether surgery is needed.

- Fluid maintenance and replacement: for most cases use small, frequent volumes of oral rehydrating solution; for severe cases that have intractable vomiting or shock, use IV fluids/electrolytes
- If there is a viral infection, use only fluid management; bacterial enteritis (positive stool culture) may need antibiotic treatment, depending on organism and patient's age
- With any decreased peristalsis or ileus (with abdominal distension), use nasogastric tube with low suction; follow electrolytes and replace losses as needed

Final Diagnosis

Pyloric stenosis

CASE 5

Chief Complaint

"My son has had belly pain and blood in his stool."

History and Physical Examination

A 2-year-old boy is brought to the emergency department by his concerned mother because he just passed a stool with red blood and mucus. He has been irritable for the last 36 hours, with intermittent attacks of belly pain, accompanied by straining efforts and loud cries. He also had some episodes of emesis, but not in the last 24 hours. He had mild diarrhea a week ago and a URI that resolved spontaneously over the last 5 days. He has no known medical problems and is growing and developing well.

Physical examination shows a pale, very irritable child with T 39.0 C (102.2 F), pulse 120/min, and BP 90/60 mm Hg. Further examination shows normal HEENT, pale skin with no rash, RRR with no murmur, and clear lungs. The abdomen is distended, and on deep palpation a slightly tender, sausage-shaped mass is felt in the right upper abdomen with its axis cephalocaudal. There is no hepatosplenomegaly. Capillary refill is 2 seconds. Neurologic exam is nonfocal and cranial nerves are intact.

Differential Diagnosis

1. Intussusception
2. Meckel's diverticulum
3. Henoch-Schönlein (anaphylactoid) purpura with possible secondary intussusception
4. Bacterial/parasitic enteritis

Clues

- Age of patient
- Stool color ("currant jelly")
- Intermittent pain
- Prior infection

Initial Management

Setting: emergency department

Diagnostic/Therapeutic Plan

- CBC
- Place IV, give bolus of 20 cc/kg NS; follow with IV hydration therapy
- Notify surgeon of case
- Abdominal flat plate, followed by air contrast enema (diagnostic and therapeutic)

CLINICAL PEARL

In a young child, abdominal pain with blood in the stool is intussusception until proven otherwise.

CLINICAL PEARL

A tender, sausage-shaped mass is a pathognomonic physical finding.

Test Results

- WBC: 14,000/mm^3 with neutrophils 85% (bands and segmental); hemoglobin 10 g/dL; platelets 230,000/mm^3

- Abdominal flat plate: density in RUQ; no free air; air contrast enema diagnostic for intussusception; radiologist will attempt reduction

Patient Safety Note

Air contrast enema is now preferred to barium enema because it has a significantly lower rate of perforation. Enema is contraindicated if there is any evidence of intestinal perforation.

Assessment

The following findings are diagnostic for intussusception. They typically occur a week after a nonspecific viral illness.

History

- Acute, severe, paroxysmal attacks of abdominal pain
- Severe irritability and straining
- Adopts lateral recumbent position, with hips and legs flexed
- May have bloody stool or can present early without any bleeding
- Most have vomiting

Physical Examination

- Toxic appearing, febrile
- Often unconsolable
- Tender, sausage-shaped cephalocaudal mass in RUQ; abdominal distension
- Typical currant jelly stool

Diagnostic Findings

- Plain film nonspecific; obtain prior to air contrast to make sure that there is no perforation; if there is perforation, do immediate surgery

- Air contrast enema shows sudden interruption of air into a coil-like intestine.
  - Portion of proximal bowel telescopes into distal
  - Most are ileocolic or ileoileocolic

Treatment

- Do not do hydrostatic reduction if there are signs of shock/perforation/peritoneal irritation; give IV resuscitation as needed and immediate surgery

- Success rate of air contrast reduction under fluoroscopy or U/S is 70–90% if performed within first 48 hrs of symptoms, and 50% after 48 hrs

- If surgical manual operative reduction is not possible or if any bowel is not viable, then resection with end-to-end anastomosis

> **CLINICAL PEARL**
>
> U/S is the imaging modality of choice for the diagnosis and exclusion of intussusception showing a target-like mass ~3 cm in diameter. This, therefore, is indicated in the stable patient immediately after the history and physical and prior to any radiographic intervention for reduction.

Discussion

Initial studies for any GI bleeding include stool guaiac, CBC, platelets, reticulocytes, PT/PTT, bleeding time, comprehensive metabolic panel. Consider microbiologic studies if suggested by history.

Workup of rectal bleeding in a child age >3 mos is detailed below.

Melena

- Suspect Meckel diverticulum ("brick-red" blood)
  - **Yes, suspect:** perform Meckel scan
    - Positive: Meckel diverticulum
    - Negative: upper GI barium study (upper GI imaging) or endoscopy
  - **No, don't suspect:** perform UGI or endoscopy
    - Normal or unable to perform: bleeding scan or angiogram
    - Abnormal: peptic ulcer disease; GERD/esophagitis; Mallory-Weiss syndrome; varices; volvulus; intestinal duplications; vascular malformations; tumor

Hematochezia

Does examination show fissures or hemorrhoids? If no, then consider microbiologic studies if suggested by history. After that:

- Suspect Meckel diverticulum
  - **Yes, suspect:** as above for melena
    - **No, don't suspect:** colonoscopy or barium enema
    - If normal, perform UGI
    - If abnormal, consider fissures; polyps; hemorrhoids; colitis; vascular malformation; vasculitis (e.g., Henoch-Schönlein purpura); IBD; hemolytic uremic syndrome; tumor
- Suspect intussusception: plain film followed by air contrast reduction (if not contraindicated)
  - Normal: colonoscopy as above
  - Abnormal: intussusception

Final Diagnosis

Intussusception

CLINICAL PEARL

Intussusception is the most common cause of intestinal obstruction age 3 mos to 6 yrs. Most of the differential diagnoses are not very common.

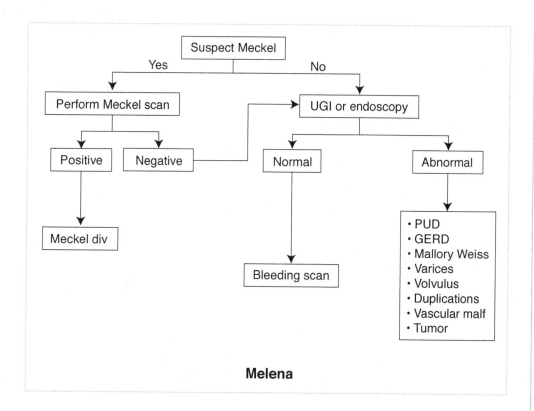

Melena

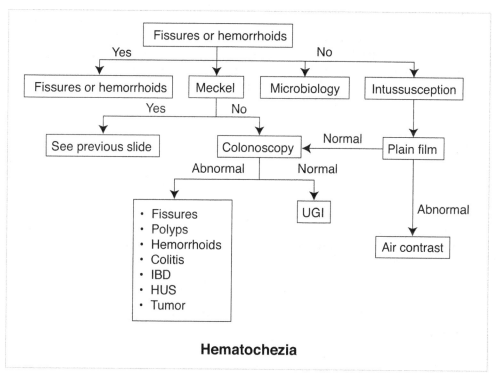

Hematochezia

CASE 6

Chief Complaint

"Why is my child so short?"

History and Physical Examination

A 7-year-old boy is brought to the office because of parental concern about his growth. His mother had an uneventful pregnancy and delivery was via NSVD. Both the mother and newborn left the hospital within 2 days, and the child was breastfed for the first 6 mos. He sat up at age 7 mos and walked with assistance at age 11 mos. All developmental milestones were WNL; however, he was found on the growth chart to be at the fifth percentile during early childhood and has remained there until this time. There was no prior history of any systemic illness, and he has a good appetite, being at the 30th percentile for weight. There are 2 other siblings, a brother (age 2) in good health and at the 15th percentile for height. His sister (age 12) is in good health. His father is 183 cm (6 feet) tall, and his mother is 165 cm (5 feet 5 inches) tall. His father, on questioning, states that he was generally shorter than his friends in school until age 14. There is no history of headache, vomiting, visual disturbance, anorexia, or diarrhea. There is also no history of polyuria or polydipsia. The patient appears to be in no acute distress and is very cooperative and friendly. His short stature is the only obvious abnormality.

Physical examination shows:

HEENT: head is normocephalic, atraumatic; pupils equally reactive to light, anicteric sclera, pink conjunctiva; fundi without any gross abnormalities; no frontal bossing or flat nasal bridge; nasal septum is in midline; no nasal polyps; bilateral external ear canals WNL; tympanic membranes with positive light reflex bilaterally; oral cavity shows moist mucosa without any exudates; mild tonsillar hypertrophy bilaterally without any midline approximation

Neck: supple, with full ROM; no adenopathy is appreciated; no thyroid masses; trachea is in midline

Lungs: clear to auscultation bilaterally

Cardiovascular: S1, S2 regular; no murmurs appreciated

Abdomen: positive bowel sounds, no tenderness, no organomegaly appreciated, no truncal fat deposition

Genitalia: Tanner stage I, testicles descended bilaterally; no inguinal adenopathy

Extremities: full ROM, no cyanosis, clubbing, or edema; pulses +2 symmetrically bilaterally

Neurology: no focal deficits

Differential Diagnosis

1. Constitutional growth delay

2. Familial short stature

3. Short stature due to chronic disease (chronic infection, rheumatic disease, chronic anemia)

4. Short stature due to endocrine disease (growth hormone deficiency, hypothyroidism, diabetes)

5. Deprivational short stature (failure to thrive)

6. Genetic/syndromic short stature (Turner syndrome, Down syndrome)

Clues

- Normal development, normal growth velocity
- Parents of normal height

Initial Management

Setting: outpatient

Initial Diagnostic Plan/Results

1. Examine growth curve	Normal velocity but growing along the fifth percentile
2. Request bone age, i.e., x-ray of left hand and wrist	Bone age seen is consistent with patient age 5

Diagnostic/Therapeutic Plan

- None; follow growth and pubertal development; give reassurance to patient and family

Assessment

Based on the history, this is a clear case of constitutional delay, i.e., a delay of growth and pubertal maturation until later in adolescence.

- History of at least 1 parent is the same as that of patient
- End-growth will be normal based on parents' heights
- Biggest concern is typically delayed pubertal development

A careful history and physical examination is warranted.

- Exclude nutritional issues: examine weight attainment and weight for height
- Examine psychosocial/environmental issues
- Perform thorough past medical history and review of systems for any evidence of undiagnosed illness
- Perform complete and careful physical exam, including neurologic; look for any dysmorphic features

CLINICAL PEARL

The particular history of the father's growth is very important. Be sure to ask about both parents' growth and measure the heights of both parents.

CLINICAL PEARL

Both parents will be short with familial short stature.

CLINICAL PEARL

Failure to thrive secondary to decreased nutrient intake, absorption, or utilization, or increased caloric expenditure. Look for psychosocial and environmental issues.

CCS NOTE

With the history presented, no other tests would be required at this stage. One could even make a point of not performing the bone age now in light of the positive family history.

Examine the growth curve. Is the child growing normally along a growth percentile or has there been a "flattening" or "falling off" of the curve? In other words, is there normal versus abnormal growth velocity?

Discussion

Do a workup of short or tall stature. First, define growth:

- Accurate measurements of weight, height, occipital-frontal head circumference
- Growth curve
  - Measurements should be plotted at each well-child visit and ideally at each sick visit as well.
  - Growth velocity (GV) = yearly increments of growth (**most sensitive indicator of child's growth**) (normal versus abnormal)
- Chronological age (CA) of patient = actual age, in yrs and mos
- Bone age (BA) = plain radiograph of left hand and wrist
- Definition of short stature is growth below 3rd percentile
- Definition of tall stature is growth above 97th percentile

The ideal (i.e., perfectly average) situation is CA = BA, with normal GV.

Short Stature	
CA > BA	Normal GV: diagnosis = constitutional growth delay
	Abnormal GV: diagnosis = chronic systemic/endocrine disease or nutritional problem
CA = BA	Normal GV: diagnosis = familial short stature; small for gestational age (SGA) infants
	Abnormal GV: diagnosis = genetic/chromosomal/syndrome

Tall Stature	
CA < BA	Normal GV: obesity, familial tall stature
	Abnormal GV: diagnosis = precocious puberty; hyperthyroidism; growth hormone excess; congenital adrenal hyperplasia; certain genetic/syndrome illnesses

Final Diagnosis

Constitutional growth delay

CLINICAL PEARL

The radiologist interprets the bones of the hand and wrist, comparing them with 'normals' for the age. The report will then state the bone age as consistent with a particular age, e.g., as normal, delayed, or advanced for that age.

Differential Diagnosis and Therapy of Short Stature

	Panhypo-pituitarism	Constitutional Delay	Familial Short Stature	Deprivational Dwarfism	Turner Syndrome	Hypothyroidism	Chronic Disease
Family history	Rare	Frequent	Always	No	No	Variable	Variable
Sex	Both	Males > females	Both	Both	Female	Both	Both
Dentition	Delayed	Slight delay	Normal	Variable	Normal	Delayed	Normal
Facies	Immature or dysmorphic	Normal	Normal	Normal	Turner facies or normal	Cretin	Normal
Sexual development	Delayed	Delayed	Normal	Delayed	Prepubertal	Usually delayed, may be precocious	Delayed
Bone age	Delayed	Delayed	Normal	Usually delayed; growth arrest lines	Slight delay	Delayed	Delayed
Hypoglycemia	Variable	No	No	No	No	No	No
Chromosomes	Normal	Normal	Normal	Normal	45,XO or partial deletion of X chromosomes or mosaic	Normal	Normal
T_4	Low or normal	Normal	Normal	Normal or low	Normal: hypothyroidism may be acquired	Low	Normal
Growth hormone	Low	Normal	Normal, rarely biologically active GH	Low	Normal, occasionally low	Low	Variable
Insulin-like growth factor	Low	Normal for maturation	Normal	Low	Normal	Low	Low or normal
Tests	Stimulated GH secretion, cranial CT	None specific	None specific	Observation in controlled environment	Karyotype	T_4, TSH	Specific for organ system abnormalities
Therapy	Replace cortisol, T_4, and GH deficits as indicated	Reassurance; testosterone to initiate secondary sex changes in selected patients	None: GH therapy is controversial	Improve environment	Sex hormone replacement, GH/oxandrolone appears useful	T_4	Reverse malnutrition and organ failure (dialysis, transplant, cardiotonic drugs, insulin)

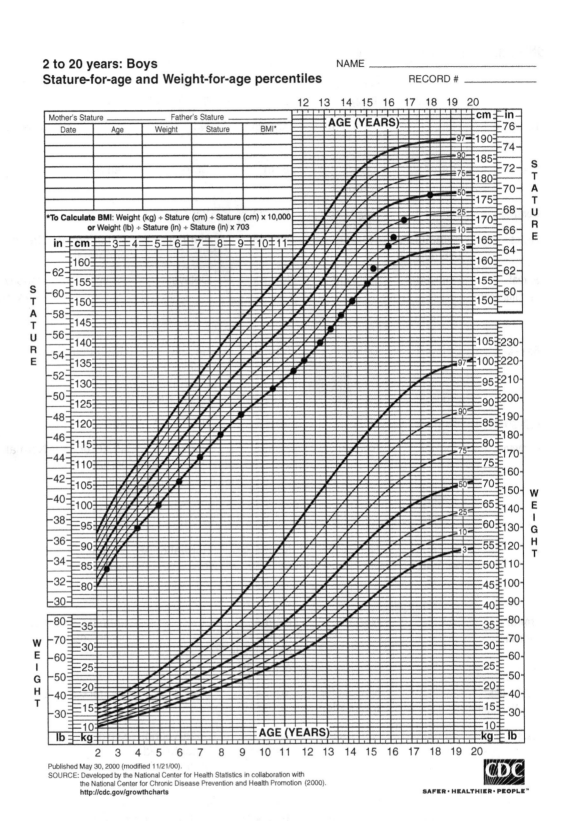

2 to 20 years: Boys
Stature-for-age and Weight-for-age percentiles

NAME _____

RECORD # _____

Growth Curve: Relative Short Stature but at a Normal Growth Velocity
Consistent with Constitutional Delay

CASE 7

Chief Complaint

Newborn with tachypnea and duskiness

History and Physical Examination

The pediatrician on call is notified by one of the newborn nursery nurses that a neonate whom he has not seen is now breathing fast and has a dusky appearance. It is an 11-hour-old male infant who was born at 37 wks' gestation to a 19-year-old G1P1 woman who had no prenatal care. According to the mother, her pregnancy went well and without problems. She had an NSVD. The baby weighs 6 lb and has Apgar scores of 7 and 8. Only stimulation is required in the delivery room.

The baby is taken to the newborn nursery and starts to bottle-feed shortly after admission. He takes the first 3 feedings without difficulty; prior to the next feeding he is examined by the nurse. Vital signs are respirations 60/min, pulse 160/min, and BP 80/40 mm Hg in the left arm. Compared with his previous color, he now appears to be somewhat dusky. It is at this time that the nurse calls the pediatrician. A physical examination is conducted, revealing the following:

General: patient is awake and alert with vigorous respiratory pattern (60/min) and mild subcostal retractions

Skin: dusky overall with cyanosis of fingers and toes

HEENT: circumoral cyanosis and mild nasal flaring

Chest: there is good bilateral air entry. There are no adventitious sounds. The chest is symmetric, with mild subcostal retractions.

Cardiovascular: heart rate and rhythm are regular; S1 is normal and S2 is soft and single; grade IV/VI SEM is heard at mid to upper left sternal border with a thrill felt at midsternal border; pulses are 1+ and symmetric; capillary refill is 2+

Abdomen: soft without mass; liver edge is palpated 2 cm below right costal margin; spleen is not palpated, and kidneys feel normal

Genitourinary: patient is a normal male with bilaterally descended testes.

Extremities: cyanosis and perfusion are noted as above; no gross malformations or deformations

Neural: patient is alert, reactive to painful stimuli; tone is symmetric but mildly decreased; DTRs are 1+ and symmetric

Differential Diagnosis

1. Cardiac disease
2. CNS disease/depression
3. Primary pulmonary disease
4. Pulmonary artery hypertension

CLINICAL PEARL

- The presence of a thrill denotes at least a grade IV murmur; a thrill is always abnormal.

- A single S2 occurs in pulmonary or aortic atresia or severe stenosis, truncus arteriosus, and often in transposition (as the aorta is to the right and anterior to the pulmonic valve, thus obscuring the sound of pulmonic closure).

Clues

- Age of patient
- Duskiness (cyanosis)
- **Murmur, single S2 (therefore, severe pulmonary stenosis)**

Initial Management

Setting: inpatient, wellborn nursery

Initial Diagnostic and Treatment Plan	Results
1. Pulse oximetry	68%
2. Prepare to put baby in 100% oxygen	Done
3. Arterial blood gas in room air	pH 7.42, pCO_2 38 mm Hg, PaO_2 43 mm Hg, base deficit −1
4. Start peripheral IV and IV fluids with 10% dextrose; also start PGE1 drip	Done
5. Repeat arterial blood gas in 100% oxygen	pH 7.43, pCO_2 37 mm Hg, PaO_2 48 mm Hg, Base deficit 0
6. Blood work:	
CBC, differential, platelets	Hb 17.3 g/dL, Hct 55, WBC 11,300/mm³, 66% polys, 8% bands, 20% lymphocytes, 6% basophils, platelets 230,000/mm³
Blood culture	Done
Urine culture	Done
Urinalysis	SG 1.019, dipstick negative, no WBC or RBC
Serum glucose	70 mg/dL
Serum calcium	9.2 mg/dL
7. Chest radiograph	Decreased lung markings; heart is normal size with apex lifted off diaphragm
8. EKG	Right ventricular hypertrophy and right axis deviation
9. Start IV ampicillin and gentamicin	Done

CLINICAL PEARL

Always perform a sepsis workup and start antibiotics in any sick neonate. Also, check serum glucose and calcium for hypoglycemia and hypocalcemia, respectively.

CCS NOTE

If a congenital cyanotic heart lesion is suspected, always initiate a PGE1 drip to keep the ductus arteriosus open and allow for pulmonary blood flow, as you do not initially know if it is a ductal-dependent lesion).

Basic Science Correlate

- Hypoxia causes pulmonary vasoconstriction in an effort to shunt blood to ventilated areas.

- Pulmonary artery hypertension may be secondary to hypoxia or may be primary (idiopathic). Increased pulmonary vascular resistance usually is responsive to oxygen, hypocarbia, alkalosis, and pulmonary vasodilators.

Assessment

For the initial evaluation of a cyanotic infant, use the following guidelines.

- Breathing pattern
  - Weak, irregular, and weak suck = CNS disease
  - Vigorous or labored with tachypnea = primary respiratory or cardiac disease
  - Clinical appearance suggests either primary respiratory or cardiac disease
- Hyperoxia test: arterial blood gases first in room air, then in 100% oxygen
  - With CNS disease, PaO_2 completely normalizes
  - With pulmonary disease, PaO_2 increases significantly as V/Q inequalities are overcome by oxygen
  - If $PaO_2 > 150$ mm Hg in 100% oxygen, intracardiac shunt is usually excluded
  - The results are most consistent with a fixed intracardiac shunt, i.e., a congenital cyanotic heart lesion

New differential diagnosis:

- Tetralogy of Fallot
- Transposition of the great arteries
- Truncus arteriosus
- Tricuspid atresia
- Total anomalous venous return
- Ebstein anomaly
- Hypoplastic left heart
- Other complex congenital heart disease

Decreased lung markings on chest radiograph suggest a lesion producing decreased pulmonary blood flow. The combination of heart appearance, EKG and clinical findings suggests tetralogy of Fallot.

CLINICAL PEARL

To rule out pulmonary artery hypertension, the patient should be ventilated to attain mild hypocarbia and alkalosis.

Further diagnostic and treatment plan	Results
1. Cardiologist arrives and performs an echocardiogram	Pulmonary valve and infundibular stenosis; unrestricted ventral septal defect with overriding aorta and right ventricular hypertrophy
2. Transport is arranged to nearest tertiary care facility	Done

CLINICAL PEARL

Familiarity with fetal circulation is important in anticipating results of diagnostic tests on the exam (e.g., EKG, chest x-ray, echo).

Discussion

Congenital heart disease occurs in 0.5–0.8/100 live births.

- Most lesions occur between 15–80 days gestation.
- Fetal oxygenation takes place at placental level.
- Foramen ovale and ductus arteriosus are necessary in utero for proper blood flow.
- At delivery with first breath, pulmonary vascular resistance begins to drop, ductus arteriosus starts to close in response to oxygen tension, and normal circulatory patterns are achieved.
- Ductus dependent lesions require prostaglandin initially pending definitive treatment.
- Echocardiogram is the best test for the diagnosis of congenital heart disease.
- Surgery is the definitive treatment.

Illustration is for review only.

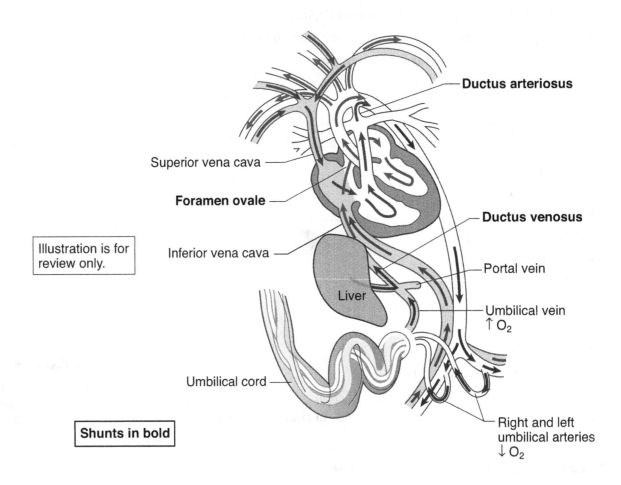

Shunts in bold

Fetal Circulation

Tetralogy of Fallot is the most common cyanotic congenital heart lesion (5–7% of all), while ventricular septal defect is most common overall (25–30%). Presentation of cyanosis depends on the severity of pulmonic stenosis and, therefore, the degree of right-to-left shunting. Diagnosis may not be established until after ductus arteriosus closes. The chest radiograph appearance with significant stenosis is that of a "**boot-shaped heart.**" This represents the apex of the heart lifted off the diaphragm due to significant right ventricular hypertrophy (also seen on EKG).

The most common cyanotic lesion presenting in immediate newborn period (first day of life) is transposition of the great arteries (3–5%).

Common lesions with decreased pulmonary blood flow (darkened lung fields) are indicative of tetralogy of Fallot, tricuspid atresia, and Ebstein anomaly; others have increased pulmonary blood flow (increased lung markings). Significant murmur (i.e., ≥grade III) generally suggests a heart lesion. The presence of a thrill (grade IV) is always abnormal. A diastolic murmur should also be considered abnormal.

Definitive diagnosis of a congenital heart lesion is established by echocardiography.

Treatment

Transfer to an appropriate facility, depending on the severity of pulmonary stenosis and subsequent shunting.

- Medical management is warranted until definitive surgical correction
- Systemic to pulmonary shunt (modified Blalock-Taussig shunt) is palliative
- Hypercyanotic (Tet) spells are indication for surgery

Final Diagnosis

Tetralogy of Fallot

CASE 8

Chief Complaint

Fever and a rash

History and Physical Examination

A 3-year-old boy has a 6-day history of fever up to 38.0° C (100.4° F), irritability, and a rash. For the last 24 hrs he has had diarrhea and vomiting after eating. He is noncooperative and irritable. Heart rate is 140/min.

Physical examination shows bilateral conjunctival injection, fissured lips, a strawberry tongue, and diffuse injection of oral and pharyngeal mucosa. Tender cervical lymphadenopathy is present. Cardiovascular exam reveals tachycardia, normal rhythm, and no murmurs. The lungs are clear to auscultation and the abdominal exam is benign. There is swelling of the hands and feet with reddening of the palms. Neurologic exam is nonfocal.

Differential Diagnosis

1. Kawasaki's syndrome
2. Systemic viral illness
3. Streptococcal disease
4. Systemic onset juvenile rheumatoid arthritis

Initial Management

Setting: inpatient

Clues

- Fever
- Conjunctivitis
- Oral findings
- Adenitis
- Hand findings

Initial diagnostic plan and treatment	Results
CBC with differential, platelets	Leukocytosis (30,000 cells/mm^3), hematocrit 32%, platelets 500,000
ESR	45 mm/hr
Comprehensive metabolic panel: electrolytes, BUN, creatinine, glucose, liver enzyme	Na 134, Cl 104, CO_2 23, BUN 18, Cr 0.9, glucose 80, AST 90, ALT 50
Urinalysis	Proteinuria
Admit to hospital with presumptive diagnosis of Kawasaki's	Done
Start IV fluids for rehydration and maintenance	Done
Begin IVIG infusion and start high-dose ASA orally in divided doses	Done
Chest x-ray	Normal
Electrocardiogram	Prolonged PR-QT intervals, abnormal Q wave, and low-voltage ST-T changes
Two-dimensional echocardiogram	Pericardial effusion

Assessment

Fever ≥5 days and the **presence of 4 of 5** of the following fit the criteria for diagnosis of Kawasaki's disease.

- Conjunctival infection
- Oral manifestations
- Skin rash
- Adenopathy/adenitis
- Hand findings

The other potential diagnoses can be ruled out based on the history and physical. In febrile illnesses with multiple findings, always get a thorough history of exposures to other persons with illnesses, travel history, history of exposure to animals (pets and farm animals), recent dietary intake, and history of anyone else at home or in the community with a similar illness.

Further Treatment Plan

Beginning on day 2, start high-dose salicylate therapy (80 to 100 mg/kg/day) and continue until afebrile for at least 48 hrs. Switch to low-dose salicylate therapy (5 to 10 mg/kg/day) for remainder of illness (4 to 6 wks) **and** until there is no evidence of coronary aneurysms, and platelet count and CRP normalize.

After an initial baseline echocardiogram, repeat at wks 2–3 of illness, again at wks 4–6, and then every 2–3 mos if there continues to be any evidence of aneurysm.

Follow the platelet count.

CLINICAL PEARL

Do not make the diagnosis of Kawasaki's disease until the criteria are met. Kawasaki's is always managed on an inpatient basis.

Discussion

Characteristics of Kawasaki's disease (mucocutaneous lymph node syndrome [MCLNS]) are as follows:

- **Must present with fever**
  - Abrupt and high-spiking
  - Initially unresponsive to antipyretics
  - Mean duration if untreated—11 days
  - Universal irritability
- **Must have 4 of 5 of the following:**
  - **Conjunctival infection**
    - Bulbar injection
    - No purulent discharge
    - Resolves in 7–10 days
    - Also early anterior uveitis
  - **Oral manifestations**
    - Dry, fissured lips
    - Strawberry tongue
    - Diffuse, intraoral erythema
    - No enanthem, stomatitis, or exudative pharyngitis
  - **Extremities**
    - Early induration of hands and feet
    - Erythema of palms and soles
    - No discrete lesions
    - Desquamation of fingers and toes in late phase
  - **Lymphadenopathy (up to 70% of patients)**
    - Large (>1.5 cm)
    - Painful, erythematous
    - Usually unilateral
  - **Skin rash**
    - Polymorphous

Other characteristic findings are:

- Cardiovascular: resting tachycardia, early myocarditis, pericardial effusion
- GI: hydrops of gallbladder
- Renal: sterile pyuria, proteinuria
- Orthopedic: arthritis of large, weight-bearing joints
- Neurologic: irritability, lymphocytic pleocytosis
- Anemia
- Leukocytosis with left shift
- ESR, CRP must be elevated
- Increasing thrombocytosis
- Elevated hepatic transaminases

Cardiovascular complications are:

- Myocarditis early, aneurysms later (beginning at wks 2–3)
- Platelets rise in wks 2–3: may lead to thromboses
- Cardiology follow-up: baseline echocardiogram; repeat at wks 2–3 and again at wks 4–6; long-term, low-dose acetylsalicylic acid if there are aneurysms (50% resolve within 1 year)

Final Diagnosis

Kawasaki's disease

CLINICAL PEARL

Be aware of the differences with respect to streptococcal pharyngitis.

CLINICAL PEARL

Consider other diseases with hand/palm and foot/toe findings.

CLINICAL PEARL

During the first 1–2 wks, we see the acute inflammatory findings.

CASE 9

Chief Complaint

Irritability, malaise, and abdominal pain

History and Physical Examination

A 4-year-old boy is referred to the office by his nursery school teachers who are concerned about his increasing irritability, poor attention span, and lethargy. He also has been vaguely complaining of recurrent bellyaches. He has otherwise been healthy, lives in a crowded pre-World War II building in Chinatown, and has a history of pica. According to his mother, he has a poor appetite and has been constipated. No dyspnea or fever is reported. He is noncooperative, pale, and afebrile, with BP 90/60 mm Hg, pulse 120/min, and respirations 18/min.

Physical examination shows HEENT to be benign and the neck supple. Cardiovascular exam shows a normal rate and rhythm and II/VI systolic ejection murmur, nonradiating. Lungs are clear to auscultation. The abdomen has no masses or hepatosplenomegaly but mild diffuse tenderness is noted on deep palpation. The extremities have a full ROM with no joint tenderness. Neurologic exam is nonfocal.

Differential Diagnosis

1. Lead poisoning
2. Iron deficiency anemia
3. Hepatitis
4. Parasitic infection
5. Hypothyroidism
6. Attention-deficit disorder

Clues

- Behavioral issues
- Abdominal pain
- Environment
- Pica

CLINICAL PEARL

Because the diagnosis appears to be straightforward, no other lab studies are warranted at this point. Check the serum lead level and evaluate the degree of anemia.

Initial Management

Setting: outpatient

Initial diagnostic plan	Results
1. CBC and smear	WBC 9,600/mm³, hemoglobin 7.3 g/dL, platelets 230,000/mm³
2. Serum lead level	50 mg/dL (normal <10)

Assessment

Lead poisoning suggested by:

- Microcytic, hypochromic anemia with basophilic stippling on smear
- GI findings: poor appetite, constipation, abdominal pain/tenderness
- Behavioral/neurologic findings: irritability, lethargy
- Poor attention span
- Personality changes
- Encephalopathy: vomiting, ataxia, seizures, papilledema, impaired consciousness

Evaluate possible sources:

- Old buildings, peeling lead paint, lead plumbing joints
- Lead-glazed pottery
- Lead-based cosmetics
- Proximity to factories using lead
- Household member working in lead factory
- Fumes from burning batteries

Further Management Plan

Get a referral from the Department of Health, and then evaluate and remove sources. Educate the family. Because the lead level here is 44–70 μg/dL, indicated treatment is oral chelation therapy with dimercaptosuccinic acid. Monitor lead levels closely to ensure normalization.

Discussion

The evaluation of anemia of underproduction (reticulocytes <2%) is as follows:

- **Mean corpuscular volume (MCV) low:** consider iron studies, hemoglobin electrophoresis, bone marrow aspirate
  - Iron deficiency
  - Thalassemia trait
  - Lead poisoning
  - Anemia of chronic disease
  - Copper deficiency
- **MCV normal:** consider iron studies, serum creatinine, thyroid and liver tests, bone marrow aspirate
  - Isolated anemia: iron deficiency anemia, acute infection, transient erythroblastopenia, anemia of chronic disease, renal disease, liver disease, hypothyroidism
  - Pancytopenia: leukemia, malignancy, aplastic anemia

- **MCV high:** consider serum vitamin B12 and folate, thyroid and liver function, bone marrow aspirate

  - Megaloblastic anemia

  - Diamond-Blackfan anemia

  - Fanconi anemia

  - Liver disease

  - Hypothyroidism

The approach to anemia is as follows:

- Blood loss

  - Acquired: trauma, upper/lower GI bleed, disseminated intravascular coagulation

  - Inherited: von Willebrand. hemophilia A, hemophilia B

  - Acquired platelet disorder: platelet dysfunction, immune thrombocytopenic purpura

- Impaired production of red blood cells (RBCs)

  - Specific deficiency: iron, folate, vitamins B6/B12, vitamin C, malnutrition, anemia of chronic disease

  - Marrow failure: inherited, acquired

- Excessive destruction of RBCs

  - Acquired: autoimmune hemolytic anemia, secondary to autoimmune disease

  - Inherited: membrane defects (spherocytosis), enzyme defects (G6PD), qualitative globin defects (sickle cell), quantitative globin defects (thalassemia)

Chelation therapy for lead poisoning (serum lead level >10 µg/dL):

- **Lead level 5–14 µg/dL:** evaluate sources and remove them; educate family; repeat level within 3 mos

- **Lead level 15–19 µg/dL:** same as above, and Department of Health referral; repeat level within 2 mos

- **Lead level 20–44 µg/dL:** same as above; repeat level within 1 month

- **Lead level 44–70 µg/dL:** same as above; treat with single drug, preferably dimercapto-succinic acid (succimer, oral)

- **Lead level >70 µg/dL:** same as above; immediate hospitalization and drug treatment

  - Without encephalopathy: ethylenediaminetetraacetic acid (EDTA) (versenate, IV) + either dimercaptosuccinic acid or British anti-Lewisite (BAL) (IV, dimercaprol)

  - With encephalopathy: EDTA + BAL

Final Diagnosis

Lead poisoning

CASE 10

Chief Complaint

Altered consciousness after falling off the bed

History and Physical Examination

A 2-year-old boy is bought to the emergency department by his mother for evaluation after falling off the bed several hours ago and sustaining trauma to the left side of the head. The mother is an 18-year-old single parent who did not graduate from high school and now works part-time to support her child. The child was at the babysitter's house at the time of the fall, along with the mother's boyfriend who occasionally helps to babysit as well.

The child was delivered via normal spontaneous vaginal delivery, and the mother had sporadic prenatal care. The newborn and mother left the hospital within 3 days, and the child was formula-fed from birth. Development milestones were appropriate for age, with height and weight at the 40th percentile. As explained by the mother today, the 18-month booster immunization was lacking due to an ongoing viral illness. The child last saw the pediatrician at age 20 mos for an acute respiratory illness.

Upon questioning about the fall a few hours ago, the mother states that her boyfriend told her that, while asleep, the child rolled over in bed and fell off. The mother was not present at that time. The bed was about 2.5 feet from the floor, and the child hit the ground on the left side, making contact with his left arm, head, and flank. The boyfriend told the mother that the child cried immediately and was easily consoled.

The mother arrived home about 3 hrs after the incident to find the child asleep in bed. When she asked about feeding, her boyfriend stated that the child had not had any formula for the last several hours. When she tried to wake the child for a feeding, he was barely arousable. At that time, EMS was called, and the child was brought to the emergency department for further evaluation. The mother denies any history of prior trauma and is hesitant to answer questions about her relationship with her boyfriend.

Physical examination shows the child to be very quiet and lethargic. No acute respiratory distress is noted. The child is not responsive to verbal stimuli. There is a left temporal hematoma, 5 × 4 cm. The right arm has an ecchymotic area and the right-upper quadrant region shows an old resolving bruise. The lower lumbosacral area has several areas of mild, yellowish discoloration in a transverse linear distribution. Skin turgor is good. Sclera is anicteric, and conjunctiva is pink. Further examination shows:

Fundi: possible right retinal hemorrhage at 3 o'clock position

Oral: moist mucosa, no lesions

Ears: tympanic membranes with positive light reflexes bilaterally, external canals WNL bilaterally; no evidence of bleeding in the canals

Neck: supple, passive ROM; minor, old, right-sided cervical abrasion noted; no cervical adenopathy, no thyroid masses

Lungs/chest: decreased respiratory effort with shallow respirations; lungs clear to auscultation; left lower costal margin healed contusion

Cardiovascular: S1, S2 regular, no murmurs

Abdomen: positive bowel sounds, minimal response to gentle palpation; possible right flank discomfort with palpation; lower lumbosacral area with several areas of yellowish discoloration as described

Genitalia: Tanner stage 1, testicles descended bilaterally; no inguinal masses

Extremities: passive ROM present bilaterally; no cyanosis, clubbing, or edema; upper right arm ecchymotic area; bilateral infrapatellar minor abrasions without any significant discoloration.

Neurology: child lethargic, not responsive to verbal stimuli; pupils reactive to light bilaterally but sluggish (L > R); deep tendon reflexes present bilaterally but somewhat decreased symmetrically

Patient Safety Note

Regardless of cause, this patient's neurologic status suggests an emergency situation. Always address the ABCs first.

Differential Diagnosis

1. Child abuse

2. Infection: sepsis, meningitis

3. Trauma: accidental injury

4. Metabolic: rickets

5. Congenital: osteogenesis imperfecta, Mongolian spots, minor skeletal anomalies

6. Immunologic: Henoch-Schönlein purpura, immune thrombocytopenic purpura

7. Hematologic: leukemia, hemophilia, von Willebrand disease

Clues

- Physical exam not consistent with history
- Bruising in various stages of healing
- Delayed immunizations (may indicate neglect)
- Social/environmental red flags

Initial Diagnostic and Treatment Plan	Results
• Intubate, and place on ventilator for airway and respiratory control	Done
• Check breath sounds, heart rate, pulse, and BP	Breath sounds clear bilaterally; HR 100/min; pulses full and equal; BP left arm 90/54 mm Hg
• Start IV with maintenance fluids	Done
• Emergency CT scan	Subdural hematoma in left temporal region; no midline shift
• Notify neurosurgeon	Done
• Document physical findings and other injuries	
• Notify child protective services and law enforcement	
• Discuss with parents	
• Move child to surgery and then place in child protective custody pending legal proceedings	

Assessment

The extent and pattern of injuries do not fit the description relayed by the boyfriend (multiple bruises in various stages of healing). The risk factors for abuse in this case are teenage and single parent, low level of education, no reliable child-care, uncertain relationship with the boyfriend, behind on immunizations, and hesitation of mother to discuss relationship with boyfriend.

Lab results show no evidence of bleeding diathesis. Increased liver enzymes are suggestive of blunt abdominal trauma. Elevated CPK is probably from old injuries.

A major management issue is to recognize the emergent nature of this obtunded child.

- Intubation and ventilation are warranted.
- Emergency CT scan of head is needed.
- Neurosurgeon needs to be notified.

When abuse is suspected, notify the hospital on-call person for this service (it may be a social worker), along with child protective services or the police.

Further Diagnostic Plan/Results

Skeletal survey	Several areas of bony injury, including healed left rib fracture and right arm metaphyseal fracture

Treatment

Drainage of subdural hematoma by neurosurgeon

Discussion

Head trauma requires an immediate physical examination (including neurologic), with child-hood Glasgow coma assessment.

- Resuscitate per airway, breathing, circulation
- Significant head trauma standard of care: head CT
  - Focal, evacuable hemorrhage: immediate neurosurgical intervention
- Minor closed head trauma
  - American Academy of Pediatrics (AAP) recommendations
    ○ **With no loss of consciousness:** observe for 24 hrs at home, under competent caregiver
    ○ **With loss of consciousness** <1 min: observe in hospital or do CT scan (no skull x-ray)

If you suspect **child abuse**, use the following general guidelines:

- **History**
  - Does the history fit the examination?
  - What is the past history if there are injuries?
  - Was there an unexpected delay in seeking medical care?
  - Is the child developmentally capable of causing a self-inflicted injury?
- **Physical examination**
  - Multiple systems involved
  - Multiple injuries at different stages of healing
  - Unexplained injuries
  - Patterned injuries

Skin injuries are the most common manifestation of physical abuse.

- **Bruises:** look for different stages of healing
  - Few are pathognomonic for abuse
  - May be external indicator of more serious internal injury
- **Inflicted burns:** children age <5 yrs at highest risk
- **Immersion burns**
  - Accidental: splash marks, varying burn depths, indistinct borders, and multiple areas of burn (struggling)
  - Deliberate: uniform depth, unvaried appearance, distinct borders
- **Contact burns**
  - Hot solids burn by contact

- Accidental: brief contact with small portion of object and thus small burn area with slurred margins

- Abuse: prolonged, steady contact with large portion of object and thus symmetric, deep imprints with crisp margins

Regarding fractures, **several single fractures** are diagnostic of abuse.

- Suspicious: fractures in multiple stages of healing and spiral fractures in nonambulatory children

- Skeletal survey is indicated for all children age <2 yrs with a suspicious fracture or other suspicious injuries; not universally recommended for children age 2–5 yrs; not recommended for children age >5 yrs

- Bone scan may be used as adjunct for more subtle injuries.

Nonaccidental head trauma (shaking, blunt impact, or both) is a major cause of mortality and morbidity.

- Perpetrators are usually a caregiver

- Infants are more frequent victims than toddlers

- Hallmarks are subdural hemorrhage, retinal hemorrhage, brain injury

- All head trauma requires ophthalmologic examination

- CT imaging is initial method of choice, possibly followed by MRI

Retinal hemorrhages are **not pathognomonic** of abuse. They are seen in 30% of newborns delivered via vaginal route but usually resolve within several days (though they can last 5–6 wks).

- Outside newborn period, severe accidental and inflicted injuries are leading causes

- May also be seen with increased intracranial pressure, severe hypertension, carbon monoxide poisoning, meningitis, and coagulopathy

If you suspect child abuse, take the following steps:

- Create thorough documentation; add drawings and dimensions of injuries

- Report to social services, child protective services, police

- With the parents:

  - Hold private discussions.

  - Focus on well being and safety of child.

  - Review findings.

  - Ask them if they feel anybody is abusing the child.

  - Inform them of the need to file a report with child protective services.

  - Do not apportion blame.

  - Explain your ethical and legal obligation to conduct investigation.

Final Diagnosis

Child abuse, subdural hematoma

CLINICAL PEARL

Tap water causes a large percentage of abusive burns and only a small percentage of accidental burns in children.

CASE 11

Chief Complaint

Painless abdominal mass

History and Physical Examination

A 3½-year-old boy is brought to the office for evaluation of a painless abdominal mass that the child's mother noted while bathing him. According to her, he has been acting and playing as usual. She reports regular bowel movements, no vomiting, no change of appetite, and no trauma. Prenatal routine sonogram was remarkable for horseshoe kidney on the right side.

Physical examination shows an afebrile, playful child, with BP 120/75 mm Hg and pulse 90/min. Normal HEENT, clear skin, and supple neck. Heart rate is regular with no murmur and lungs are clear to auscultation. Extremities are normal and there is no adenopathy in the nodes. The abdomen is soft, and a nontender, tennis-ball-sized hard mass is noted on deep palpation, slightly to the right at the level of the umbilicus. The liver and spleen are not palpable, and no bruits or pulsations are appreciated.

CLINICAL PEARL

On the exam you will not be expected to know different BPs for different ages. You will be given obviously high BP.

Differential Diagnosis

1. Wilms tumor
2. Neuroblastoma
3. Choledochal cyst
4. Ectopic or horseshoe kidney
5. Renal vein thrombosis
6. Teratoma
7. Fecal material
8. Pancreatic cyst

Initial diagnostic plan	Results
CBC	WBC 8,200/mm³, hemoglobin 15.5 g/dL
Comprehensive metabolic panel	WNL
Urinalysis	Dip negative for blood
Abdominal sonogram	8- to 10-cm mass arising from lower pole of the right kidney, which is horseshoe-shaped; great vessels patent; no evidence of renal vein invasion
Urinary catecholamines	Vanillylmandelic acid and homovanillic acid WNL

Assessment

This is a very typical presentation.

Combined clinical, lab, and radiographic pictures in a child of this age are consistent with Wilms tumor.

- Painless abdominal mass noted while bathing
- No other symptoms present
- History of a renal abnormality (horseshoe kidney)
- Acute elevation of BP
- Nontender mass on palpation, paraumbilical
- Noncalcified renal mass

Further Diagnostic Plan

After the diagnosis is made, further workup is needed to define the extent and prognosis.

1. MRI of the abdomen to verify extent of the disease
2. Examine for renal vein, contralateral kidney, and liver or node involvement
3. CT of the chest to rule out metastatic disease
4. Echocardiogram to detect tumor in the right atrium and to evaluate pretreatment cardiac function
5. Coagulation studies
6. Laparotomy and ideally complete excision of tumor
7. Surgical specimens to be sent for chromosomal studies (11p13 is pathognomonic)

Further Management Plan

- Surgical removal of mass
- Radiation therapy only if tumor has unfavorable histology or is stage III, IV
- Chemotherapy regimen if staging requires

Discussion

It is important to distinguish Wilms tumor from neuroblastoma.

Final Diagnosis

Wilms tumor

Wilms Tumor	
Nephroblastoma	• Mixed embryonal neoplasm of kidney • Second most common malignant abdominal tumor • May involve both kidneys: bilateral in 7% of patients • Usually age 2–5 yrs
Associations	• Hemihypertrophy (Beckwith-Wiedemann syndrome) • Aniridia • Other anomalies, usually genitourinary
Most are sporadic	• 1–2% with family history (autosomal dominant) • Favorable and unfavorable histology (ectopia, anaplasia)
Clinical: abdominal mass	• Mother usually notices while bathing or physician during well-child exam • Smooth and firm, may cross midline • May have abdominal pain and vomiting • Hematuria not common • Hypertension secondary to renal ischemia
Diagnosis	• CBC, liver function test, renal function test • Tumor markers (chromosomal) • Abdominal flat plate, U/S, CT, MRI; detect intrarenal origin • Extent: examine inferior vena cava prior to surgery (angiography); bone scan; CXR, chest CT
Stages	• Stage I: confined to kidney • Stage II: kidney, but penetrates capsule • Stage III: postsurgical residual nonhematogenous extension confined to abdomen • Stage IV: hematogenous metastases; liver, lungs • Stage V: bilateral renal
Treatment	• Surgery: patency of inferior vena cava prior to surgery; if not patent, then preoperative chemotherapy • Chemotherapy, radiation • If inoperable: chemotherapy, partial resection, radiation • If bilateral: unilateral nephrectomy and partial contralateral
Prognosis	• 2–year 56–98% • 4–year 54–97%

Neuroblastoma	
Embryonal cancer of peripheral sympathetic nervous system	• 8% of childhood malignancies • Most frequent tumor of neonates • Median age is 2 yrs (90% age <5 yrs) • Succession of mutation events prenatally and perinatally • Environmental and genetic factors • Familial: 1–2%
Most arise in abdomen, either adrenal or retroperitoneal sympathetic ganglia	• Firm, nodular, palpable mass at flank or midline • Calcification or hemorrhage
30% originate from cervical, thoracic, or pelvic ganglia	
Most common metastases: long bones, skull, bone marrow, liver, lymph nodes, skin	
Increase in vanillylmandelic acid (VMA) and homovanillic acid (HVA) in urine in 95%	
Stages	• Stage I: confined to organ of origin • Stage II: beyond organ but not across midline • Stage III: beyond midline • Stage IV: disseminated • Stage IV-S: age <1 year with disseminated disease, but no bone involvement and primary tumor that would otherwise be stage 1 or 2; usually regresses in observation

CASE 12

Chief Complaint

Worsening behavioral problems in a 3-year-old girl

History and Physical Examination

A 3-year-old girl is brought to the office because of worsening behavioral problems over the last 2 yrs. Her grandmother is the legal guardian and has been taking care of her since age 2 mos. Her mother is age 24 and has been in a drug rehabilitation program for the last 2.5 yrs with mixed results. Immunizations are up-to-date. The child has no significant past medical history. Her mother used cigarettes, alcohol, and sporadic illegal drugs during the pregnancy. Prenatal care was sporadic at best. The child was born at term, was small for gestational age, and spent 1 week in the hospital for observation.

She appears to be very active, impulsive, and outgoing. Her height is at the fifth percentile for age. The head appears to be small. There are increased epicanthal folds and a low nasal bridge. The maxillary areas are underdeveloped with a thin upper lip. Physical examination shows supple neck and with no masses. Lungs are clear and the abdomen shows positive bowel sounds with no organomegaly. Cardiovascular examination reveals S1, S2, mild pectus excavatum, and physiologic splitting of S2. The extremities show no cyanosis/clubbing, a short fifth finger on both hands, and bilateral limited movement of fingers and elbows. Neurologically, problems with coordination are observed. The child is hyperactive and alert, and very easily startled

Differential Diagnosis

1. Fetal alcohol syndrome (FAS)
2. Failure to thrive

Clues

- Behavioral problems
- Social issues
- Small for gestational age
- Small postnatal
- Dysmorphic

Initial Diagnostic Plan

1. No specific tests for FAS

CLINICAL PEARL

An exact diagnosis often can be made via careful dysmorphic evaluation.

CLINICAL PEARL

"Small for gestational age" means there was intrauterine growth retardation (with several possible causes the case presented here).

Treatment Plan

Physical therapy, occupational therapy; special education program; psychosocial counseling

Assessment

The findings are characteristic for FAS.

- Mother used alcohol during pregnancy
- Intrauterine growth retardation
- Behavioral abnormalities
- Small postnatal stature
- Dysmorphic features: microcephaly, epicanthal folds, low nasal bridge and thin upper lip, underdeveloped maxillae, pectus excavatum, short fifth fingers, and limited movement of fingers and elbows
- Neurologic abnormalities

Discussion

The etiology of FAS is ethanol or byproducts. The least significant defect, seen at 2 drinks per day, is slight, small gestational age. It is not until 4–6 drinks per day that other features become evident. The most significant cases of FAS are seen in those whose mothers who have had $\geq$8–10 drinks per day.

Basic Science Correlate

Alcohol causes irreversible CNS effects in utero throughout pregnancy. The fetus does not eliminate alcohol as effectively as the mother, and is also re-exposed by swallowing amniotic fluid containing ethanol.

The risk of having a serious problem (mostly mental deficiencies) in children born to alcoholic women is 30–50%.

Diagnostic criteria for FAS is a confirmed phenotype, with or without evidence of maternal alcohol exposure.

- Face: abnormal facial features consistent with FAS or 2 of following:
  - Short palpebral fissures
  - Abnormal philtrum (maxillary hypoplasia)
  - Thin upper lip
  - Other facial features: epicanthal folds, micrognathia
  - Smooth philtrum
- CNS: any one of the following
  - Occipital frontal circumference <10% at birth or at any age
  - Standardized measure of intellectual function $\leq$1 standard deviation below mean
  - Standardized measure of developmental delay $\leq$1 standard deviation below mean
  - Developmental delay or intellectual disability diagnosed by qualified examiner
  - ADHD

- Growth: symmetrical IUGR plus any one of the following:
  - Intrauterine height or weight corrected for gestational age <10%
  - Postnatal weight or height <10% for age
  - Postnatal weight or height <10%
- Cardiac (not present in all patients): primarily septal defects
- Minor limb and joint abnormalities
  - Some restriction of movement
  - Altered palmar crease pattern
  - Brachydactyly

Natural history of FAS:

- May be tremulousness in neonatal period
- Postnatal linear growth remains retarded with thin adipose tissue; often looks like failure to thrive
- Infants tend to be irritable and later hyperactive as children
- Usually more social as young adults
- Often dental malalignment, malocclusion, eustachian tube dysfunction, and poor visual-spatial coordination

Therapy for FAS is supportive, with counseling for reoccurrence.

Prognosis of FAS:

- Severity of maternal alcoholism and extent and severity of pattern of malformations are most predictive of ultimate prognosis
- At age 18 yrs, average functioning at fourth grade level
- Abnormal behaviors: poor judgment, distractibility, difficulty recognizing social cues

Patient Safety Note

Since there is no known safe limit of alcohol intake during pregnancy, it should be avoided altogether.

Final Diagnosis

Fetal alcohol syndrome

CASE 13

Chief Complaint

Failure to gain weight

History and physical exam

An 11-month-old boy is seen in the office for failure to gain weight. He was born at term to a 24-year-old primigravida after an unremarkable pregnancy, labor, and delivery. Birth weight was 7 pounds 10 ounces, Apgar scores of 8 and 9.

The patient's first bowel movement was at 36 hrs of age, consisting of thick meconium. Since then, he has had poor weight gain despite adequate caloric intake. His mother describes bulky greasy stools. She also relates repeated episodes of wheezing and persistent coughing, and states that he tastes salty when she kisses him. On physical examination his weight is 17 pounds. He is thin with little adipose tissue or muscle mass. Lung exam is remarkable for scattered crackles and wheezes.

Differential Diagnosis

1. Cystic fibrosis (CF)

2. Celiac disease

3. Bronchiolitis

4. Asthma

5. Immotile cilia syndrome

6. Shwachman-Diamond syndrome

Clues

- Failure to thrive despite adequate calories

- Thick meconium, delayed production

- Bulky, greasy stools

- Repeated respiratory symptoms

- Salty

Initial Management

Setting: outpatient workup and treatment

Diagnostic/Therapeutic Plan

- Chest x-ray

- Complete chemistry profile

- Sweat chloride

Test Results

- Chest x-ray: hyperinflation, evidence of diffuse obstruction

- Hypoalbuminemia

- Sweat chloride: 75 mEq/L Cl

Assessment

- Always plot height and weight on growth charts when evaluating failure to thrive, and attempt to obtain previous medical records that may have recorded growth parameters.

- Document the caloric intake.

- Associated respiratory symptoms should raise suspicion of CF.

- Additionally, nasal polyps or rectal prolapse in a child should raise suspicion of CF and prompt you to obtain a sweat chloride test. (Sweat test should be delayed until infant age $\geq$2 wks and weight $\geq$2 kg.)

- Clubbing is associated with CF.

- Look for GI symptoms associated with introduction of foods (e.g., gluten and celiac disease).

Further Management Plan

- Repeat sweat chloride (done 2x on separate days)

- Treat respiratory symptoms

- Parental counseling and education

Follow-up Management

The goal is to **clear airway secretions and control infections**. This is done using the following:

Bronchodilators	Albuterol/saline
Antibiotics	Cover for *Pseudomonas, Staph aureus, Burkholderia cepacia* Oral, IV, aerosolized *Pseudomonas* requires 2 antibiotics to reduce resistance
Steroids, recombinant DNase	
Chest physical therapy	

Nutrition plays a role in CF.

- Over 85% of cases have exocrine pancreatic insufficiency, resulting in inadequate digestion of fats and proteins.

- Stools are frequent, bulky, and greasy.

- Patients fail to gain weight and often require diet adjustment with pancreatic enzyme replacement and vitamin replacement (ADEK).

- Patients lose excessive amounts of salt, so fluid replacement is essential when exercising (especially during warm weather); hypochloremic alkalosis is common.

- Parents may notice a salt "frosting" of the skin or a salty taste when they kiss their child.

Education of the patient and parent is important. Do follow-up evaluations every 2–3 mos.

Basic Science Correlate

- Autosomal-recessive condition
- Defect is on chromosome 7, CFTR (cystic fibrosis transmembrane conductance regulator) gene mutation, which affects chloride secretion
- Most common mutation is delta F508
- Common respiratory pathogens: *Pseudomonas aeruginosa, Staph aureus, Burkholderia cepacia* complex
- Sweat chloride test is pilocarpine iontophoresis

Discussion

CF is the most common lethal recessive inherited disease in whites. Failure to clear mucous secretions is hallmark of disease, resulting in primarily respiratory manifestations. However, it is a multisystem disease, which also has GI, endocrine, exocrine, and reproductive manifestations.

The sweat chloride test is the **gold standard for diagnosis (>60 mEq/L)**. However, the new diagnostic criteria for CF include:

Presence of any of the Following	*Plus* Any of the Following
Typical clinical features (respiratory, GI, GU)	2 positive sweat chloride tests on 2 days
History of a sibling with CF	Identification of 2 CF mutations
Positive newborn screen	Increased nasal potential difference

Two positive sweat chloride results are required—the first for diagnosis and the second for confirmation.

Multiple organ systems can be affected with CF.

- Respiratory: bronchiolitis, bronchiectasis, nasal polyps, atelectasis, pneumothorax, clubbing
- GI: meconium ileus (**commonly first manifestation** found in newborns); malabsorption; bulky, fatty stools; failure to thrive; rectal prolapse
- Endocrine: pancreatic insufficiency (exocrine and endocrine)
- GU: delayed sexual development, azoospermia, decreased fertility
- Sweat glands: salty taste, propensity to salt depletion with exercise, hot weather

CF requires aggressive antibiotic therapy, chest physical therapy, and clearing secretions.

Final Diagnosis

Cystic fibrosis

CASE 14

Chief Complaint

Toe walking

History and Physical Examination

A 2-year-old boy is seen by the primary care provider because he walks on his toes. He was born at term to a 26-year-old G2P2. Pregnancy was complicated by a maternal UTI. Newborn screen was normal. The patient did not start walking until 18 mos. Physical exam reveals a small left hand and left foot pointed downward. Ankle clonus is present, and deep tendon reflexes are increased.

Differential Diagnosis

1. Cerebral palsy (CP)
2. Degenerative diseases
3. Metabolic disorders
4. Spinal cord tumor
5. Muscular dystrophy

Clues

- Delayed motor milestones
- Contracture of foot
- Ankle clonus and increased DTRs

Initial Management

Setting: outpatient

Diagnostic/Therapeutic Plan

- Spinal MRI
- Brain MRI
- Serum creatine kinase

Test Results

- Spinal MRI: normal
- Brain MRI: atrophic cerebral hemisphere on the right
- Serum creatine kinase: normal

There is no best test for the diagnosis of CP. It is a diagnosis of exclusion.

Assessment

Most children with CP have normal labor and delivery. Around 80% of cases have antenatal insult, causing abnormal brain development. Intrapartum asphyxia occurs in <10%.

Look for intrauterine exposure or maternal infection. There is increased prevalence in low birth weight <1000 grams, usually secondary to intraventricular hemorrhage or periventricular leukomalacia.

Genetic evaluation is warranted if there are congenital anomalies or metabolic disorders. Check newborn screen.

Treatment Plan

CP requires a team approach: occupational therapy, physical therapy, speech therapy, social work, surgery, and pediatric neurology.

- Teach special parenting skills secondary to abnormal muscle tone
- Provide orthotics, walkers
- Use heel cord releases, spinal rods
- Decrease spasticity: dantrolene, benzodiazepines, baclofen, and botulinum toxin
- Offer feeding devices
- Treat other underlying problems, e.g., seizures

Discussion

CP describes a myriad of motor syndromes. It has a wide range of causes: developmental, genetic, metabolic, ischemic, and infectious.

CP results as an injury to the developing brain. It is a static encephalopathy, which means the injury itself is non-progressive. Clinical changes in the patient give the appearance of progression of the disease, but these are merely physical manifestations of the prior injury. CP can be associated with seizures, abnormalities of speech, vision, and intellect.

There are 3 types of CP. With **spastic hemiplegia**, there is decreased spontaneous movement on affected side.

- Early hand preference
- Delayed walking, toe walkers (spasticity)
- Seizures in 1/3, intellectual disability in 1/4
- MRI is most sensitive test

With **spastic diplegia**, there is bilateral spasticity legs > arms. The prognosis is excellent for normal intellectual development with low seizure risk.

- Legs drag when crawling

- Bilateral Babinski

- Scissoring of legs

- Walking delayed, toe walkers

- Disuse atrophy of muscles

With **spastic quadriplegia**, the most severe form of CP, all of the extremities are affected. There is a high association with intellectual disability and seizures.

- Swallowing problems lead to aspiration

- Increased tone, spasticity, contractures, increased deep tendon reflexes

Final Diagnosis

Cerebral palsy

CASE 15

Chief Complaint

Recurrent ear infections

History and Physical Examination

A 2-year-old boy is seen for an ear infection. According to his chart, this is his 4th infection of the year. In addition, he had 3 episodes of otitis media last year, as well as 2 hospitalizations for pneumonia. He is an only child and is cared for at home by his mother. Maternal uncles have a history of pneumonia. Physical exam reveals a small boy, <5% for weight and height. Both tympanic membranes are red and bulging. Tonsils are not visible and no cervical lymph nodes are palpable. The rest of the exam is normal.

Differential Diagnosis

1. Bruton's agammaglobulinemia (X-linked)
2. Transient hypogammaglobulinemia of childhood
3. Common variable immunodeficiency
4. IgA deficiency
5. DiGeorge's syndrome
6. Severe combined immunodeficiency (SCID)
7. Wiskott-Aldrich syndrome
8. Recurrent otitis media

Clues

- Male sex
- Recurrent infections
- No real exposures
- Lymphoid hypoplasia

Initial Management

Setting: outpatient workup and treatment; referral to infectious disease or immunology colleagues will be warranted after initial evaluation

Diagnostic/Therapeutic Plan

- CBC
- Serum immunoglobulins

Test Results

- CBC normal
- Serum immunoglobulins: decreased IgG, IgA, and IgM

Assessment

Suspect immunodeficiency syndromes when:

- ≥1 systemic bacterial infection (sepsis, meningitis)
- ≥2 serious respiratory or documented bacterial infections (cellulitis, draining otitis media, pneumonia)
- Serious infections at unusual sites
- Infections with unusual pathogens
- Common infections of unusual severity
- Also: ≥8 otitis media/year, ≥2 serious infections/year

Features:

- Failure to thrive
- Rash-eczema, telangiectasia
- Diarrhea, malabsorption
- Recalcitrant thrush
- No lymph nodes, tonsils especially when ill
- Weight loss, fever
- Less common: lymphadenopathy, hepatosplenomegaly, recurrent meningitis

Always look for multiple infections, patterns. Ask for family history of recurrent infections. Look for other non-immune features of immunodeficiency (e.g., facial features and DiGeorge's).

Defect	Type of Infection	Organisms
T-cell	Fungal, viral, parasitic	CMV, herpes, varicella, *Pneumocystis, Candida*
B-cell	Bacterial, esp. encapsulated	*Strep pneumoniae, H. influenzae., N. meningitidis*
Complement	Bacterial, esp. encapsulated	*N. meningitidis*
Phagocytic	Bacterial, fungal	*Staph aureus, E. coli, Candida, Pseudomonas*

Further Management Plan

1. Treat otitis media with antibiotics
2. Monthly administration of IV immunoglobulin (IVIG)

Discussion

Basic Science Correlate

The immune system originates from embryonic gut-associated tissue:

- Primary lymphoid organs
  - Thymus
  - Bone marrow
- Secondary lymphoid organs
  - Spleen
  - Lymph nodes
  - Tonsils
  - Peyer's patches

The components of the above are T, B, and NK cells, antibody production, cellular immunity, phagocytes, and complement.

Screening Test for Immunodeficiencies

Most immune deficiencies can be evaluated initially at minimal cost with proper screening tests.

- CBC with manual differential
  - Normal platelets exclude Wiskott-Aldrich
  - Normal absolute neutrophil count excludes neutropenia, leukocyte adhesion defects
  - Normal absolute lymphocyte count excludes severe T-cell defects
  - Markedly increased neutrophils in absence of signs of infection; think of leukocyte adhesion defect
  - Absent Howell-Jolly bodies exclude congenital asplenia
- *Candida* skin test: most cost effective test of T cell function
- ESR: normal excludes chronic bacterial or fungal infection
- Serum immunoglobulin levels: IgG, IgA, IgM

CLINICAL PEARL

Leukocyte adhesion defects are associated with delayed separation of the umbilical cord.

Suspected Deficiency	Clinical Presentation	Initial Labs	Definitive
B cell	• Encapsulated bacteria • Enterovirus, hepatitis	• Quantitative Ig • Normal IgA excludes most	• Flow cytometry • Molecular Dx if no FH
T cell	• Opportunistic infections • Chronic diarrhea • FTT	• Absolute lymphocyte count • Normal precludes Dx • If low, *Candida* skin test • Normal precludes all	• Mitogen stimulation • Flow cytometry • Molecular Dx if no FH
Phagocytic	• *Staph* and gram-negative	• Respiratory burst assay with rhodamine • Flow cytometry	• Molecular Dx
Complement	• Pyogenic infections • Life threatening septicemia • *Neisseria* infections	• CH50	• Specific complement assay • Molecular Dx

Bruton's (X-linked hypogammaglobulinemia)

- Clinically normal until 6 mos; maternal antibody protects
- Then, recurrent pyogenic infections: bacterial otitis media, bronchitis, pneumonia, meningitis
- Look for *Strep pneumoniae, H. influenzae* B
- Approximately 20% have affected male maternal relatives
- No lymphoid tissue
- Treat with IVIG
- 50% survival by age 50

Final Diagnosis

Bruton's X-linked hypogammaglobulinemia

CASE 16

Chief Complaint

Routine health supervision visit for 1-year-old girl

History and Physical Examination

A 1-year-old child is seen in your office for a routine health supervision visit. The mother has no concerns at this time. The patient is eating table foods and starting to walk unassisted. She is using 1–3 words. Immunizations are up-to-date.

On physical examination she is at the 50th percentile for weight and 75th percentile for height. HEENT is normal. She has 8 teeth. Lungs are clear to auscultation. Heart is without murmur, and she has good capillary refill and no pulse lag. Abdomen is soft to palpation without organomegaly. Genitalia is healthy female Tanner 1. She is ambulating in the exam room.

Discussion

This is a normal 1-year-old child. The health supervision visit is an excellent opportunity to assess the nutrition, growth and development of the patient, as well as administer immunizations. It is also a time to evaluate interactions between the parents and child. In addition to addressing any concerns on part of the parents (and the child if age appropriate), anticipatory guidance and advice on patient safety should be given. It is the model for preventive care medicine.

Car seats (AAP recommendations): children should be placed in an appropriate-sized car seat. All occupants of the car should be wearing seat belts.

- Age 0-4: children should be placed in a car seat that is rear-facing and set in the back seat (never in the front seat with an air bag); child should stay rear-facing until at least age 2

- Age 4 to age 8: children should be placed in a booster seat

- Age ≥13: children can safely ride in the front seat

Water safety: children should never be left alone near a pool or spa. Pools, spas, buckets, and tubs should be drained when not in use.

- An adult should be within arm's reach of all toddlers near water. Children should never swim alone.

- Swim lessons can be started as early as age 1 year; however, do not assume the child is "drown proof" simply because lessons have been provided.

- Pool fences should be at least 4 feet high around all sides of the pool; they should not be "climbable."

- Pool gates should be self-closing and self-latching, and should open "out" from the pool.

- Rescue equipment (preferably fiberglass or another non-conducting material) should be kept nearby.

Sun safety: children age <6 mos should be kept out of the sun and dressed in lightweight clothes that cover the skin. For all other children:

- Cover up: hats, sunglasses, tightly woven clothes

- Stay in shade during peak hrs of 10 AM-4 PM

- Use sunscreen with SPF 15 or greater; reapply every 2 hrs, after swimming or sweating

Firearm safety: guns should preferably not be kept in the home, but if they are present, they should be unloaded and locked up. Always inquire about possible guns at playmate's homes.

Environmental safety: homes should be "childproofed."

- Set gates at stairs and guards on windows higher than first floor

- Cover outlets

- Close doors

- Face all pot handles in

- Set water heater no more than 120° F

- Discourage the use of walkers

- Keep poison center phone numbers handy

Bike safety: children should use properly fitting helmets and appropriately sized bikes.

Screening

- Newborn screen

- Age 12 and 24 mos: lead screen

- Age 9–11 yrs and 17–21 yrs: dyslipidemia

- Each health supervision visit: development

- Age 11–21 yrs: depression

Adolescence

- – Sexually related behavior

- – Tobacco, alcohol and other drug use

- – Intentional/unintentional injuries

- – Violence, bullying

- – Mental health

CASE 17

Chief Complaint

"Why is my baby yellow?"

History and Physical Examination

A 30-year-old woman, estimated gestational age 40 wks, comes to the labor and delivery floor with contractions of 3 mins and spontaneous rupture of membranes for 2 hrs. She has gestational diabetes, which is diet-controlled. Her blood type is A-positive. Pelvic examination reveals 4 cm of dilation and 90% effacement and the vertex at −2 station. Labor is augmented with oxytocin and progresses without complications. A girl (Apgar score 9 at 1 min and 9 at 5 mins) is delivered, forceps assisted, over a right mediolateral episiotomy. Her birth weight is 3,800 g. The newborn is examined by the pediatrician and noted as appropriate for gestational age. She is breast-feeding without difficulty upon discharge from the hospital.

Two days after discharge, the mother brings the newborn to the office because she notes her baby appears to be "yellow." Physical examination is WNL, except for the clinical jaundice, especially in the face.

Clues

- The A+ blood type in the mother rules out Rh and most ABO isoimmunization. There is still a possibility of minor-blood-group incompatibility.

- An early cause of jaundice is lack of calories secondary to poor breast-feeding (it may occur with formula-fed infants, as well). This is not the same as breast-milk jaundice.

CCS NOTE

Although isoimmunization is unlikely, the direct Coombs test is a good idea for an initial screen if there is an ABO and or Rh setup with anemia.

Differential Diagnosis

1. Physiologic jaundice
2. Pathologic jaundice: direct hyperbilirubinemia; indirect hyperbilirubinemia

Initial diagnostic plan	Results
1. Bilirubin (total, conjugated, unconjugated)	9 mg predominantly unconjugated
2. CBC	Normal hemoglobin, normal WBC (not suggestive of infection)
3. Coombs test	Negative

Basic Science Correlate

Bilirubin is the byproduct of heme metabolism. Bilirubin itself is conjugated by the enzyme uridine uridine diphosphate glucuronosyl transferase (UGT1A1), resulting in bilirubin diglucuronides, which are soluble and then secreted into the bile. Enterohepatic circulation of bile refers to the uptake of unconjugated bilirubin via absorption through the intestines, and then transported back into the biliary system.

Breast milk jaundice refers to jaundice that occurs after the first week of life and lasts for 3–12 wks. Breast milk causes increased intestinal absorption of bilirubin due to increased enterohepatic circulation.

Anticipatory guidance: continue to encourage and support mothers in their decision to breastfeed; recommend exclusive breastfeeding for the first 6 mos of life and appropriate frequency: 8–10×/24 hrs, and continued monitoring of frequency of urine diapers — minimum of 6 per 24 hrs.

Assessment

Physiologic jaundice (**very common**) is caused by an increased RBC mass with a subsequent increased level of RBC metabolism in the presence of immature hepatic enzymes, leading to hyperbilirubinemia. Characteristics include:

- Rate of rise <5 mg/dL in 24 hrs
- Jaundice visible on days 2–3 of life
- Bilirubin peaks on days 2–4 of life; total bilirubin decreases to <2 mg/dL days 5–7 (very few infants will have bilirubin >12.9 mg/dL)

Search for the cause (possible pathologic jaundice):

- Appears in first 24 hrs of life
- Rate >5 mg/dL in 24 hrs
- Total bilirubin >12 mg/dL in full-term infant or >10 to 14 mg/dL in preterm
- Persists >10–14 days
- Direct bilirubin >2 mg/dL at any time

Indirect hyperbilirubinemia is increased unconjugated bilirubin and is the most common hyperbilirubinemia. Direct hyperbilirubinemia is conjugated (with glucuronide), defined as direct bilirubin >2 mg/dL.

Basic Science Correlate

Phototherapy converts bilirubin to lumirubin by structural isomerization.

Further Management Plan

In this case, we would simply monitor the bilirubin levels and ensure good feeding. Ask about the number of wet diapers and stools per day.

With higher levels of bilirubin, phototherapy is commonly used. There are no universal standards for its use, but it is based on bilirubin level, day of life, gestational age at birth, and infant risk assessment.

- Consider when total bilirubin is approximately 2/3 of the exchange level.

- Expect exchange level to be 25–30 mg/dL in an otherwise healthy term infant, and much lower for preterms and ill neonates.

- There is increased risk of kernicterus (indirect bilirubin crossing the blood-brain barrier and affecting basal ganglia) with total bilirubins persistently >30 mg/dL.

Continue phototherapy until there is a consistent decrease to <12 to 14 mg/dL. Bilirubin follow-up levels are needed to ensure return to lower levels.

Discussion

Workup for pathologic hyperbilirubinemia starts with the question, **Is bilirubin direct versus indirect** (conjugated vs. unconjugated)?

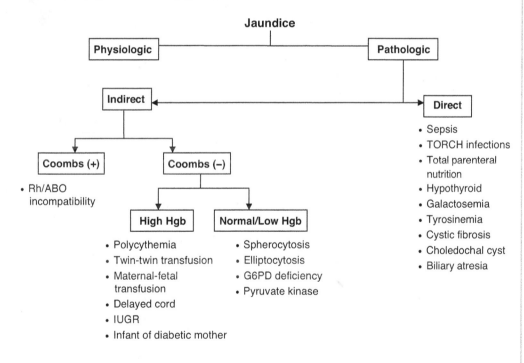

Jaundice Workup

Direct

- Infectious: sepsis, intrauterine infection (TORCH)

- Anatomic: congenital hepatitis (biliary atresia); choledochal cyst

- Endocrine/metabolic: hypothyroidism; galactosemia; cystic fibrosis; alpha-1 antitrypsin deficiency; prolonged total parenteral nutrition

CCS NOTE

- If sepsis is suspected, do a septic workup.

- Check lab results for any questionable prenatal screens.

- Check IgM-specific titers for TORCH (urine culture × 3 for CMV, PCR of any fluid for herpes).

- Look for reducing substance in urine for galactosemia.

- Start with U/S of liver and bile ducts; cholangiography/biopsy may be needed for biliary atresia.

Indirect: Coombs test

- Positive: isoimmunization (ABO, Rh, minor blood groups)

- Negative:

  - [Hb] **high = polycythemia**: delayed cord clamp; maternal-fetal transfusion; twin-twin transfusion (monozygotic); intrauterine growth retardation; infants of diabetic mothers

  - [Hb] **normal or low**

    ○ **Reticulocyte count increased:** characteristic RBC morphology spherocytosis; elliptocytosis; noncharacteristic RBC morphology G6PD deficiency; pyruvate kinase deficiency

    ○ **Reticulocytes normal, nonspecific RBCs:** enclosed hemorrhage (cephalohematoma); increased enterohepatic circulation; asphyxia

Final Diagnosis

Physiologic hyperbilirubinemia

CASE 18

Chief Complaint

Mild pain in right groin and inner thigh

History and Physical Examination

An 8-year-old boy is brought to the office because of a limp of the right leg for 3 months. He states that he limps intermittently after activity, but for the last 2 days it has been constant. He also complains of mild pain in the right groin and inner thigh. He is afebrile, has normal vital signs, and appears well. Physical examination shows normal HEENT; neck is supple with no lymphadenopathy; and the abdomen is benign. The lungs are clear to auscultation bilaterally. Cardiovascular exam reveals normal rhythm, no murmurs. The extremities show decreased ROM of right hip in abduction and internal rotation. Neurological exam reveals nonfocal, cranial nerves II–XII intact, normal muscular tone, no clonus; reflexes 2+ and symmetric.

Differential Diagnosis

1. Joint disease

2. Infection

3. Trauma

4. Connective tissue disease

5. Neoplastic disease

6. Other orthopedic disorders: leg length inequality, vertebral disorders, osteoid osteoma (neck of femur common)

Clues

- Knee pain may indeed be due to referred pain from hip pathology or as is suggested here, localized to the soft tissue around the hip.

- Pertinent negatives include no joint swelling, erythema, or tenderness.

- The presence of a limp for 3 mos rules out significant infection, i.e., septic arthritis or osteomyelitis.

Initial Management

Setting: outpatient

Diagnostic/Therapeutic Plan

- X-rays: standing anteroposterior and frog-leg lateral of pelvis

- CBC

- ESR

CCS NOTE

This is always a good initial workup to evaluate a limp, especially if the hip is suspected. Otherwise, x-rays of specific bones can be ordered. In this case it is clear this cannot be a septic hip or osteomyelitis. In evaluating the hip, the combination of the standing AP x-ray and frog-leg gives the radiologist the information needed to appropriately interpret any abnormalities of the hip joint.

Test Results

- X-rays: complete collapse of femoral head
- CBC: normal
- ESR: normal

Assessment

Presentation in a prepubertal boy with a chronic limp, referred pain to groin and inner thigh, normal CBC and ESR, and the characteristic pelvic x-ray translates to Legg-Calvé-Perthes disease (avascular necrosis of femoral head).

Discussion of Differential Diagnosis:

- Slipped capital femoral epiphysis (SCFE) (**most common adolescent hip disorder**) is commonly seen in obese or tall males with rapid growth spurts; with acute and acute-on-chronic SCFE often presenting with a history of minor trauma. Pain is often referred to the knee and x-rays show a widening of growth plate with or without slip. Treatment is in-patient bed rest, and then in situ pinning of the epiphysis and displaced femoral head.

- Developmental dysplasia of the hip (DDH): Risk factors in a neonate are breech positioning in utero, positive family history, female sex

- Infection

  - Osteomyelitis or septic arthritis: acute with systemic illness; may be toxic-appearing; significant pain and tenderness to palpation; elevated WBC with left shift and increased ESR (and CRP)

  - Transient synovitis: age 3–8 yrs; affected joint is usually of the hip; pain preceded by nonspecific viral illness (URI); no fever or mild temperature elevation, no systemic findings; mild WBC and ESR elevations; no abnormal x-ray findings; resolves in 7–10 days

- Connective tissue disease: juvenile idiopathic arthritis (JIA) (**most common**) does not typically involve the hip initially; search for other joint swelling, erythema, and tenderness; consider ESR, CRP, rheumatoid factor, and ANA as screens

- Neoplastic disease (**most common primary orthopedic malignancies in decade 2 of life**); use initial plain x-ray to evaluate tumor versus trauma

  - Ewing sarcoma: plain x-ray shows "onion-skin" pattern

  - Osteogenic sarcoma: plain x-ray shows "sunburst" pattern

  - Other malignancies may present with joint or bone pain: leukemia, lymphoma, metastatic neuroblastoma

Patient Safety Note

Generally with trauma, a history often can be elicited from the child or caregiver.

CLINICAL PEARL

Always consider systemic disease as an etiology, especially if a child has bilateral SCFE, though the presentation may be asynchronous (occur at different times). An endocrine workup should be obtained, e.g., to rule out hypothyroidism or growth hormone deficiency if there is clinical evidence of this. Other risk factors for SCFE include renal failure and irradiation.

Treatment Plan

The aim is to contain the femoral head within the acetabulum in order to maintain the natural shape of the hip joint, thereby preserving normal function. This may be accomplished by nonsurgical containment with bed rest and abduction exercises.

In a child with a limp, use the following guidelines:

- **Limp that is painful**
  - History of trauma: yes
    - Abnormal x-rays: fracture, SCFE
    - Normal x-rays: non-bony injury
  - History of trauma: no
    - Positive fever with acute systemic symptoms: check CBC, ESR/CRP, x-rays, ± bone scan, U/S, MRI
      - Abnormal results: osteomyelitis, septic arthritis, transient synovitis, rheumatic disease
      - Normal results: transient synovitis, rheumatic disease
    - No fever or acute illness: consider x-rays
      - Trauma, abuse
      - Transient synovitis
      - Legg-Calvé-Perthes disease, slipped capital femoral epiphysis
      - Rheumatic disease
      - Malignancy
      - Neuromuscular disorders
- **Limp that is not painful**
  - First noticeable when patient started to walk (age ~1 year): no
    - Refer to No history of trauma above
  - First noticeable when patient started to walk (age ~1 year): yes
    - Careful neurologic exam
      - Normal: developmental hip dysplasia; leg length inequality; foot abnormality (e.g., clubfoot)
      - Abnormal: cerebral palsy; anatomic spinal abnormality; other neuromuscular disease

Discussion

Legg-Calvé-Perthes disease presents age 3–12, and is defined as idiopathic osteonecrosis or avascular necrosis of the hip. There are, however, known causes that may cause avascular necrosis as well, e.g., systemic glucocorticoid use or renal failure.

For diagnosis, x-rays may be initially performed, but they may appear normal in the early stages. Other findings that can be visualized are an irregular physis or a widened medial joint space. If x-rays are normal, do a bone scan or MRI.

Treatment is orthopedic referral and non-surgical containment of the femoral head.

Final Diagnosis

Legg-Calvé-Perthes disease

CASE 19

Chief Complaint

Rash

History and Physical Examination

A 6-year-old boy has not been feeling well for the last week. He has had a low-grade temperature, joint pains, and abdominal pain with occasional vomiting. His mother became more concerned this morning when she noticed a rash on the backs of his legs. He appears tired but in no acute distress.

Vital signs are T 38.1 C (100.6 F), pulse 100/min, respirations 20/min, and BP 96/60 mm Hg. Eyes are anicteric, and tympanic membranes are normal. Nares are without discharge; his throat is pink without lesions or exudate and his neck is supple without adenopathy. Lungs are clear. Heart sounds are normal, and there is no murmur. His abdomen is soft with active bowel sounds and mild diffuse tenderness; no mass or organomegaly; no guarding, rigidity, or rebound is present. Extremities are without cyanosis, clubbing, or edema. There are well-defined hyperemic macules scattered over the legs and buttocks, with a rare lesion on the back of the arms. Some are raised and palpable, and none blanch with pressure.

Differential Diagnosis

1. Henoch-Schönlein purpura (HSP)
2. Rocky Mountain spotted fever (RMSF)
3. Kawasaki disease
4. Meningococcemia
5. Systemic juvenile idiopathic arthritis

Clues

- Location of rash
- Description of rash
- Abdominal pain, vomiting
- Examination showing diffuse tenderness

Initial Management

Setting: inpatient workup and treatment

Diagnostic/Therapeutic Plan

CCS NOTE

The occult blood in the stool and abnormal urinalysis are very significant for this case, and will change the location of management of this patient.

- Stool for occult blood
- ESR
- CBC
- Urinalysis
- Hospital admission for close monitoring: abdominal findings for possibility of acute abdomen; urine, electrolytes, and renal function (obtain renal consult if no improvement or worsening); IV hydration and possible IV steroids for abdominal pain (but effectiveness not clear); pain control with acetaminophen

Test Results

- Stool: positive
- ESR: 18 mm/h
- CBC: WBC 9,900/mm³, hematocrit 42%, platelets 320,000/mm³
- Urinalysis: 2+ protein with RBC and WBC casts

Assessment

With RMSF, the rash commonly starts on the hands and feet, and then spreads to the rest of the body. It becomes purpuric. This patient does not meet the criteria for Kawasaki disease, nor is this the pattern of rash seen in meningococcemia (by the time the rash appears, the patient is usually obtunded).

Clinical diagnosis of HSP is based on the following:

- Constitutional symptoms
- Joint pain
- Characteristic rash in dependent areas, e.g., legs, buttocks, lower back, back of arms; begins as hyperemic macules and progresses to purpura and petechiae
    - May initially be confused with immune thrombocytopenic purpura (ITP) but normal platelet count rules this out
    - There is a misconception that purpuric rash only appears on the backs of lower parts of body; that is not always the case
- Abdominal findings
- Renal findings

CCS NOTE

The presence of abdominal and/or renal findings in HSP warrants hospitalization.

Discussion

HSP (anaphylactoid purpura) is the most common cause of nonthrombocytopenic purpura in children. It typically follows an upper respiratory infection.

- Vasculitis of small vessels
- Most cases are in winter or spring; not common in summer
- Males > females

Clinical:

- Low-grade fever and fatigue
- Rash begins as erythematous maculopapules
- Petechiae and then PALPABLE (diagnostic criteria) purpura follows, evolving from red to purple and then to rust-brown before fading and may reappear up to 4 mos after initial appearance
- Occurs in crops that last 3–10 days
- Rash is non-pruritic and present on dependent areas
- Arthritis: usually localized to knees and ankles

Edema and damage to vessels of GI tract (**most common acute complication**):

- Colicky abdominal pain
- Diarrhea, vomiting

- Occult blood (or gross) in stool

- Hematemesis

- Intussusception

- Perforation

Renal involvement (25–50% of patients; can present up to 6 mos after initial diagnosis):

- Proteinuria

- Interstitial nephritis

- Glomerulonephritis

- Renal insufficiency/failure

Labs are neither specific nor diagnostic:

- Moderate thrombocytosis and leukocytosis (acute-phase reactants)

- Acute GI blood loss, leading to anemia

- Abnormal urinalysis

Further Management Plan

Treatment is symptomatic with bed rest at home and pain control if there are only constitutional symptoms plus rash and joint pain. The presence of GI or renal symptoms requires hospitalization.

- For GI symptoms, use IV steroids for severe pain and/or symptoms

- For renal symptoms, follow renal function, BP, chemistries, urinalysis

If there is no improvement with other symptoms or if condition worsens, consider a renal biopsy and treatment per specific pathology.

Basic Science Correlate

The pathologic characteristic of HSP in the GI tract is bowel wall edema and even hemorrhage. This is due to an immune-mediated vasculitis resulting in IgA deposition. The bowel wall edema and inflammation can be the means for a lead point for intussusception, as well as ischemia and then perforation.

Because of the bowel wall edema, IV steroids will be absorbed better than PO. Major complications of HSP are renal failure and bowel perforation or intussusception in the GI tract.

Follow-up Management and Prevention

Patients with HSP should be followed closely after discharge from the hospital. Renal involvement can manifest up to 6 mos after initial presentation. Patients should be seen every 1–2 wks for the first 2 mos, and then every 1–2 mos for 1 year. Obtain BP at each visit, as well as urinalysis and monitoring for proteinuria and hematuria. If either BP or urinalysis is abnormal, draw serum BUN and creatinine (to monitor renal function) and refer to a nephrologist.

Final Diagnosis

Henoch-Schönlein purpura

CASE 20

Chief Complaint

Fever and irritability for a couple of days

History and Physical Examination

A 19-month-old girl is brought to the office because of a sudden-onset fever of 40.2 C (104.4 F) and right ear pain. She has generally been in good health but has recently attended a day care center. Two days ago she developed a low-grade temperature with colorless rhinorrhea and some irritability. She seemed slightly better with over-the-counter decongestant medications. This morning, she was much more irritable than previously, pulling at her right ear. She appears easily consoled by her mother.

Physical examination shows that the anterior fontanelle is closed. The left tympanic membrane is normal, and the right tympanic membrane is erythematous and bulging. Nares have minimal watery discharge with colorless crusting. The throat is slightly hyperemic without lesions or exudate, and the neck is supple without adenopathy. Lungs are clear. Heart sounds are normal with 1/6 systolic ejection murmur at the left sternal border. The abdomen is soft, not tender, with no mass or organomegaly appreciated. Extremities are without cyanosis, clubbing, or edema.

CLINICAL PEARL

The ear canals must be cleared of cerumen to obtain a good view of the tympanic membranes. Always perform pneumatic otoscopy to determine the degree of tympanic membrane movement.

Differential Diagnosis

Acute otitis media of bacterial or viral etiology

Initial Management

Setting: outpatient workup and treatment

Initial diagnostic plan	Results
Usually diagnosed by history and exam.	
Insufflation on pneumatic otoscopy	Diminished mobility on the right

Assessment

This presentation fits the criteria for acute otitis media:

- Acute onset of signs and symptoms
- Presence of middle ear effusion: bulging or fullness, limited or absent mobility, air fluid level or bubble, otorrhea
- Signs and symptoms of middle ear inflammation: tympanic membrane bulging or full, and either distinct tympanic membrane erythema or otalgia

Treatment Plan

1. Pain relief is essential: acetaminophen, NSAIDs (except acetylsalicylic acid because of risk of Reye syndrome)

2. Initial observation for older child if nonsevere (mild pain, T <39.0 C [102.2 F] and uncertain acute otitis media (ensure a follow-up in 48 hrs); for clinical failure at 48–72 hrs, start antibiotics

3. Amoxicillin, high-dose (**drug of choice**): for age <5 yrs and severe, give 10-day course, divided bid; for age >5 yrs and mild, give 5–7-day course; for clinical failure at 48–72 hrs, change antibiotics (amoxicillin-clavulanate, cefuroxime axetil, cefdinir, intramuscular ceftriaxone)

Discussion

Otitis media is a general term that describes inflammation of the middle ear.

- **Acute suppurative otitis media** (peak prevalence 6–20 mos)

  - Heritable component

  - Inverse prevalence with socioeconomic factors, i.e., less common in those who were breast-fed and more common in those whose mothers smoked during pregnancy; who are exposed to other children (day care)

  - More common in cold months in temperate climates

  - More common in those with congenital facial/neck/airway abnormalities

  - Many cases involve both bacteria and viruses: most common pathogenic bacteria isolated from middle ear fluid are *S. pneumonia*, nontypeable *H. influenza*, and *Moraxella catarrhalis*

  - Pathogenesis is Eustachian tube obstruction; impaired middle ear ventilation; subtle immune defects; and craniofacial anomalies

- **Otitis media with effusion** (*chronic* if effusion ≥3 mos)

  - Test hearing and continue to monitor

  - Antibiotics not recommended, nor are antihistamines/decongestants

  - Tympanostomy tubes recommended after 4–6 mos of bilateral otitis media with effusion with any bilateral hearing defect

Evaluation of ear pain: **tympanic membrane and canal normal**?

- **Yes**: referred pain, temporal mandibular joint disease, tonsillitis/pharyngitis, herpes zoster, dental condition (abscess, tooth eruption)

- **No**:

  - Positive external ear findings (localized tenderness/swelling in outer third of canal = furuncle; pain on movement of pinna or tragus, swollen and erythematous canal ± discharge (otitis externa, foreign body)

  - Positive middle ear findings (tympanic membrane red and bulging, decreased mobility, effusion = acute otitis media; tender swelling of skull posterior to auricle = mastoiditis; tympanic membrane smooth and noninflammatory, decreased mobility = otitis media with effusion; sac-like structure behind or adjacent to tympanic membrane ± discharge = cholesteatoma)

Final Diagnosis

Otitis media

CASE 21

Chief Complaint

Rash, joint pain of the hands

History and Physical Examination

A 17-year-old girl has a 2-day history of facial erythema and rash, which also appeared today over the trunk. She also noted some swelling of her hands, which is painful when she tries to clutch objects. These symptoms were preceded by low-grade fever not exceeding 38.7 C (101.7 F), runny nose, and pink eyes for the last 2 days. She had previously been in good health. Her immunization record is up to date, except for the MMR vaccine, which she received at age 14 mos. Vital signs are T 38.2 C (100.8 F), pulse 92/min, and BP 115/75 mm Hg. Physical examination shows:

HEENT: discrete erythematous maculopapules involving the entire face, extending behind the ears; some confluent erythematous areas; mild bilateral conjunctivitis and pharyngeal erythema notable, along with retroauricular, postoccipital, and posterior cervical lymphadenopathy; no photophobia

Skin: rash over entire trunk similar to the face, but larger areas of confluence; minimal itching, no desquamation

Neck: supple

CV: RRR, no murmurs

Lungs: clear to auscultation

Abdomen: benign, no hepatosplenomegaly

Extremities: full ROM with mild swelling of the small joints of the hands bilaterally

Neurology: nonfocal, cranial nerves intact

Differential Diagnosis

1. Rubella
2. Measles
3. Scarlet fever
4. Infectious mononucleosis
5. Juvenile idiopathic arthritis, systemic onset

Clue

- Patient didn't receive a second dose of MMR

Initial Management

Setting: outpatient workup and treatment

Diagnostic/Therapeutic Plan

- CBC

Test Results

- WBC: 6,000/mm^3
- Lymphocytes: 60% (none are atypical)
- Hemoglobin: 12.5 g/dL
- Platelets: 230,000/mm^3

Assessment

There is no necessary test here. This case is based on clinical diagnosis. Evaluation of child-hood exanthematous illnesses is done as follows:

- Prodromal symptoms: 2-day history of low-grade fever, rhinorrhea, and pink eyes
- Nature of rash: erythematous, maculopapular
- Initial location of rash: face and behind ears
- Description of rash spread: craniocaudal
- Enanthem: none
- Lymphadenopathy: yes (retroauricular, posterior cervical, occipital)
- Other associated signs and symptoms: swelling of hands, mild swelling of small joints of hands
- Known exposures/other information: no known exposures/no second MMR

With these clinical findings, the diagnosis is rubella.

Further Diagnostic Plan

Ask about any possibility of pregnancy. No other lab analyses are warranted. This is a clinical diagnosis.

Treatment Plan

There is no specific treatment for infection with rubella. Care is supportive. Amantadine is effective in vitro but it is not in infants with congenital rubella.

Discussion

Some common rashes include:

- **Petechial or purpuric: CBC, differential, platelets, consider PT/PTT, blood culture, CSD**
  - Viruses: enteroviruses, congenital rubella, cytomegalovirus, atypical measles, hemor-rhagic varicella, HIV

- – Bacteria and *Rickettsia*: sepsis, endocarditis, *Pseudomonas aeruginosa*, Rocky Mountain spotted fever, endemic typhus
  - – Others: Henoch-Schönlein purpura, vasculitis, thrombocytopenia
- **Macular or maculopapular**
  - – Viruses: roseola, measles, rubella, fifth disease, Epstein-Barr, adenovirus, enteroviruses, hepatitis B
  - – Bacteria and *Rickettsia*: *Mycoplasma pneumoniae*, scarlet fever, leptospirosis, meningococcal (early), Lyme disease, Rocky Mountain spotted fever (early), typhus
  - – Other: Kawasaki disease, *Coccidioides immitis*
- **Diffuse erythroderma**
  - – Scarlet fever
  - – Other streptococci
  - – Toxic shock syndrome
  - – Staphylococcal scalded skin
- **Urticarial**
  - – Viruses: Epstein-Barr, hepatitis B, HIV, enteroviruses
  - – Bacteria: *M. pneumoniae*, group A strep
  - – Other: parasites, insect bites, drug reaction
- **Vesicular, bullous, pustular**: consider Gram stain and culture of lesion, Tzanck preparation, PCR testing
- **Erythema nodosum**: consider strep culture or antigen detection tests, hepatitis B serology, purified protein derivative test, chest x-ray
  - – Viruses: Epstein-Barr, hepatitis B
  - – Bacteria: group A strep, TB, *Yersinia*, cat-scratch disease
  - – Fungi: coccidioidomycosis, histoplasmosis
  - – Other: sarcoidosis, IBD, systemic lupus erythematosus, Behçet disease
- **Distinctive rashes**
  - – Ecthyma gangrenosum → *Pseudomonas aeruginosa*
  - – Erythema chronicum migrans → Lyme disease
  - – Necrotic eschar → *Aspergillosis*, mucormycosis
  - – Erysipelas → group A strep
  - – Koplik spots → measles
  - – Erythema marginatum → rheumatic fever

Final Diagnosis

Rubella

Common Childhood Infections With Exanthems

	Measles	Rubella	Mumps	Varicella	Fifth Disease	Roseola	Scarlet Fever
Virus	RNA-Paramyxo	RNA-Rubivirus	RNA-Paramyxo	Neurotropic herpes	DNA-erythro	Human herpes 6&7	Group A strep—erythrogenic exotoxin
Incubation	8–12 days	14–23 days	16–18 days	14–16 days	4–14 days	9–10 days	2–5 days
Prodrome	Cough, coryza, conjunctivitis; high fever	Mild constitutional symptoms	Hepatitis A, fever, malaise, muscle pain	Low-grade fever, malaise, URI symptoms	Mild URI symptoms	URI symptoms, abrupt onset. High fever, then breaks	Sore throat
Enanthem	Koplik spots	Forchheimer spots	Glandular swelling	None	None	None	Exudative pharyngitis, strawberry tongue
Exanthem	Macules—hairline, face, neck, then to trunk and extremities	Similar to measles; posterior cervical and auricular nodes	Swollen parotid and submandibular glands	Crops of papules, vesicles, crusts at same time; central to peripheral	Slapped cheeks, then to trunk, and then central clearing—lacy	Fever falls rapidly, then fine macular rash on trunk and spreads to extremities	Fine maculopapular rash; feels like sandpaper; especially in antecubital and inguinal area; Pastia lines
Complications	Pneumonia, encephalitis; subacute sclerosing panencephalitis	Congenital rubella—teratogenic	Encephalitis, orchitis, pregnancy-aqueductal stenosis; pancreatitis	Superinfection, zoster, pneumonia, hepatitis, encephalitis, congenital varicella	Aplastic anemia	Pneumonia	Acute renal failure, glomerulonephritis
Return to School	At least 2 wks after appearance of rash	7 days after onset of rash	9 days after onset of parotid swelling	After all lesions have crusted	Once rash develops, no longer infectious	No control measures	24 hrs after start of antibiotics

CASE 22

Chief Complaint

Fever and difficulty breathing

History and Physical Examination

A 2-month-old boy is brought to the office during the winter with a 2-day history of a fever of 38.3 C (100.9 F) and difficulty breathing. His mother reports that he also has a poor appetite and clear nasal discharge. His 4-year-old sibling has a "cold." The patient has an unremarkable birth history and no past medical history. He appears to be active but in mild respiratory distress. His pulse is 160/min, respirations 60/min, and temperature 37.0 C (98.6 F).

Physical examination shows a supple neck; bilateral expiratory wheezing, subcostal retractions; normal heart rate and rhythm with no murmurs; benign abdomen; no cyanosis and good perfusion in the extremities; and clear skin with no rashes.

Basic Science Correlate

Wheezing is primarily expiratory and occurs in the intrathoracic airways. Upon expiration, the intrathoracic airways become smaller and the extrathoracic airways enlarge.

Differential Diagnosis

1. Respiratory syncytial virus (RSV)

2. *Chlamydia trachomatis* pneumonia

3. Bacterial pneumonia

4. Asthma

Initial Management

Setting: emergency department

Diagnostic/Therapeutic Plan

- Chest x-ray
- CBC

Test Results

- X-ray: air trapping with hyperexpansion; peribronchial thickening and interstitial pneumonia
- CBC: WNL

CCS NOTE

With a history of poor oral intake and concern about the child's hydration status, consider ordering a chem 7 and urinalysis as well.

Assessment

Bronchiolitis is a clinical diagnosis, and the most common etiologic agent is RSV. The RSV season is usually November to April. Other less common organisms are rhinovirus, parainfluenza virus, adenovirus, human metapneumovirus, and influenza.

Look for the following:

- Initial nonspecific upper respiratory tract infection; often household contact with URI
- Usually low-grade fever, may go higher
- Cough becomes worse with onset tachypnea, dyspnea, and wheezing
- Can occur with respiratory syncytial viral pneumonia

If in doubt of diagnosis, obtain a nasopharyngeal swab for rapid antigen detection of respiratory syncytial virus, and chest x-ray (if concerned about pneumonia). The need for hospitalization depends on the need for monitoring respiratory distress; hypoxia, dehydration with poor oral intake, and level of comfort of caregivers.

Treatment Plan

Admit inpatient for observation and symptomatic treatment. Consider a trial of beta-2 agonist and/or racemic epinephrine. If child worsens with concern for impending respiratory failure and needs intensive care, first consider non-invasive ventilation, e.g., continuous positive airway pressure (CPAP).

Discussion

Bronchiolitis is mostly caused by respiratory syncytial virus. Evaluation includes the following:

- **Past medical history**
  - Prematurity
  - Chronic lung disease
  - Congenital heart disease
  - Immune-deficient states
- **Current severity of illness**
  - Fever, irritability
  - Oral intake, hydration status
  - Breath sounds, air movement
  - Wheezing
  - Work of breathing, degree of distress
  - Pulse oximetry

Consider hospitalization if:

- Hypoxemia
- Work of breathing interfering with oral intake
- Rapidly worsening course
- High-risk patient

CLINICAL PEARL

Use of CPAP currently lacks sufficient data.

Treatment

- Beta agonists (for some patients)
- Inhaled racemic epinephrine (for airway edema relief in some patients)
- **Aerosolized hypertonic saline**
- **Do not use steroids**
- Supportive care
- Oxygen as needed

Follow-up Management

- There is an increased risk for recurrent wheezing after an infection with RSV.
- It is not predictive of asthma unless other predictive indices exist.

Prevention

- Palivizumab (monoclonal antibody against an RSV glycoprotein) is administered via intramuscular injection 1× month during respiratory syncytial virus season to specific high-risk populations only, e.g., children age <2 who are premature, who have chronic lung disease, and who have significant congenital heart disease.
- Handwashing at all times; in addition, in hospital setting, maintain contact and droplet precautions including gloves, gown, and mask
- Eliminate exposure to cigarette smoke
- As much as possible, prevent exposure to other children with URIs, especially if the children are in high risk category

Final Diagnosis

Respiratory syncytial virus bronchiolitis

CLINICAL PEARL

Bronchodilators may or may not be effective. A trial is warranted. If ineffective, discontinue.

CASE 23

Chief Complaint

Cough and shortness of breath for 5 days

History and Physical Examination

A 5-year-old boy is brought to the emergency department because of a cough and shortness of breath, progressive over the last 5 days. About 3 days ago, he was noted to have upper respiratory symptoms with a low-grade temperature and rhinorrhea. He developed a nonproductive cough with an increased respiratory rate and exercise intolerance. This is the first time the child has experienced these symptoms. He appears alert and cooperative. Vital signs are T 37.7 C (99.9 F), pulse 120/min, respirations 36/min, and BP 90/50 mm Hg.

Physical examination shows anicteric sclera, normal tympanic membranes, watery nasal discharge, and nontender sinuses. His throat is pink without lesions or exudate, and the neck is supple without adenopathy. There is mild accessory muscle use. Lungs have diffuse expiratory wheezes without crackles or egophony. Heart sounds are normal without murmur. Abdomen is soft, not tender, with no mass. Extremities are without edema, and nail beds are pink.

Differential Diagnosis

1. Asthma

2. Foreign body aspiration

3. Allergic reaction

4. Bronchiolitis

5. Pneumonia

6. URI

7. Congenital heart disease with increased pulmonary circulation

8. Cystic fibrosis

9. Chronic aspiration

10. Immunodeficiency

11. Ciliary dyskinesia

12. Congenital airway anomaly

13. Extrinsic airway compression (e.g., vascular ring or sling)

Initial diagnostic and treatment plan	Results
1. Pulse oximetry	Oxygen saturations are 91% on room air
2. Peak expiratory flow measurement	70% of predicted
3. Oxygen by nasal cannula	
4. Albuterol nebulizers	
5. Oral prednisone	
6. Chest x-ray	

Assessment

Because this is the initial presentation, a baseline chest x-ray is warranted.

Acute asthma most typically presents the first time after a viral upper respiratory infection.

- Worsening of symptoms: cough, respiratory distress with development of wheezing

- No description of stridor; therefore differential involves intrathoracic airway processes

- Always consider foreign body aspiration: look for asymmetry

- Examination shows mild respiratory distress: mild accessory muscle use with diffuse expiratory wheezes; no description of focal or unilateral decrease in breath sounds; no crackles (rales)

- Lack of previous atopic history or positive family history goes against atopic asthma (IgE-mediated); symptoms most likely to regress from early childhood to adolescence

- Pulse oximetry in room air shows borderline saturations and peak expiratory flow are moderately reduced

  - No routine use of ABG

  - Perform ABG if continued hypoxia on oxygen; deterioration; air leak (pneumothorax) AAP states no ROUTINE use of ABG (severe cases)

Treatment for any acute flare-up is a short-acting beta-2 agonist (albuterol) by inhalation, along with PO or IV corticosteroids e.g., prednisone 3–7 day course. Observe in the emergency department or office for any post-treatment rebound; also, monitor closely at home and schedule follow-up visit.

Discussion

Asthma is defined as the chronic inflammatory disorder of airways. It includes recurrent episodes of wheezing, breathlessness, chest tightness, coughing. There is widespread but variable airflow obstruction, which is reversible. Asthma is (1) hyperresponsiveness of airways, which is at least partially reversible, and (2) acute and chronic inflammation.

Classification and Treatment

Intermittent asthma: rule of 2's

- Daytime symptoms no more than 2x per week
- Nighttime awakenings no more than 2x per month
- Exacerbations are brief
- Step 1 therapy: PRN use of inhaled short-acting beta-2 agonists; if >1 canister per month, need to increase therapy; no regularly scheduled daily use; treat flares with a course of systemic steroids

Mild persistent asthma

- Symptoms >2x per week but <1x per day
- Nighttime symptoms 3 to 4x per month
- Worsening of symptoms may cause minimal interference in activity
- Step 2 therapy: long-term control with low-dose inhaled corticosteroids (preferred) in all age groups; alternate is nebulized cromolyn (less effective than inhaled corticosteroids)

Moderate persistent asthma

- Daily symptoms and use of inhaled short-acting beta-2 agonists
- Nighttime symptoms >1x per week, though not every night
- Symptoms affect activity
- Step 3 therapy:
  - Age 0–4 yrs: increase the inhaled corticosteroid to medium-dose
  - Age ≥5 yrs: low-dose inhaled steroid + long-acting beta agonist (salmeterol), combined into one metered-dose inhalant; alternate is medium-dose or low-dose inhaled steroid + leukotriene receptor antagonist (montelukast)

Severe persistent asthma

- Continual symptoms: frequent nighttime symptoms; frequent exacerbations, limited physical activity
- Step 4 therapy: Medium-dose inhaled steroid + long-acting beta agonist (or leukotriene receptor antagonist)
- Step 5 therapy: High-dose inhaled steroid + long-acting beta agonist (or leukotriene receptor antagonist)
- Step 6 therapy: High-dose inhaled steroid + long-acting beta agonist (or leukotriene receptor antagonist) + oral corticosteroids
- Make repeated efforts to reduce systemic steroids and maintain control with high-dose inhaled steroids

Severity Classification and Treatment

Class	Daytime Symptoms	Nighttime Symptoms	PFTs	Treatment
Intermittent	$\leq 2\times$/ week	$\leq 2\times$/ month	$FEV_1 \geq 80\%$ predicted; PEF variation $<20\%$	Short-acting β agonist PRN
Mild persistent	$>2\times$/ week	$>2\times$/ month	$FEV_1 \geq 80\%$ predicted; PEF variation 20–30%	Inhaled steroids β agonist for breakthrough
Moderate persistent	Daily	$>1\times$/ week	FEV_1 60–80% predicted; PEF variability $>30\%$	Inhaled steroids Long-acting β agonist Short-acting β for breakthrough Leukotriene-receptor
Severe persistent	Continual; limited activities; frequent exacerbations	Frequent	$FEV_1 \leq 60\%$ predicted; PEF variability $>30\%$	High-dose inhaled steroid Long-acting β agonist Short-acting β agonist Systemic steroids Leukotriene-receptor

The goals of asthma management are to achieve minimal or no chronic symptoms day or night, and minimal or no exacerbations. Additionally:

- No limitation on activities
- Maintain near normal pulmonary function
- Minimal use of short-acting beta agonists ($<1x$ per day, <1 canister per month)
- Minimal or no adverse effects from medications

Final Diagnosis

Acute asthma exacerbation

CLINICAL PEARL

Along with these therapies, don't forget to reassess allergic triggers and make efforts to control the child's environment, as well as address second-hand smoke exposure if any.

CLINICAL PEARL

Written immunization records are valid if the vaccine, date of administration, interval between doses, and patient's age are appropriate for a comparable vaccine in the United States.

CASE 24

Chief Complaint

"My child needs shots, but I'm unsure which ones."

History and Physical Examination

A 5-year-old boy who immigrated to the United States from Ecuador 6 mos ago is brought to the office by his mother before he starts school. The mother has lost his immunization card and is unsure which immunizations he was previously given in Ecuador. Physical examination shows a benign HEENT exam, a supple neck, an average heart rate and rhythm with no murmurs, clear lungs, and a benign abdomen. He has full ROM in the extremities and no rashes on the skin.

Assessment

With no immunization documentation, this patient would be considered to be unimmunized. For this 5-year-old, the recommended catch-up schedule would be:

- DTaP, HBV, MMR and IPV (no Hib or PCV if age ≥5 yrs and a normal child)
- 1 month later: DTaP and HBV
- 2 mos after first visit: DTaP, IPV
- At least 8 mos after first visit: DTaP, HBV, IPV
- At age 11–12: MMR
- 5 yrs after last DTaP: Td and then every 10 yrs
- Single dose of varicella vaccine

Discussion

The following is what we really need to know about childhood immunizations. Go to **cdc.gov** for details about childhood immunizations.

Classification of vaccines

- **Live attenuated:** viral (e.g, MMR, varicella, nasal influenza, oral rotavirus) and bacterial (e.g., BCG, oral typhoid)
- **Inactivated** (killed):
  - Whole: viral (polio)
  - Fractional
    - Protein-based: subunit (hepatitis B, influenza, acellular pertussis) or toxoid (diphtheria, tetanus)
    - Polysaccharide-based: pneumococcal 23-valent, meningococcal conjugate: Hib, pneumococcal 13 valent

Contraindications and precautions of vaccines

- Absolute contraindications

  - Severe allergy/anaphylaxis to a prior dose of a vaccine or a component

  - Encephalopathy following pertussis vaccine (now rare with DTaP, but can happen; even more reactogenic with any FULL-DOSE pertussis given after age 7 yrs, so is contraindicated (partial dose pertussis is okay, i.e., the Tdap).

- Relative contraindications

  - Pregnancy: okay to give 1 dose of Tdap vaccine if patient is due vaccine or unimmunized

  - Immunosuppression: in general, give no live viral vaccines except for MMR and varicella with HIV if (a) no AIDS-related illnesses, and (b) CD4 >15% total lymphocytes at the time of the vaccine

Do not reduce dosage or change schedule for preterm infant; immunize as one would for a full-term infant. The only exception is a first dose of hepatitis B in infants <2000 g.

Hepatitis B vaccine (HBV): recommendations as per the CDC

- **If mother is HBsAg-negative**

  - Give first dose at birth, prior to leaving the birth hospital.

  - Give next 2 doses at age 1–2 mos and 6–18 mos.

- **If mother is HBsAg-positive**

  - Give first dose with hepatitis B immune globulin (HBIG) within first 12 hrs after birth, administered at different injection sites.

    ○ Up to 95% rate in prevention of perinatal transmission

    ○ Complete schedule with 2 more doses of HBV given at 1 and 6 mos

    ○ Test infants for HBsAg and anti-HBs 1–2 mos after completion of series and at age 9–18 mos

- **If mother's hepatitis B status is unknown**

  - Draw blood on mother for HBsAg testing; while waiting for results, administer HBV to newborn within 12 hrs of birth. If mother is HBsAg-positive, administer HBIG to newborn as soon as possible but no later than age 7 days.

Diphtheria, tetanus, acellular pertussis (DTaP)

- Acellular pertussis introduced due to concern about encephalopathy with previous pertussis vaccine but rarely may still occur (see above)

- May give vaccine with minor illnesses and fever

- Five doses of DTaP;

- The childhood tetanus (Tdap) is given **one time** ideally at age 11–12 visit. If missed, give once anytime up to age 65 (an attempt to decrease incidence of pertussis, which has increased to epidemic proportions since the late 1990s)

- The following individuals should receive tetanus prophylaxis (Td and tetanus-immune globulin):

  - Those with wounds at increased risk of contamination with dirt, feces, saliva; wounds with necrotic or gangrenous tissue; frostbite; crush and avulsion injuries; and burns

CLINICAL PEARL

There is no evidence linking vaccines for MMR or any other neurologic/degenerative disease to autism. The CDC states that vaccines are safe, and the issue has now been put to rest.

- If <3 doses or status of tetanus immunization is unknown: with clean, minor wounds, give Td only; all other wounds give both Td and TIG

- If ≥3 doses of tetanus immunization: clean, minor wounds do not need Td or TIG unless last Td was given >10 yrs ago; if so, give Td. All other wounds do not need Td or TIG, unless it has been more than 5 yrs since last Td. If so, then give Td.

Tetanus Prophylaxis in Wound Management

History of Doses of Tetanus Toxoid	Clean, Minor Wounds		All Others*	
	Td	TIG	Td	TIG
<3 or unknown	Yes	No	Yes	Yes
≥3	No†	No	No†	No

TIG, tetanus immune globulin; Td, tetanus and diphtheria vaccine.

*All other wounds = increased risk of tetanus: dirt, saliva, feces, avulsions, frostbite, puncture, crush, burns, and missiles.

†Unless >10 years from last dose.

†Unless >5 years from last dose.

Inactivated polio vaccine (IPV) has taken the place of oral polio vaccine (previous subclinical polio-like illnesses)

- 4 doses; last booster is given at age 4–6 yrs, before starting school

Haemophilus influenzae **type b conjugate vaccine (Hib)**

- 4 doses; last booster is given age 12–18 mos

- If child is unvaccinated and receives first dose after age 15 mos, only 1 dose of Hib vaccine is required

- No dose in a normal child after age 5 yrs if under- or nonvaccinated

Measles, mumps, rubella (MMR) is grown in chick embryo fibroblast cultures, thus is safe in egg-allergic children (may vaccinate without testing).

- Give first dose at or after age 12 mos

- Second dose is recommended at age 4–6 yrs, but may be given any time if at least 4 wks have elapsed after first dose; if second dose has not been received, complete by age 11–12

- The following individuals should receive immune globulin for measles:

  - Susceptible people as prevention or modification within 6 days of exposure

  - Susceptible household contacts of patients with measles, of age, pregnant women, and the immunocompromised

  - Infants in first 6 mos of life **if** mother has no evidence of immunity. Can give vaccine from 6–12 mos for postexposure prophylaxis **but still** need the normally-timed 2 (more, so 3 total) vaccines

If immune globulin was received after exposure, then measles vaccine should be given 6 mos after immune globulin administration, if patient is at least age 12 mos.

Patient Safety Note

Do not administer to patients with known allergy or anaphylaxis to neomycin or gelatin, both of which are present in the vaccine.

Measles

Age	Management (post-exposure)
0–6 mo	Nothing, unless mother is not immune (if not immune, immunoglobulin only)
6–12 mo	Immunoglobulin plus vaccine
>12 mo	Vaccine only within 72 hours of exposure for susceptible individuals
Pregnant or immunocompromised	Immunoglobulin only

Varicella

- At any visit at or after age 12 mos with no reliable history of chickenpox
- Give 2 doses (4 wks apart)
- Fully (100%) protective against severe disease (mild varicella is still visible)
- Live vaccine contraindications:
  - Moderate to severe acute illness
  - Malignancy or T-cell defect, including HIV with CD4 counts <25%
  - High-dose steroid treatment
  - Pregnancy
  - Component allergy
- Who should receive varicella-zoster immune globulin (VZIG)?
  - Immunocompromised children (and adults) without history of varicella or varicella immunization
  - Susceptible pregnant women
  - Newborns whose mother had onset of chickenpox from 5 days before delivery to <48 hrs after delivery
  - Hospitalized premature infants of ≥28 wks' gestation, whose mother lacks reliable history of chickenpox or serologic evidence
  - Hospitalized premature infants <28 wks' gestation or whose birth weight ≤1000 g, regardless of mother's history or serologic status

Pneumococcal vaccine (PCV): 2 types

- 13-valent PCV
  - Recommended for all children aged 2 to 23 mos
  - Give 4 doses; fourth dose by age 15 mos

- 23-valent PCV, PP SV23

  - In addition to PCV for high- and moderate-risk groups (SS, HIV, immune deficiency, chronic cardiopulmonary disease, chronic renal insufficiency, DM, day-care, African American/American Indian/Alaskan Native descent)

  - PPSV23: protective antibody responses to the most common pneumococcal serotypes in children age ≥2 yrs; given at age 24 mos and 5 yrs after first dose for patients who are immunocompromised or those with asplenia (functional or anatomic)

Meningococcal conjugated vaccine-MCV4

- Active immunization against serotypes A, C, Y and W-135

- Recommended for travelers to areas with high rates of infection; first-year college students living in dormitories; military; and those with asplenia/high-risk conditions.

Influenza vaccine

- Recommended annually for ALL children age 6 mos to 18 yrs at the beginning of each annual influenza season. Certain children are at high risk and should be vaccinated first during season if inadequate supply of vaccine. All adults age >50 yrs and all women who are pregnant or may be pregnant during influenza season should receive the vaccine early on, i.e., October or first half of November.

Both intramuscular injection and nasal-influenza vaccine are grown in embryonated eggs and thus have a potential problem with egg allergy.

Patient Safety Note

- Patients who have had a severe allergic reaction to the influenza vaccine should not receive it in the future.

- However, patients who have had an allergic reaction to egg (including having received epinephrine or having had respiratory distress or angioedema) may still receive the influenza vaccine if administered in a controlled setting, i.e., with qualified personnel who can identify and manage immediate anaphylaxis.

Nasal influenza vaccine is live attenuated (need live viral vaccine precautions). Dosing for patients age 2–49 yrs is as follows:

- All children age ≤8 yrs receive 2 doses, 4 wks apart, for first immunization only and 1 dose yearly thereafter

- Children age 6–36 mos receive half-dose (0.25 mL)

- All others receive 0.5-mL dose (i.e., those age ≥3 yrs)

Final Diagnosis

Catch-up immunization

CLINICAL PEARL

PPD (purified protein derivative) may be given the same day as the MMR but if given separately, give the PPD ≥4 weeks after the MMR so that the measles vaccine does not suppress the reactivity to the PPD.

CASE 25

Chief Complaint

Sore throat of 1 day's duration

History and Physical Exam

A 6-year-old girl is brought to the office with a 1-day-history of abrupt onset of sore throat and fever. She has had 2 episodes of vomiting. She denies cough or rhinorrhea. Physical exam is remarkable for T 38.8 C (102 F), erythematous, enlarged tonsils with exudates, and palatal petechiae. Enlarged, tender anterior cervical lymph nodes are palpable. A diffuse, erythematous, sandpaper-like rash is present, more prominent in the flexural areas.

Differential Diagnosis

1. Streptococcal pharyngitis (group A streptococcus [GAS], strep pyogenes) GABHS (group A, beta-hemolytic strep)

2. Viral pharyngitis: adenovirus, coronavirus, rhinovirus, respiratory syncytial virus (RSV), coxsackievirus

Clues

- Abrupt onset

- Exudative pharyngitis without ulceration

- Abdominal pain, along with nausea and vomiting; however, diarrhea is not common with streptococcal pharyngitis

- Headache

Initial Management

Setting: outpatient workup and treatment

Initial diagnostic plan	Results
1. Rapid streptococcal antigen test	Positive

Assessment

Some overlap can be found between the clinical presentations of viral and bacterial pharyngitis. **Group A strep** usually has a more acute onset, and is more common in late autumn, winter, and spring. When Group A strep is associated with an erythematous macular/papular, i.e., sandpaper-like rash, that is called scarlet fever. The rash of scarlet fever progresses in a craniocaudal direction, culminating in desquamation of the hands and feet, with sparing of the palms and soles. Notably, the rash is more prominent in the flexural areas, called Pastia's lines.

Viral pharyngitis has a more gradual onset, associated with upper respiratory infection, and is more common in fall, winter, and spring.

Adenovirus should be considered for patients presenting with pharyngitis and conjunctivitis.

CLINICAL PEARL

The presence of cough, rhinorrhea, and/or conjunctivitis points toward a viral etiology:

- Mononucleosis (EBV)

- Other bacteria: *Arcanobacterium haemolyticum, Mycoplasma pneumoniae, Corynebacterium diphtheriae*

Coxsackievirus (herpangina) is characterized by fever, sore throat, dysphagia and ulcerative lesions on the anterior tonsillar pillars, soft palate, uvula, tonsils, and posterior pharyngeal wall. Odynophagia is a common presenting symptom, and as such, supportive care should include pain management along with IV fluid administration if the child is unable to drink fluids, in order to prevent dehydration.

Mononucleosis (EBV) is associated with fever, fatigue, significant lymph gland swelling and exudative tonsillitis, muscle aches, rash, and hepatosplenomegaly. Approximately 5% of cases of EBV-associated infectious mononucleosis have a positive throat culture for group A strep which represents pharyngeal streptococcal carrier state. Infectious mononucleosis should be suspected in a patient diagnosed with group A strep who fails to respond to treatment after 48–72 hrs or who develops a diffuse macular erythematous rash if amoxicillin was given (interaction of amoxicillin with EBV).

Corynebacterium diphtheriae has a unilateral or bilateral leather-like adherent tonsillar membrane that can extend to affect the uvula, soft palate, posterior oropharynx, hypopharynx, and glottic areas. Underlying soft tissue edema and enlarged lymph nodes can cause a bull-neck appearance. The lack of fever and dysphagia helps to differentiate *C. diphtheriae* from group A strep and EBV infections.

Further Diagnostic Plan

The antigen screen has high specificity. However, a negative result requires a backup throat culture (gold standard).

Treatment Plan

Prevention of rheumatic fever is the primary goal of treatment. Penicillin is the drug of choice, but amoxicillin is often preferred because of palatability. Clinical recovery is hastened by antibiotic treatment but by only 12–24 hrs. The main reason for the Rx is prevention of ARF; it will be prevented if started within 9 days of the start of illness.

However, if the antigen screen is negative and a backup throat culture is required, one should wait for the results of the throat culture prior to initiating antibiotic treatment.

Penicillin effectively prevents primary attacks of rheumatic fever, even when initiated as long as 9 days after the acute onset of the illness. Therefore, a brief delay of 24–48 hrs for processing the throat culture prior to starting antibiotic therapy does not increase the risk of rheumatic fever. With penicillin allergy, use an oral macrolide. However, there has been increasing resistance to macrolides due to overuse of these drugs, so depending on the previous reaction, a first-generation cephalosporin may be an alternative.

Indications for treatment include the following:

- Symptomatic pharyngitis and a positive rapid strep test, or positive throat culture
- Clinical diagnosis of scarlet fever (sore throat, sand-paper type rash, Pastia's lines, circumoral pallor, strawberry tongue, enlarged tonsils)
- Household contact with documented strep pharyngitis
- Recent history of acute rheumatic fever in a family member

The patient is no longer contagious after 24 hrs of therapy. Repeat the throat culture only if sore throat or mild fever persists after antibiotic treatment.

Discussion

Viral pharyngitis predisposes to bacterial otitis media. GAS pharyngitis complications include peritonsillar abscess, retropharyngeal abscess, rheumatic fever, and glomerulonephritis.

Viral Versus Bacterial Pharyngitis

	Viral	Bacterial
Age (in years)	<5, >10	5–10
Onset	Gradual	Acute
Upper respiratory infection	+++	−
Rash	+	+++
Exudate	+	+++
Ulcers	+++	−
Rapid strep screen	−	+++
Throat culture	−	+++++
Vomiting/Abdominal pain	+	++
Lymph nodes	++	++
Conjunctivitis	++	−
Palatal petechiae	+	+++

Final Diagnosis

Group A beta-hemolytic streptococcal pharyngitis (scarlet fever)

CASE 26

Chief Complaint

Burning on urination

History and Physical Examination

A 5-year-old girl comes in with complaints of burning on urination for 3 days. She has had fever for 1 day's duration. She denies vomiting or diarrhea. She has a history of taking bubble baths. Past medical history is remarkable for a urinary tract infection 1 year ago. Her T is 38.7 C (101.7 F) and BP 128/90 mm Hg. Physical exam is remarkable for mild right-sided CVA tenderness. A mass is palpable in the right upper quadrant. Urinalysis shows 25–50 WBCs per high power field. The next day, the urine culture grows 100,000 colonies of *E. coli* and she is treated with antibiotics.

Differential Diagnosis

1. Vesicoureteral reflux (VUR)
2. Urinary tract infection (UTI)
3. Hypertension
4. Hydronephrosis

Initial diagnostic plan	Results
1. Renal U/S	Enlarged kidney on right
2. Voiding cystourethrogram (VCUG)	Dilated tortuous ureter on right with reflux to enlarged right kidney

Assessment

For UTI, diagnose with urine culture (**gold standard**). In young children, think of renal causes for hypertension (e.g., renal parenchymal disease due to chronic pyelonephritis, or chronic glomerulonephritis, ureteral obstruction, renovascular disease, renal trauma, etc.).

For VUR, the voiding cystourethrography (VCUG) system is used to diagnose and grade.

- **Grade I**: reflux into non-dilated ureter
- **Grade II**: reflux into upper collecting system without dilatation
- **Grade III**: reflux into dilated ureter and/or calyceal blunting
- **Grade IV**: reflux into grossly dilated ureter
- **Grade V**: massive reflux, tortuous ureter, hydronephrosis

Treatment Plan

Treat UTI with antibiotics such as cephalosporins, amoxicillin-clavulanate, or trimethoprim-sulfamethoxazole (TMP-SMZ). Clinicians should be aware of local susceptibility patterns. If pyelonephritis, use broad spectrum antibiotics. If dehydrated, vomiting, or <1-month-old, use IV antibiotics (ceftriaxone or ampicillin/gentamicin for <1-month-old).

Perform renal U/S to rule out congenital anatomic abnormalities, hydronephrosis, abscess formation. Also perform VCUG if:

- Recurrent febrile UTI or UTI with complications
- U/S shows renal abnormality; e.g., hydronephrosis, scarring, or concern for VUR

Discussion

VUR is an abnormal backflow of urine from the bladder to the ureter and renal pelvis. This backflow of urine aids in transporting bacteria from the bladder to the upper urinary tract, causing a predisposition to UTI, i.e., pyelonephritis, and as a consequence, if persistent or worsening, renal scarring, poor renal growth and decreasing renal function

Five Grades of Vesicoureteral Reflux

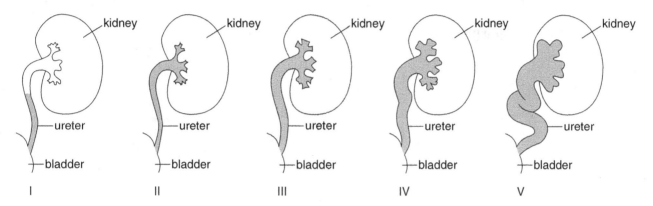

Extensive scarring leads to hypertension. A higher reflux grade has a higher likelihood of renal injury. Reflux can be due to an abnormal ureterovesicular junction (primary VUR), or secondary to anatomic abnormalities (posterior urethral valves); or a neuropathic bladder (myelomeningocele).

If hydronephrosis is noted on the prenatal U/S, one should consider VUR as an etiology. Reflux may also be discovered during evaluation of a UTI. After VUR is diagnosed, upper tract imaging should be done to determine renal size and scarring. This can be done using U/S to monitor for the presence of renal scarring, or renal scintigraphy. If scarring is present, follow the creatinine.

- First, U/S for anatomy
- Then, VCUG for pathophysiologic reason for recurrent UTI, i.e., VUR
- Finally, if clinically significant VUR (II-V), a radionuclide scan (best test for renal size, scars and function); IVP is rarely performed in children any longer

Further Treatment Plan

Recent studies show that grades I–III VUR in children usually resolves with time; follow with VCUG and radionuclide scan. Studies also now show (and the policy has been adopted by the AAP) that antibiotic prophylaxis is not effective. The best management is to follow carefully for any sign of UTI and screen with urine cultures; early aggressive therapy is the best treatment for the prevention of long-term complications and slow resolution of the natural history over time. Voiding dysfunction is a comorbidity and should be managed with behavioral therapy/bladder training in order to obtain the best possible outcome.

For grades IV–V, surgical re-implantation of ureters is the mainstay of treatment and may be considered if there is a breakthrough UTI, new renal scars, or worsening of reflux or renal function.

Patient Safety Note

UTI in a child must be treated promptly. Once diagnosis has been made, parents should be instructed to watch for fever (which requires immediate medical care with a urinalysis and urine culture). Each episode of UTI will place the child at risk for increased scarring, loss of healthy parenchymal tissue, and future renal complications, such as high BP and decreased renal function.

Final Diagnosis

Vesicoureteral reflux

CASE 27

Chief Complaint

Small jaundiced baby

History and Physical Examination

You are called to the newborn nursery to evaluate an 8-hour-old infant. The patient was born at 37 wks' gestation to a 21-year-old primigravida. Mother is blood type A positive, group B strep negative, VDRL negative, rubella status unknown. Pregnancy was remarkable for a fever and rash in the first trimester. A low-grade fever was reported during labor. Birth weight was 4 pounds 7 ounces, Apgars 8/9.

Physical exam reveals a small neonate with little subcutaneous fat. He is noticeably jaundiced, with several purpuric lesions scattered about. HEENT is remarkable for bilateral cataracts. Lungs are clear; heart exam is positive for a to-and-fro machinery murmur. Abdominal exam reveals an enlarged liver. Rest of the physical examination is normal.

Differential Diagnosis

1. Congenital rubella syndrome
2. Toxoplasmosis
3. Syphilis
4. Congenital cytomegalovirus
5. Herpes
6. Group B streptococcal sepsis
7. Hepatitis
8. Physiologic jaundice

Clues

- Maternal fever and rash in first trimester
- Newborn with jaundice, purpura, cataracts, machinery murmur, hepatomegaly

Initial Management

Setting: newborn nursery

Initial diagnostic plan	Results
1. CBC	Normal
2. Complete chemistry profile	Elevated liver function tests and liver enzymes (they are 2 different things)
3. Bilirubin	Elevated direct and indirect (this is an LFT)
4. Blood culture	Pending
5. Urine culture	Pending
6. Blood type, Rh, Coombs	A+, negative

Treatment Plan

Give empiric antibiotics, e.g., ampicillin and gentamicin, pending the culture results; no other treatment is necessary. Also immunize the mother.

Assessment

Prenatal history is the baby's past medical history: maternal exposures, immunization status, infections, medications all affect the fetus. Jaundice in the first 24 hrs of life is always pathologic and should be investigated. Always fractionate bilirubin (direct/indirect) to help with the differential diagnosis. Blood type, Rh, and Coombs tests are essential in the evaluation of jaundice as well.

TORCH titers (IgM) help to differentiate congenitally acquired infections and are the best screening test. Significant overlap exists in presentation of TORCH infections. Sequelae are most common if the infection occurs in the first trimester. Best for CMV are 3 separate urine CMV cultures; for herpes it is PCR of bodily (vesicular) fluid.

Further Diagnostic Plan/Results

- Rubella IgM titers: elevated
- Echocardiogram: patent ductus arteriosus
- Hearing screen: abnormal

Discussion

Infection results from transplacental infection with rubella virus. Rubella in pregnancy is generally a mild illness, presenting usually with a macular rash that spreads craniocaudal, starting on the face and eventually reaching the feet. The rash resolves in the same direction as well. Other symptoms include:

- Nerve deafness (most common finding)
- Patent ductus arteriosus (PDA) (most common cardiac finding)
- Cataracts (common)
- Intrauterine growth retardation; low birth weight (common)
- Purpura ("blueberry muffin" rash)
- Chorioretinitis ("salt and pepper" appearance to retinal surface)
- Panencephalitis, intellectual disability

The most common diagnostic test is rubella IgM assay. The result may be a false positive due to competing IgG antibodies, so obtain a PCR or culture to confirm. In addition, persistent IgG rubella antibody may also signify congenital rubella syndrome.

Therapy is supportive: cardiac, audiologic, ophthalmologic, neurologic consultation/follow-up. Prevent with immunization prior to pregnancy. There is no antiviral treatment.

CLINICAL PEARL

Patients with congenital rubella syndrome are at increased risk for developing insulin-dependent diabetes mellitus in older childhood and adulthood.

Manifestations of Congenital Infections

Pathogen	Manifestation
Rubella	Cataracts, heart defects, hydrocephalus, microcephaly, microphthalmia, petechiae, purpura, thrombocytopenia, retinitis, seizures, deafness, intellectual disability
Toxoplasmosis	Hydrocephalus, intracranial calcifications, microcephaly, retinitis, thrombocytopenia, seizures, eye pathology, intellectual disability
Syphilis	Anemia, hepatosplenomegaly, osteitis, snuffles, rhagades, dental
Cytomegalovirus	Periventricular calcifications, microcephaly, hepatitis, petechiae, purpura, retinitis, thrombocytopenia, seizures, deafness, intellectual disability
Herpes	Hydrocephalus, microcephaly, encephalitis, hepatitis, skin lesions, vesicles

Final Diagnosis

Congenital rubella syndrome

PART II

OBSTETRICS AND GYNECOLOGY

CASE 1

Chief Complaint

"I am 2 months late for my period."

History and Physical Examination

A 20-year-old G0 P0 woman comes to the office stating that her last menstrual period was 2 months ago. She previously has had regular menses. She became sexually active a couple of months ago and had been using a diaphragm for contraception irregularly. She is not in a stable relationship and has multiple sexual partners. She states she has been diagnosed with some sexually transmitted disease but does not remember what it was. She has experienced severe nausea and vomiting for the past week. Also, she has noticed fullness in her breasts with increased tenderness for a few weeks. She also complains of constantly feeling fatigued even after she has had adequate sleep. Vital signs are stable.

General physical examination is unremarkable. Vital signs are stable. Abdomen is flat, soft and non-tender. Visual inspection of external genitalia shows normal perineum. Speculum exam shows a well estrogenized vaginal mucosa and normal appearing cervix. Bimanual exam reveals a non-tender, anteverted uterus enlarged to approximately 10 weeks' size.

Differential Diagnosis

1. Secondary amenorrhea probably due to pregnancy

2. Hyperemesis gravidarum

Initial Management

Setting: outpatient office

Diagnostic/Therapeutic Plan

- Qualitative urine β-hCG

- Urine dip for ketones and specific gravity

- Patient's weight

CLINICAL PEARL

When patients complain of severe nausea and vomiting in the first trimester, it is imperative to rule out other etiologies before attributing it to normal pregnancy. Molar pregnancies and hyperthyroidism can also present with nausea and vomiting.

CLINICAL PEARL

The most common cause of secondary amenorrhea in the reproductive years is pregnancy. Always get a pregnancy test.

Test Results

- Urine β-hCG positive

- Urine dip positive for trace ketones; specific gravity 1.015

- Weight 120 lbs (unchanged from past few months)

Assessment

Probable intrauterine pregnancy; hyperemesis is ruled out

Basic Science Correlate

Pregnancy tests detect levels of human chorionic gonadotropin (hCG), which is composed of an α-subunit and a β-subunit. The β-hCG subunit is specific for trophoblastic tissue. A negative test virtually rules out pregnancy. The test can be qualitative (positive or negative) or quantitative (measures levels). The urine test is always qualitative with a sensitivity threshold minimum of 25–50 IU/L. The serum test can be either quantitative or qualitative, with the latter having a sensitivity threshold minimum of β-hCG is 5–10 IU/L. Although the more sensitive method for detecting β-hCG is serum, a positive urine β-hCG usually suffices and is more cost-effective.

Urine ketones assess the degree of carbohydrate starvation. Urine specific gravity is a simple way of assessing adequacy of fluid intake. Values >1.030 indicate possible dehydration. Serial changes in patient weight are the best indicator of long-term changes in fluid status.

Further Management Plan/Results

• Vaginal obstetric U/S	• Normal-appearing intrauterine singleton pregnancy, crown-rump length of 10 wks; fetal cardiac motion present 145/min
• TSH and free T4	• Within normal range for pregnancy

Final Assessment

Normal-appearing intrauterine pregnancy, size equals dates

Discussion

Pregnancy should be suspected whenever a woman in her childbearing years misses a menstrual period. Common signs and symptoms include amenorrhea, nausea, fatigue, breast tenderness and frequent urination. The symptoms of nausea and vomiting usually resolve by end of first trimester. An office urine pregnancy test is an easy quick tool to assess for possible pregnancy. β-hCG is highly specific for trophoblastic villi and pregnancy.

Once pregnancy is confirmed the next step in management is to determine gestational age. Using the woman's LMP and Naegele's rule the EDD (estimated due date) can be determined by subtracting 3 months and adding 7 days. Pregnancy wheels are used to calculate the EDD when the LMP is known. However, remember these calculations assume a 28-day menstrual cycle with conception occurring at day 14. Most women will have a cycle length more or less than 28 days so the EDD may need to be adjusted either forward or backward.

Obstetric U/S can determine if pregnancy is intrauterine or extrauterine, gestational age, as well as assess for viability. The uterus is a pelvic organ up to 12 wks. In the first trimester, a vaginal U/S gives much better visualization and resolution than an abdominal U/S. A gestational sac can be visible at 4.5–5 wks and a yolk sac around 5–6 wks. A fetal pole with cardiac activity can be detected around 5.5–6 wks.

Follow-up Management and Prevention

- Obtain routine prenatal lab tests.

  - CBC (anemia)

  - Urinalysis (UTI), urine culture (UTI)

  - Blood type and Rh (need for RhoGAM)

  - Atypical antibody screen (alloimmunization)

  - RPR (syphilis)

  - Rubella IgG titer (need for postpartum immunization)

  - Hepatitis B surface antigen (carrier for HBV)

  - HIV screen (HIV)

  - Gonorrhea and chlamydia PCR/culture (screen for cervical infection)

  - Pap smear if indicated (cervical dysplasia)

  - Screen for lead exposure

- Discuss first-trimester genetic screening at wks 11–13: U/S for nuchal translucency along with serum free β-hCG and pregnancy-associated plasma protein-A (PAPP-A)

- General pregnancy counseling

  - Avoidance of cigarette smoking, alcohol, use of drugs, changing cat litter box, consuming undercooked or raw meats, and environmental/work hazards

  - Appropriate weight gain

  - Use of seat belts

  - Infection precautions

  - Review of safe medications

- Nutritional counseling: increase calorie intake by 300/day

- Nausea and vomiting counseling: encourage frequent small meals, try bland foods (such as toast, apple sauce, rice), avoid fried foods

- Return prenatal visits: every 4 wks up to 28 wks, then every 2 wks up to 36 wks, then every wk until delivery

- Start iron and folic acid nutritional supplementation

Final Diagnosis

Normal pregnancy

CCS NOTE

To order pregnancy counseling, press the ORDER icon and type in "counseling." When the drop-down menu appears, select "counsel patient, pregnancy."

CCS NOTE

The order "prenatal labs" is not recognized by the CCS software. It does not appear in the drop-down menu. Because each component would need to be ordered separately, this case simulation is unlikely to appear on the CCS part of the exam.

CASE 2

Chief Complaint

"I'm pregnant and have vaginal bleeding."

History and Physical Examination

A 24-year-old primigravida woman at 8 weeks' gestation by dates presents to your office because of vaginal bleeding and minimal lower abdominal cramping for 1 day. She denies trauma, nausea, vomiting and dysuria. Her last sexual intercourse was 2 weeks ago. This was a planned pregnancy but took 8 months to conceive after discontinuing OCP. She is very anxious and worried about what is happening.

Today she is afebrile with stable vital signs. Her abdomen is soft, non-distended with minimal suprapubic tenderness. Inspection of external genitalia shows normal labia minora and majora but there is old blood on the perineum. Speculum examination reveals a small amount of dark red blood in the vagina. The external cervical os is closed and no lesions are seen. Bimanual examination shows an 8-week sized enlarged, symmetrical non-tender uterus. No cervical motion tenderness is noted and no adnexal mass is palpated.

Differential Diagnosis

1. Threatened abortion
2. Missed abortion
3. Inevitable abortion
4. Incomplete abortion
5. Completed abortion
6. Hydatidiform mole
7. Unruptured ectopic pregnancy

Initial Management

Setting: outpatient workup and treatment

Diagnostic/Therapeutic Plan

- **Quantitative serum β-hCG titer for a baseline if pregnancy viability is uncertain.** It is important to know the serum titer if early pregnancy viability is in question. The titer should double every 2–3 days with a normal intrauterine pregnancy. It is also necessary if ectopic pregnancy is a possibility.

- **CBC to assess for anemia.** It is important to have a baseline hemoglobin in any patient who is bleeding

- **Vaginal speculum exam.** Assesses if any lower genital bleeding lesions are present as well as whether the cervix is closed or open.

- **Vaginal U/S to assess for intrauterine pregnancy and viability.** The sorting out of the differential diagnosis is dependent on whether the vaginal U/S shows an intrauterine pregnancy and whether it is viable.

CLINICAL PEARL

- LEEP is an outpatient office procedure performed under local anesthesia, so is less expensive.

- CKC is an in-hospital operating room procedure performed under anesthesia, so is more expensive.

Choose a cost-effective procedure when possible.

- **Blood type and screen to assess if RhoGAM is indicated.** RhoGAM may be given if a D&C is required in management.
- **Atypical antibody screen** (indirect Coombs test) to rule out alloimmunization

Test Results

- Serum β-hCG titer is 46,000 mIU
- Hemoglobin: 12 g/dL; Hematocrit: 37%; WBC 6,300/dL
- Vaginal speculum exam: no lower genital lesions and cervix is closed
- Vaginal U/S: normal appearing intrauterine pregnancy with a single grossly normal appearing embryo with crown-rump length consistent with 8 wks' gestation. Cardiac motion is noted.
- Blood type is A+
- Atypical antibody screen is negative.

Assessment

This case is consistent with **threatened abortion**. This diagnosis occurs in approximately 20–25% of all pregnancies with only about 1/2 of these pregnancies ending in complete abortion. About 80% of all spontaneous abortions occur in the first trimester. The following criteria must be met:

- Early pregnancy bleeding with no tissue has been passed vaginally.
- Speculum exam reveals there are no lower genital tract lesions or cervical dilation.
- Vaginal U/S reveals a normal appearing viable embryo.

Diagnostic modalities. The etiology of early pregnancy bleeding is assessed by:

- First, a **vaginal speculum exam** to determine if lower genital tract lesions (vagina or cervix) are present and if the cervical canal is open or closed
- Second, a **vaginal U/S** to visualize whether or not the patient has a viable intrauterine pregnancy

Basic Science Correlate

- The majority of early pregnancy losses are due to aneuploidy (cytogenetic abnormalities of the embryo). This includes autosomal trisomies and Turner syndrome. Lethal Mendelian dominant or recessive syndromes can also cause early losses.
- Gestational dating in very early pregnancy can be performed by measuring the diameter of the gestational sac by vaginal U/S. However, the most accurate first trimester pregnancy dating is obtained by measuring the crown-rump length of the embryo/fetus. The accuracy of crown-rump length dating in the first trimester is +/−5 days.
- If the difference in gestational age using menstrual dating compared with the vaginal U/S dating is within the +/−5 days, then the menstrual dating should be used. If the difference between those ages is >5 days, the U/S dating should be used.

Treatment Plan

1. Reassure patient of the favorable prognosis, in light of the positive fetal cardiac activity
2. Routine follow-up: instruct her to call if she has worsening pain, bleeding, fever, chills, or passage of tissues

Discussion

Approximately 15–20% of all pregnancies terminate in clinically recognized abortions. Once there is fetal HR activity detected by U/S, there is only a 5% first trimester loss rate.

The following are almost always **first-trimester diagnoses** and should be considered in patients with early pregnancy bleeding:

- **Missed abortion** is diagnosed with or without early pregnancy bleeding with no tissue passed. On speculum exam there are no lower genital tract lesions or cervical dilation. Vaginal U/S shows a non-viable pregnancy (either absent fetal pole or no cardiac motion). Management in a stable patient is largely determined by her choice. There are 3 options:
  - Wait to see if the POC will be spontaneously expelled
  - Administer misoprostol vaginally to induce contractions leading to POC expulsion
  - Be scheduled for a suction dilatation & curettage (D&C)

- **Inevitable abortion** is diagnosed with early pregnancy bleeding with no tissue passed. On speculum exam no lower genital tract lesions are seen but the internal cervical os is open (admits the tip of a ring forceps without resistance). Vaginal U/S findings may show either a viable or non-viable pregnancy. Management in a stable patient is largely determined by her choice. There are 3 options:
  - Wait to see if the POC will be spontaneously expelled
  - Administer misoprostol vaginally to induce contractions leading to POC expulsion
  - Be scheduled for a suction dilatation & curettage (D&C); heavy bleeding would indicate an emergency D&C

- **Incomplete abortion** is diagnosed with early pregnancy bleeding with some tissue POC passed vaginally. However, some POC remain in the uterus as demonstrated by vaginal U/S. Speculum exam shows no lower genital tract lesions but internal cervical os is open. Management in a stable patient is largely determined by her choice. There are 3 options:
  - Wait to see if the POC will be spontaneously expelled
  - Administer misoprostol vaginally to induce contractions leading to POC expulsion
  - Be scheduled for a suction dilatation & curettage (D&C); heavy bleeding would indicate an emergency D&C

- **Completed abortion** is diagnosed with early pregnancy bleeding and a previously confirmed intrauterine pregnancy. Speculum exam shows no lower genital tract lesions and cervical canal is closed. Vaginal U/S reveals an empty uterus without gestational sac with a thick endometrial stripe. There is only 1 option: conservative management.

- **Hydatidiform mole** is a placental tumor diagnosed by obstetrical U/S, which shows the classic "snow-storm" appearance and multiple small sonolucent areas corresponding to the "grape-like" vesicles seen on gross pathology. The serum β-hCG is markedly elevated, usually >100,000. Management is suction D&C to remove the POC, which are sent to pathology to identify benign versus malignant findings.

- **Unruptured ectopic pregnancy** is diagnosed in stable patients when vaginal U/S shows the absence of intrauterine pregnancy in the presence of a quantitative serum β-hCG >1500 mIU. Management is medical with parenteral methotrexate in early gestations but is surgical with laparoscopy in advanced gestations.

It is important to administer RhoGAM for Rh-negative patients who undergo a D&C.

Final Diagnosis

Threatened abortion

CASE 3

Chief Complaint

"I'm worried that my baby won't be healthy because I am so old."

History and Physical Examination

A 39-year-old multigravida woman at 12 weeks' gestation comes to the clinic for a routine prenatal visit. She has 15-year history of idiopathic seizure disorder successfully controlled with valproic acid. Her obstetric and gynecologic histories are otherwise unremarkable. A distant relative and a friend have both delivered children with Down's syndrome after conceiving in their early 40s, and she is worried about her own risk. She prefers to avoid invasive prenatal diagnostic procedures. General physical examination is unremarkable. Uterus is 12-week size. Gestational age is confirmed by a 9-week sonogram.

Differential Diagnosis

1. **Advanced maternal age**

   - Patient meets criteria for AMA by obstetric terms, given that she is age >35

2. **Chromosome abnormality**

   - Patients with AMA are at increased risk for chromosomal abnormalities especially trisomy 13, 18, or 21

3. **Open neural tube defect**

   - Patient takes valproic acid, which increases the risk of open neural tube defects

   - At this point in the pregnancy the neural tube is closed (closure occurs at 5th and 6th wk of gestation), but it is too early to screen for an abnormality with maternal serum alpha-fetoprotein or view with a second-trimester anatomy U/S. This will have to be done later in the pregnancy.

Initial Management

Setting: outpatient workup and treatment

Diagnostic/Therapeutic Plan

- U/S to measure fetal nuchal translucency (NT)

- Serum free β-hCG

- Pregnancy-associated plasma protein-A (PAPP-A)

Test Results

- U/S to measure fetal NT: thickened nuchal translucency

- Serum free β-hCG: elevated

- PAPP-A: low

Assessment

- Abnormal NT and serum markers
- First trimester screening yields a 1:20 risk for Down's syndrome for the patient

Further Management Plan/Results

• Genetic counselor meeting to discuss valproic acid-related increased risk of neural tube defects and AMA increased risk of trisomy 21	• Fetal karyotype is 46,XX (normal)
• CVS was offered and patient accepted	• False-positive first-trimester screening test

The patient is still at risk for having an open NT. Testing will include a second-trimester serum alpha-fetoprotein and anatomic fetal U/S.

Discussion

This patient's fetus is at increased risk for both neural tube defects caused by valproic acid and increased risk of Down's syndrome because of her age. Patients will always have an age-related risk of Down's, which can be adjusted up or down based upon screening performed in the first- or second-trimester. In this case the pattern of serum results, as well as the nuchal translucency thickening, increases her age-adjusted risk to 1:20. The serum marker pattern for trisomy 13 and 18 seen on the first-trimester screen is a low free β-hCG and low PAPP-A.

After a positive screening test, patients should meet with a genetic counselor to discuss the results along with diagnostic and management options. Nondirective information enables the parents to balance the risks, limitations, and benefits of prenatal screening and diagnostic testing with the medical, educational and social issues involved in raising a child with Down's syndrome or pregnancy termination. Women with positive screening results are offered definitive fetal karyotype determination by chorionic villus sampling (CVS) if they present <14 wks of gestation.

Antenatal genetic screening/diagnosis: Invasive testing (CVS or amniocentesis) is offered to pregnant women age ≥35 because of the significantly increased risk for Down's syndrome (1/1,250 ages 15–19 versus 1/900 at age 30 versus 1/350 at age 35). First-trimester screening can be offered if the patient presents early enough (<13 wks). Testing includes nuchal translucency, serum hCG, and serum PAPP-A.

If the patient presents later in pregnancy, the quadruple marker screen should be offered to all pregnant women (alpha-fetal protein, hCG, inhibin A, and estriol) and neural tube defects (alpha-fetal protein). Elevated hCG and inhibin A in conjunction with decreased maternal serum alpha-fetal protein and estriol are suspicious for trisomy 21. When all 4 markers are low, it suggests either dating error or trisomy 18. Patients should be counseled regarding the considerable false-positive rate.

Etiology of genetic anomalies: Most Down's syndrome occurs because of nondisjunction. Risk increases with advancing maternal age, though most Down's syndrome babies are born to women age <35 because most babies are born to younger women. The highest risk of Down's syndrome is a balanced parental Robertsonian translocation, involving the D group of acrocentric chromosomes 13, 14, and 15 and the G group of chromosomes 21 and 22. The theoretical risk for Down's syndrome in a child from parents with this disorder is 33%.

Patient counseling: Genetic counseling should never be used to coerce a patient to undergo or forego certain tests for pregnancy management decisions. Information should be obtained and provided in a nondirective fashion so that the counselor acts in a completely objective manner, never interjecting personal opinions.

If the fetus is diagnosed with Down's syndrome, the patient may continue with the pregnancy or terminate the pregnancy by dilation and evacuation or induction of labor with vaginal prostaglandins.

If the patient elects to continue the pregnancy, a diagnostic workup should be carried out to evaluate for fetal endocardial cushion defects and duodenal atresia, both of which are increased in Down's syndrome.

Final Diagnosis

Advanced maternal age with false-positive first-trimester genetic screening

CLINICAL PEARL

Amniocentesis is the most common invasive diagnostic test performed in pregnancy and is usually done at 15–20 wks gestation. Pregnancy loss rates are 0.25–0.5%.

CASE 4

Chief Complaint

Abnormal RBC antibodies

History and Physical Examination

A 32-year-old woman, G2 P1, comes to the outpatient office for her second prenatal visit at 12 weeks gestation by dates. Her first visit was 4 weeks ago and routine prenatal laboratory tests were ordered. She has no complaints. She denies bleeding, cramping, nausea, vomiting or dysuria. Her first pregnancy was 5 years ago and her prenatal course was uncomplicated. She went into spontaneous labor at 39 weeks, undergoing an unremarkable spontaneous vaginal delivery of a healthy 3200 gram daughter who is alive and well. Her 38-year-old sister just delivered a term baby with trisomy 21.

An obstetrical U/S performed today shows a normal intrauterine pregnancy with a single fetus with crown-rump length consistent with 12 weeks gestation. Prenatal laboratory panel reveals blood type O negative. Atypical antibody titer (indirect Coombs test) is positive. She has been married for 10 years to the same husband, who is the father of both pregnancies. His blood type is AB positive. Their first child is B positive.

Differential Diagnosis

1. **Maternal alloimmunization with antibodies against either the D antigen or some other RBC antigen**

    - This is the only diagnosis possible.

    - The only question now is to identify whether the antibodies in the mother's blood pose a danger to the fetus.

Initial Management

Setting: outpatient workup and treatment

Diagnostic Testing

- Typing of the atypical antibody by the blood bank (to identify the antibody and determine whether it is associated with hemolytic disease of the newborn)

Test Results

- Antibodies are identified as anti-Kell

Assessment

The anti-Kell antibodies are associated with severe hemolytic disease of the newborn.

Basic Science Correlate

In this case, the positive atypical antibody test (indirect Coombs test) confirms the diagnosis of alloimmunization. The mixing of foreign RBCs with the patient's RBC may occur after transfusion of mismatched RBCs (rare) but most likely it is from feto-maternal bleeding in a previous pregnancy (common). We can assume that the mother's RBCs are negative for the Kell antigen because otherwise, she would be producing auto-antibodies that would hemolyze her own RBCs. This would result in an auto-immune hemolytic anemia.

The potential danger to this pregnancy is that if the fetal RBCs possess the Kell antigen, the IgG anti-Kell antibodies in the mother's circulation could cross the placenta into the fetal circulation. Those antibodies, if present in a high enough concentration, could cause hemolysis of the fetal RBCs resulting in fetal anemia. If the anemia is severe enough it could cause non-immune fetal hydrops, high-output cardiac failure, and even lead to death.

The fetus is only at risk if its RBCs are Kell antigen-positive. We can test RBCs from the baby's biological father and if they were found to be negative, the fetus would have to also be negative. Alternatively the definitive identification of fetal Kell antigen status, if paternity is uncertain, is by obtaining fetal RBCs by percutaneous umbilical blood sampling. This is an invasive procedure requiring placement of a needle into the umbilical vein.

Further Diagnostic Plan

- Determine if the father of the baby is Kell positive
- Determine the anti-Kell antibody titer

Further Test Results

- Father of the baby is Kell antigen positive
- Anti-Kell titer is 1:2

Further Treatment Plan

Follow monthly anti-Kell titers. If the antibody titer should rise to >1:8, it is essential to rule out fetal anemia by using a non-invasive test, Doppler U/S measurement of fetal arterial blood flow. The circle of Willis is easily visualized in the fetal head and the middle cerebral artery peak systolic velocity (MCA-PSV) is measured. The MCA-PSV blood flow is inversely related to the degree of fetal anemia.

Discussion

The risk of fetal anemia is predicated on presence of 5 prerequisites:

1. Mother is antigen negative
2. Father is antigen positive
3. Atypical antibodies are present in the mother's circulation
4. Antibodies are associated with HDN
5. Antibody titer is >1:8.

All 5 must be present for the fetus to be at risk. If even one is absent there is no risk.

Just because the patient is Rh negative, we cannot assume the atypical antibody is directed against the D antigen. It is important for the blood bank to specifically type the antibody and determine whether it is associated with HDN. Some antibodies, such as anti-Lewis, do not cause RBC hemolysis regardless of how high their titer might be. Since anti-Kell antibodies are associated with HDN it is important to determine the titer.

If the father had been Kell antigen negative, the fetal RBC would also be Kell antigen negative and therefore not susceptible to hemolysis from the atypical antibodies. No intervention would be needed. With the father Kell antigen positive, the first 4 prerequisites for fetal anemia are present. However, the low antibody titer means the fetus is not currently at significant risk. As long as the titer stays less than 1:8, just follow monthly titers and observe.

Prevention

To prevent isoimmunization in RhD-negative women, IM RhoGAM is given. RhoGAM contains passive IgG antibodies that are injected into the mother's bloodstream. Those anti-D antibodies search out any Rh (D) positive RBC, attach to the RBC D-antigen and the antibody-antigen reaction causes hemolysis and destruction of the foreign RBC. This hemolysis needs to take place before the mother's own lymphocytes recognize the Rh (D) positive RBCs and start to make endogenous RhoGAM.

Routine administration of RhoGAM is at 28 wks and repeated after delivery if the baby is Rh positive. Special administration is recommended after events associated with increased risk of feto-maternal bleeding, such as ectopic pregnancy, amniocentesis, D&C, abruptio placentae, and placenta previa. One vial of RhoGAM will neutralize 15 mL of fetal RBCs.

Final Diagnosis

Alloimmunization to Kell antigen

CASE 5

Chief Complaint

Abnormal quadruple-marker screen

History and Physical Examination

A 30-year-old primigravida woman comes to the clinic at 17 weeks' gestation by dates. She recently underwent quadruple marker genetic screening that resulted in a maternal serum alpha-fetoprotein (MS-AFP) value 3.0 multiples of the median, which is abnormally high.

On examination the uterus is at her umbilicus. Fetal heart tones are present at 155/min by Doppler stethoscope.

Differential Diagnosis

1. **More advanced gestational age**
   - This is the most common reason for an MS-AFP. The test is gestational-age-dependent and thus accurate dating is required to interpret the test.

2. **Neural tube defects**
   - If dating is accurate, an elevated MS-AFP is a marker for open neural tube defects or abdominal wall defects.

3. **Multiple gestation**
   - The values for MS-AFP are calibrated based upon singleton gestations. If another fetus is present and producing the protein, a false positive will result.

4. **Ventral wall defects**
   - If dating is accurate, an elevated MS-AFP is a marker for abdominal wall defects.

5. **Fetal demise**
   - Fetal death causes elevated AFP. This is not the case here given a positive FHT.

6. **Congenital nephrosis**

7. **Placental bleeding**

Initial Management

Setting: outpatient workup and treatment

Diagnostic/Therapeutic Plan

- Abdominal obstetric U/S

Test Results

- Singleton live fetus with fetal measurements (biparietal diameter, head circumference, abdominal circumference, and femur length) consistent with 17 week's gestation

- Fetal anatomy: unremarkable

- Amniotic fluid volume: normal

Assessment

With the U/S showing a fetus appropriate for dates, the most common cause of abnormal MS-AFP—dating error—is ruled out. If the U/S gestational age is significantly more advanced than dates (and no fetal anomaly is seen), no further workup is needed. Other factors which can alter the interpretation of serum alpha-fetal protein are maternal weight (protein is diluted in the larger volume of distribution of obese patients), multiple gestations (serum alpha-fetal protein is proportional to the number of fetuses), and fetal viability (fetal death raises alpha-fetal protein).

However, in the present case, correct dating of a singleton pregnancy has been confirmed. Thus, workup is offered, which includes further genetic counseling and amniocentesis. Amniotic-fluid alpha-fetoprotein (AF-AFP) has a much higher specificity than the serum AFP.

Further Management Plan/Results

CCS NOTE

The CCS software does not recognize the order "AF-AFP" or "AF-AChE." Enter: "Amniotic fluid chromosome analysis."

• Genetic counseling	
• U/S guided amniocentesis for amniotic fluid AFP and acetylcholinesterase (AChE)	• Fetal karyotype is 46,XX • AF-AFP and AF-AChE are WNL

Discussion

Termination of a pregnancy should not be recommended on the basis of MS-AFP testing alone. It is only a screening test to define who is at risk and is never a diagnostic test.

- **False-positive** test occurs when screening test is abnormal but fetus is normal
- **True-positive** test occurs when screening test is abnormal and fetus is abnormal
- **False-negative** test occurs when screening test is normal but fetus is abnormal
- **True-negative** test occurs when screening test is negative but fetus is normal

Alpha-fetoprotein is synthesized by the fetal yolk sac, GI tract, and liver. It is the major serum protein of the embryo and early fetus. Fetal urine is the major source of AF-AFP.

MS-AFP levels are drawn at 15–20 weeks' gestation and measured in ng/mL. Most positive high MS-AFP values arise because of a pregnancy dating error. Because normal ranges of MS-AFP are gestational-age related, errors in gestational age calculation result in MS-AFP values being interpreted as falsely positive high or falsely positive low, depending on which direction the error in dating occurred.

Causes: True positive high MS-AFP values occur with fetal or placental abnormalities that allow unusually large quantities of AFP to leak out and get into the maternal circulation. They include:

- Open neural tube defects (such as anencephaly and open spina bifida)
- Ventral wall defects (such as gastroschisis)
- Renal disease (such as congenital nephrosis)
- Multiple gestation (with >1 fetus generating alpha-fetoprotein)
- Placental bleeding
- Fetal demise

Workup: When an MS-AFP screening test is positive (>2.5 multiples of the median), further evaluation is required to determine if true pathology (neural tube or ventral wall defects) is present. All positive results should undergo an U/S examination to confirm gestational age, fetal viability, and number of fetuses, and to perform a detailed fetal anatomic survey. If the U/S reveals an apparently normal, singleton fetus at the correct gestational age, further evaluation is usually indicated.

Amniocentesis can assess gross cytogenetic abnormalities only through karyotyping but cannot identify single gene disorders (such as autosomal dominant or recessive diseases). Karyotyping from fetal amniocytes (cells desquamated from the fetal skin that are aspirated along with the amniotic fluid) has an error rate <1%.

AF-AFP and AF-AChE are the primary biochemical tests performed on amniotic fluid for detection of open neural tube defects.

- AF-AFP is more specific than MS-AFP

- AChE is an enzyme contained in blood cells, muscle, and nerve tissue that elevates in the event there is a neural tube defect

- Elevation of both substances is >90% accurate for detecting an open neural tube defect

Follow-up Management

At this point the patient may resume routine prenatal care.

Final Diagnosis

False-positive elevated MS-AFP screening test but normal fetus

CASE 6

Chief Complaint

"My baby is not moving as much as she used to."

History and Physical Examination

A 39-year-old woman, G4 P3, comes to the outpatient office for her return prenatal visit stating that over the past 24 hours her baby has not been moving as much as it used to. She is 32 weeks gestation by dates confirmed by a 9-week U/S. Her pregnancy is complicated by chronic hypertension, diagnosed 5 years ago and managed with oral labetalol, as well as type 2 DM, diagnosed 3 years ago and managed with 2x daily injections of NPH insulin and injections of insulin lispro before meals. Her hemoglobin A1C 2 weeks ago was 9.1 g/dL. Serial obstetric ultrasounds have shown a single female fetus with estimated fetal weight at the 5th percentile of expected. Last ultrasound was 10 days ago. Weekly umbilical artery Doppler studies have shown normal diastolic flow with the last assessment made 4 days ago. At that time the NST was reactive with 4-quadrant AFI showing 12 cm of fluid and maximum vertical pocket (VP) 4 cm.

Today, maternal BP is 135/85 mm Hg. Random glucose is 150 mg/dL and fundal height is 29 cm. Auscultation of the FHR using an obstetric Doppler device shows HR 135/min.

Differential Diagnosis

1. **Fetus is hypoxic and/or acidotic so not moving.**

   - The patient's chronic hypertension, type 2 diabetes, and IUGR put the fetus at risk for hypoxia and acidosis. However, it is important to remember that while antenatal fetal tests are highly accurate in confirming fetal well-being, they are poor predictors of fetal jeopardy.

2. **Fetus is sleeping so not moving.**

   - Fetal movements will normally decrease when the fetus is asleep. Wake-sleep cycles in the normal fetus are usually less than one hour in duration.

3. **Fetal movements are present but not perceived by patient.**

   - A fetus can be expected to normally move at least 10 times in 2 hrs. Studies comparing the maternal sensation of fetal movements with sonographically visualized fetal movements show that half the time, even though the fetus is moving, the mother may not perceive the movements.

Initial Management

Setting: outpatient workup and treatment

Diagnostic/Therapeutic Plan

Modified biophysical profile, consisting of 2 components:

- Non-stress test (NST)
- AFI and MVP

Results

- NST is initially non-reactive after observing for 30 min (no FHR accelerations seen). After vibroacoustic stimulation is applied, 3 FHR accelerations occur in the next 7 min, making the NST reactive.

- The 4-quadrant AFI is performed with obstetric U/S and noted to be 14 cm. The MVP of amniotic fluid is 3.5 cm.

Assessment

Fetal oxygenation is satisfactory, as documented by multiple fetal movements (accelerations) on the NST. Placental perfusion of the fetal kidneys is adequate, as documented by the normal fetal urination/amniotic fluid.

Basic Science Correlate

The **NST** is assessed as either **reactive** or **non-reactive** based on the presence or absence of FHR accelerations. Accelerations are the fetal response to movement and are mediated by the sympathetic nervous system.

- Accelerations are abrupt increases in FHR above the baseline lasting <2 min; they are unrelated to contractions.

- An external FHR monitoring device is used to detect the presence or absence of accelerations. If accelerations **meet criteria**, the NST is **reactive**. If they **don't meet criteria**, the NST is **non-reactive**. The criteria vary by gestational age.

  - At <32 wks, the FHR increase should be $\geq$10 beats/min lasting $\geq$10 sec
  - At $\geq$32 wks, the FHR increase should be $\geq$15 beats/min lasting $\geq$15 sec

- Accelerations occur in response to fetal movements and are always reassuring of fetal well-being. With a reactive NST, the likelihood of fetal death in the next week is <3 per 1000 if there are no changes in maternal status.

Basic Science Correlate

The **contraction stress test (CST)** assesses the ability of the fetus to tolerate transitory decreases in intervillous blood flow, which occur with uterine contractions. It uses external FHR and contraction monitoring devices.

- Fetal well-being is assessed on the presence or absence of late decelerations. Late decelerations are gradual decreases in FHR below the baseline with onset to nadir $\geq$30 sec. The deceleration onset and end is delayed in relation to contractions.

- An external FHR monitoring device is used to detect the presence or absence of accelerations. An external toco (tocodynamometer) monitoring device is used to detect the beginning and ending of uterine contractions. If 3 contractions in 10 min are not spontaneously present, they may be induced with either IV oxytocin infusion or nipple stimulation using warm towels placed on the breast.

- Late decelerations are thought to be caused by uteroplacental insufficiency. With a negative CST, the likelihood of fetal death in the next week is <1 per 1000 if there are no changes in maternal status.

Antepartum Fetal Testing Sequence

The initial fetal assessment tests should be the NST and AFI. Together these 2 tests are known as the **modified biophysical profile**. There are no contraindications to the NST/AFI.

- If the NST is reactive and AFI is normal, the testing is over. If the NST is non-reactive after 40 min, then a VAS should be used to stimulate fetal movement. If the NST becomes reactive, the testing is over.

- If the NST is persistently non-reactive in spite of VAS, then proceed to the complete BPP. There are no contraindications to the BPP. If BPP score is 8 or 10, the testing is over.

- If BPP score is 0 or 2, prompt delivery should occur. If BPP score is 4 or 6 at term, delivery should occur.

- If BPP score is 4 or 6 prior to 36 weeks, proceed to the CST. There are contraindications to the CST. If the CST is negative, the testing is over. If the CST is positive, proceed to delivery.

The **NST** indirectly assesses the frequency of fetal movements by looking for FHR accelerations.

- Reactive NST requires the presence of 2 accelerations in a 20-min window of time meeting the above criteria. This is **reassuring** and highly predictive for fetal well-being. Management is to repeat the test weekly or biweekly as indicated.

- Nonreactive NST is diagnosed when any criteria for reactivity has not been met: either the number of accelerations in 20 min or the amplitude/duration of the acceleration. Eighty percent of nonreactive NSTs are false-positives (meaning the fetus is not hypoxemic). Nonhypoxemic causes include fetal sleep, prematurity, drug effects, and CNS anomalies. Management of a persistently nonreactive NST is stimulation of the fetus with VAS to see whether there is movement and reactivity. If the NST is persistently nonreactive, perform a biophysical profile.

Vibroacoustic stimulation. Since accelerations of the fetal HR are a response to movement, the NST will not show accelerations when the fetus is sleeping and will be called nonreactive. The VAS uses an artificial larynx which is placed on the maternal abdomen where the fetal head is located. The vibrations and high-decibel sound are designed to wake the fetus out of its sleep, causing it to move and prompt an FHR acceleration. Use of the VAS in antenatal testing reduces the incidence of nonreactive NSTs as well the overall testing time.

A complete **BPP** measures **5 components of fetal well-being:** NST, amniotic fluid volume, fetal gross body movements, fetal extremity tone, and fetal breathing movements. The last 4 components are assessed using obstetric U/S.

Scores given for each component are 0 or 2, with maximum possible score 10, and minimum score 0.

- **Score of 8 or 10:** highly **reassuring** of fetal well-being. Management is to repeat the test weekly or as indicated. Fetal death rate is only 1 per 1,000 in the next week.

- **Score of 4 or 6: worrisome.** Management is delivery if fetus >36 wks, or repeat the test in 12–24 h if fetus <36 wks. An alternative is to perform a CST.

- **Score of 0 or 2:** highly predictive of fetal **hypoxia** with low probability of false-positive. Management is prompt delivery regardless of gestational age.

A modified BPP includes only the NST and amniotic fluid volume. Its negative predictive value is almost as high as a complete BPP.

The **CST** is rarely performed because of the cost and the personnel time required. The most common indication is a BPP of 4 or 6.

- **Negative CST:** requires the absence of any late decelerations with contractions. This is **reassuring** and highly indicative of fetal well-being. Management is to repeat the test weekly or as indicated.

- **Positive CST: worrisome**. Requires the presence of late decelerations associated with at least 50% of contractions. Fifty percent of positive CSTs are false-positive (meaning the fetus is not hypoxemic). They are associated with good FHR variability. The 50% of true positives are associated with poor or absent variability. Management is prompt delivery.

Contraindications: CST should never be performed when contractions would be hazardous to the mother or fetus, e.g., previous classical uterine incision, previous myomectomy, placenta previa, incompetent cervix, preterm membrane rupture, or preterm labor.

Final Diagnosis

Nonreactive NST due to fetal sleep

CASE 7

Chief Complaint

"My baby is too small."

History and Physical Examination

A 31-year-old multiparous woman comes to the outpatient clinic for a routine prenatal visit at 32 weeks gestation by dates. A first trimester U/S confirmed her gestational age. Her pregnancy is complicated by chronic hypertension managed by alpha-methyldopa. Her total pregnancy weight gain to date is 10 lb. She admits to cigarette-smoking 1 pack/day but denies alcohol and illicit drug use. Her appetite has been poor lately but she denies nausea, vomiting, or diarrhea. She reports that fetal movements are active and unchanged over the last month.

On examination today her BP is 140/90 with normal pulse and respirations. Fundal height is 28 cm, which is unchanged from what it was 4 weeks ago. Fetal heart tones could not be identified with a Doppler stethoscope.

Differential Diagnosis

1. **Gestational dating error**
   - Ruled out by gestational age confirmed by first trimester U/S

2. **Fetal demise**
   - Must always be considered when FHT cannot be obtained with Doppler
   - Intrauterine growth restriction [IUGR] Patient has risk factors: chronic hypertension, smoking

3. **Oligohydramnios**
   - Can occur when decreased placental function leads to decreased fetal renal blood flow, which results in decreased fetal urine

Initial Management

Setting: outpatient workup

Diagnostic/Therapeutic Plan

- Abdominal obstetric U/S

Test Results

- Single live fetus with composite average U/S gestational age of 29 wks; fetal HR is 145/min
- Fetal biparietal diameter and head circumference is 31 wk size
- Fetal abdominal circumference is 25 wk size and femur length is 27 wk size
- Four-quadrant amniotic fluid index (AFI) is 7 cm; MVP is 2 cm
- Gross body movement, breathing movements and extension-flexion are noted

Initial Assessment

- Fetal demise is ruled out
- Asymmetric IUGR
- Chronic hypertension reasonably controlled

Further Management Plan/Results

Modified biophysical profile (BPP)	• Reactive NST • AFI 7 cm (normal 9–24 cm) • MVP 2 cm (normal >2 cm)

Treatment Plan

- Outpatient follow-up
- Serial NSTs, AFIs and biophysical profiles to evaluate fetal well-being weekly
- Serial U/S to monitor fetal growth every 2–3 weeks
- Serial weekly umbilical artery Doppler diastolic flow assessment
- Delivery if fetal compromise evident
- Assess optimum mode of delivery (C-section vs vaginal delivery) since some compromised fetuses cannot tolerate labor

Discussion

In the last half of pregnancy, after 20 weeks, the height of the uterine fundus (measured from the pubic symphysis) should approximate (in cm) the number of weeks. In this case the gestational age by dates is 32 weeks, so fundal height should be 32 + 3 cm. The actual measurement is 28 cm, which is 4 cm less than expected.

When the difference between expected and actual measured fundal height is >3 cm, it needs to be investigated. Before assuming a problem exists with the pregnancy, however, check to see whether examiner's measurement error exists, due to maternal obesity or true gestational age being less than thought. Obstetrical U/S should be ordered to assess for actual fetal size, which can rule out a dating error.

There are 2 other possible causes of a uterus smaller than expected: **IUGR** and **oligohydramnios**.

Intrauterine growth restriction (IUGR). This obstetrical complication is defined as composite fetal size by U/S <10th percentile of expected. Accuracy of dating is critical to know what the true gestational age is. A synonym for IUGR is small for gestational age (SGA).

- **Asymmetric IUGR** is assessed when U/S findings show fetal size less than expected with the measurements of the fetal biparietal diameter and head circumference relatively **normal** but the fetal abdominal circumference is relatively **small**. This is due to decreased placental perfusion due to maternal vascular disease (e.g., chronic hypertension, lupus, type 1 diabetes). The fetus has normal growth potential but is prevented from actualizing it by a lack of nutritional substrates from insufficient placental function (most commonly from maternal hypertension as is probable in this case). The fetus preferentially shunts blood to the brain, thereby preserving the head growth. Decreased amniotic fluid may be seen in these cases and testing for fetal well-being is imperative.

- **Symmetric IUGR** is assessed when the U/S findings show a failure of **all** the fetal measurement parameters (BPD, HC and AC) to follow normal growth curves. This is consistent with an intrinsic fetal problem of long duration, which is associated with decreased growth potential. Examples include:

  - Cytogenetic abnormalities [e.g., trisomy 18, trisomy 13, Turner syndrome]

  - First trimester intrauterine infections [e.g., toxoplasmosis, cytomegalovirus]

  - Gross structural anomalies [e.g., gastroschisis, congenital heart disease]

- While most small-for-gestational-age fetuses are constitutionally small, this is a diagnosis of exclusion. Thus, it is important to monitor fetal growth and well-being to determine when to continue observing and when to intervene and deliver.

Oligohydramnios is diagnosed when the sum of the deepest vertical pockets of amniotic fluid seen by U/S in the 4-quadrants (RUQ, RLQ, LLQ and LUQ) is <5 cm. This is known as the 4-quadrant amniotic fluid index (**AFI**). AFI 5–8 cm is borderline, with 9–25 cm normal. An MVP of amniotic fluid should be >2 cm.

The main source of amniotic fluid is fetal urination. Hypertension can cause placental insufficiency, which can decrease renal blood flow leading to oligohydramnios. Decreased amniotic fluid can result from fetal anomalies involving the kidney, ureters, bladder or urethra as well as maternal medications (e.g., indomethacin and ACE inhibitors).

Umbilical artery Doppler systolic flow is used as an assessment of fetal well-being only in IUGR pregnancies. The test measures the ratio of systolic to diastolic flow in the umbilical artery. With advancing pregnancy, the vessel resistance usually decreases, resulting in an increased diastolic flow. Nonreassuring findings, which may indicate the need for delivery of an IUGR fetus, are absent diastolic flow and, even worse, reversed diastolic flow.

Final Diagnosis

Asymmetric intrauterine growth restriction

CASE 8

Chief Complaint

"I'm having abdominal pain every 8–10 minutes."

History and Physical Examination

A 24-year-old G2P1 at 28 weeks presents to the outpatient maternity unit complaining of on-and-off back pain for the past 24 hrs. She states that the back pain comes and goes every 8–10 minutes. Her prenatal course was complicated by early pregnancy bleeding at 10 weeks gestation. Obstetric U/S at that time confirmed a viable pregnancy with crown-rump length appropriate for dates. Her cervix remained closed and the bleeding spontaneously resolved. She is taking prenatal vitamins with folic acid. She denies vaginal fluid gush or leakage. She is unsure if she is having contractions.

On presentation at L&D she seems nervous and uncomfortable. General physical exam is unremarkable. Uterine fundal height is 28 cm with fetal heart tones noted in the RUQ to be in the 140s.

Differential Diagnosis

1. **Preterm labor**
   - Requires cervical dilation and/or effacement
2. **Preterm contractions**
   - No cervical dilation or effacement
3. **UTI**
   - Uterus can be irritated by bladder infection
4. **Chorioamnionitis**
   - Unlikely without membrane rupture
5. **Concealed abruption**
   - Could explain preterm contractions without bleeding

Initial Management

Setting: outpatient maternity unit

Diagnostic/Therapeutic Plan

- Maternal VS (assess fever if possible chorioamnionitis)
- Review of obstetric and medical history (assess for history of previous preterm deliveries)
- Physical exam (to assess for uterine contractions and tenderness)
- Speculum exam for fetal fibronectin (specimen must be collected before vaginal U/S or digital cervical exam)

- Test for group B streptococcus (obtain a rectovaginal swab)
- Digital cervical exam (for cervical position, dilation, effacement, consistency and fetal station)
- Bedside abdominal U/S (for presentation, placenta location, and amniotic fluid)
- Vaginal U/S for cervical length (with labor progression cervix shortens)
- Urinalysis (looking for WBC and bacteria)

Test Results

- VS: afebrile; BP 115/65 mm Hg; HR 95/min; R 18/min
- Obstetric history: first pregnancy was complicated by idiopathic preterm labor leading to a 30-week spontaneous vaginal delivery, but patient has not been receiving 17-OH-P; no pregnancy terminations; no history of surgery on cervix (LEEP or cone biopsy)
- Physical exam: abdomen is soft and non-tender; uterus is soft and non-tender
- Fetal fibronectin test: positive
- Group B streptococcus culture: pending
- Digital cervical exam: mid position, 3 cm dilated, 50% effaced, soft consistency, −2 station
- Bedside abdominal U/S: cephalic presentation, posterior placenta without previa and no retroplacental hematoma, AFI 12 cm (normal 8–25 cm), MVP is 4 cm (normal ≥2 cm)
- Vaginal U/S: cervical length 15 mm (normal ≥25 mm) with significant funneling
- Urinalysis negative with no WBC or bacteria

Assessment

The patient meets the 3 criteria for preterm labor.

1. First, assess the patient's vitals and take a targeted history. This patient has had good prenatal care and an uncomplicated prenatal course. If gestational age was unknown, a bedside U/S could determine an estimated age using parameters such as biparietal diameter and femur length.

2. Next, assess the patient for abdominal tenderness and any signs of abruption. If fetal monitoring is available, place patient on continuous fetal HR monitoring to assess fetal well-being and continuous tocometer for frequency of contractions.

3. A speculum exam should be undertaken before digital exam, given her gestational age and unknown if fetal membranes are intact. If patient is determined to be unruptured, then do a culture for group B streptococcus and fetal fibronectin. A bimanual exam can then be undertaken. These digital exams should be limited.

CLINICAL PEARL

All pregnant women should be screened for preterm delivery risk: **history** of previous preterm delivery and **cervical length** on 18–20 week U/S.

- Gravidas with previous preterm delivery and normal cervical length should be offered weekly IM 17-OH-progesterone (17-OH-P) starting 16–20 wks continuing to 36 wks.

- Gravidas with cervical length <20 mm but no preterm delivery history should be offered daily vaginal progesterone treatment until 36 wks.

Further Management Plan

- IV MgSO$_4$ infusion (for fetal neuroprotection)
- IM antenatal corticosteroids (for induction of fetal pulmonary surfactant maturity)
- Antibiotics for group B streptococcus prophylaxis (to prevent early onset of group B streptococcus sepsis)
- Tocolytic agents (to allow antenatal steroid effect)

Discussion

Preterm birth occurs in 12% of births in the United States and is responsible for 70% of neonatal morbidity and mortality. Preterm labor precedes half of preterm births. All pregnant women should be educated about the symptoms of preterm labor. They should be assessed to see if they have any of the risk factors predicting preterm birth.

Diagnosis. Preterm labor is diagnosed when **all** of the following 3 criteria are present:

- Gestational age 20–37 weeks
- Associated with regular uterine contractions ($\geq$3 in 30 minutes)
- With cervical dilation of $\geq$2 cm or a change in cervical dilation, effacement or both

Symptoms. Suspect preterm labor if a patient presents with any of the following:

- Contractions every 10 min or more often
- Change in vaginal discharge (fluid leakage or bleeding)
- Pelvic pressure (feeling that the baby is pushing down, low dull backache, menstrual-like cramping, abdominal cramps with or without diarrhea)

Risk factors. Women at greatest risk of preterm labor have 1 or more of the following:

- History of previous preterm birth
- Current overdistended uterus (e.g., multiple fetuses, polyhydramnios)
- Mullerian anomalies (e.g., didelphys or bicornuate uterus)
- History of cervical procedures (e.g., LEEP, cone biopsy)
- Current infections (bladder, vagina or chorioamnionitis)
- Current cigarette smoking and substance abuse

Fetal fibronectin is a protein matrix produced by fetal cells that acts as a biological glue, binding the trophoblast to the maternal decidua. It "leaks" into the vagina if preterm birth is likely and can be measured with a rapid test using a vaginal swab through a speculum.

- **Prerequisites.** All of the following criteria should be met:
  - 22–35 weeks gestation
  - Cervical dilation <3 cm
  - Membranes intact

- **Method**. The fetal fibronectin specimen is obtained with a swab of the posterior cervical fornix through a speculum. To avoid a false positive test, pelvic exam or vaginal U/S should be avoided for 24 hrs prior to testing.

- **Interpretation**. The main value of the test is a negative result, which predicts the chance of preterm birth in the next week is <1%. With a positive result, the likelihood of preterm birth is 50%.

Once a diagnosis of preterm labor is established, the following interventions may help decrease the neonatal morbidity and mortality:

- **IV magnesium sulfate for fetal neuroprotection**
  - May reduce the severity and risk of cerebral palsy in surviving very preterm neonates
  - Start infusion if <32 weeks gestation regardless of delivery route
  - Aim to have infusion going for >4 hrs prior to delivery to reach steady state level in fetus

- **IM antenatal corticosteroid therapy**
  - May lower the severity or frequency of respiratory distress syndrome, intracranial hemorrhage, necrotizing enterocolitis, and death
  - A single course of corticosteroids is recommended with gestational age 24–34 weeks at risk for preterm delivery within 7 days
  - A complete course is 2 IM 12-mg doses of betamethasone given 24 hrs apart

- **IV penicillin G prophylaxis**
  - May reduce the likelihood of group B streptococcus early-onset sepsis, which is increased in premature neonates
  - Obtain vaginal and rectal culture for group B streptococcus before starting antibiotics; continue antibiotics until cultures come back negative or delivery occurs
  - Administer penicillin G, 5 million units IV initial dose, then 2.5 million units IV every 4 hrs until delivery; alternatively use clindamycin, erythromycin, or vancomycin

Tocolytic agents cannot be relied on to delay preterm delivery for >48 hrs. However, this window of time allows for 2 important interventions:

- Time to administer a 48-hour course of betamethasone to enhance fetal pulmonary surfactant

- Time to transport the mother and fetus in-utero to a facility with neonatal ICU.

Oral tocolytic agents are no more effective than placebo.

- **Magnesium sulfate**
  - Tocolytic effect is from competitive inhibition of calcium
  - Clinical monitoring based on decreasing but maintaining detectable deep tendon reflexes
  - Side effects include muscle weakness, respiratory depression, and pulmonary edema
  - Contraindications include renal insufficiency and myasthenia gravis

- **β-adrenergic agonists** include terbutaline.
  - Tocolytic effect depends on the β-adrenergic receptor myometrial activity.

- – Side effects include cardiovascular side effects (hypertension, tachycardia), hyperglycemia, hypokalemia, and pulmonary edema.
- – Contraindications include cardiac disease, DM, uncontrolled hyperthyroidism
- **Calcium-channel blockers** include nifedipine.
  - – Tocolytic effect depends on decreasing intracellular calcium.
  - – Side effects include tachycardia, hypotension, and myocardial depression.
  - – Contraindications include hypotension.
- **Prostaglandin synthetase inhibitors** include indomethacin.
  - – Tocolytic effect depends on decreasing smooth muscle contractility by decreasing prostaglandin production.
  - – Side effects include oligohydramnios, in-utero ductus arteriosus closure, and neonatal necrotizing enterocolitis.
  - – Contraindications include gestational age <34 weeks

Final Diagnosis

Preterm labor

CASE 9

Chief Complaint

Abnormal 1-hour glucose screen

History and Physical Examination

A 32-year-old Latina multigravida at 29 weeks gestation comes to the outpatient clinic for a routine prenatal visit. She has just undergone a 1-hour 50 gram oral glucose tolerance test (OGTT) screening for gestational diabetes. The glucose value came back at 175 mg/dL. Height is 5' 4" (1.62 m) tall and weight is 180 lb (81.6 kg). Her pregnancy weight gain has been 25 lb (11.3 kg) thus far. Her previous pregnancy was in Mexico and she doesn't remember if she had gestational diabetes or not. She did not have any U/S exams performed and she went into labor spontaneously on her due date. Her labor was only 6 hours long and she pushed for only 30 minutes. However the male neonate weighed 4,280 grams and the baby's shoulders got stuck. It took 2 minutes to get the baby out and he had trouble moving his right arm for a few days after delivery. Her fundal height today is 33 cm. FHT are 135/min in the LLQ.

Differential Diagnosis

1. **Gestational diabetes** (GDM)

   - The development of true GDM occurs because a patient's genetic predisposition to glucose intolerance is combined with increasing human placental lactogen (hPL) levels in the last half of the pregnancy. Even though the patient's insulin levels rise during the pregnancy, the anti-insulin effect of hPL results in an inability of the patient to keep glucose levels within the normal range. Hyperglycemia is the end result.

2. **False positive diabetic screen**

   - The majority of gravidas who have a positive 1-hour 50 gram OGTT will have a negative 3-hour 100 gram OGTT. This is a reflection of the poor specificity of the test. However, the *sensitivity* of the test is more important since we do not want to miss those patients who truly do have GDM.

Initial Management

Setting: outpatient workup and treatment

Diagnostic/Therapeutic Plan

- 3-hr 100 gram OGTT

Test Results

- FBS 106 mg/dL (high)
- 1 hr: 190 mg/dL (high)
- 2 hr: 160 mg/dL (high)
- 3 hr: 120 mg/dL

Assessment

Gestational diabetes is diagnosed when at least 2 of 4 values are above the upper limits of normal. In this case, 3 of the 4 values are abnormal. Generally speaking, while 15% of all gravidas have a positive 1-hour screening test, only 15% of women with a positive 1-hour screening test will be found to have gestational diabetes. Therefore a positive 1-hour screening test must be followed up with a 3-hour 100 gram OGTT.

Treatment Plan

- Education of the patient regarding a diabetic diet
- Education of the patient regarding the importance to the fetus of glucose control
- Home blood glucose monitoring
- Weekly prenatal office visits
- Monthly U/S for fetal growth

Discussion

All pregnant women are at risk for glucose intolerance. Since screening for diabetes using risk factors alone results in 50% of women with gestational diabetes being missed, the current recommendations are for universal screening of all women with a 1-hour 50 gram glucose load at 24–28 wks followed up with a definitive test, the 3-hour 100 gram OGTT.

Gestational diabetes (GDM) is diagnosed with 2 abnormal values on a definitive 3-hour 100 gram oral glucose tolerance test performed after a fast of 9–14 hrs following 3 days of unrestricted carbohydrate loading. Any glucose intolerance diagnosed in pregnancy is diagnosed as gestational diabetes, even though some patients will have new onset type 1 or type 2 diabetes that just happened to start during pregnancy.

Overt diabetes is diagnosed when pre-gestational glucose intolerance is present. Type 1 diabetes (or **juvenile onset** diabetes) is characterized by insulinopenia due to pancreatic islet-cell destruction. Type 2 diabetes (or **adult-onset** diabetes) is characterized by insulin resistance.

The primary methods for assessing success of glycemic control are home blood glucose testing with target values (a) fasting blood glucose <90 mg/dL, and (b) 1-hour postprandial values <140 mg/dL. All GDM patients should have a trial of diet therapy before giving medications.

Basic Science Correlate

The mechanism of pregnancy-induced glucose intolerance largely involves hormonal factors. The main factor is the anti-insulin effect of high levels of human placental lactogen; levels start low in pregnancy and steadily increase as pregnancy progresses. This explains why GDM is mostly diagnosed in the last half of pregnancy. Other contributors include placental insulinase which degrades insulin, and elevated free cortisol and progesterone which antagonize insulin.

Genetic predisposition is a major factor with GDM, with Latina women at 3:1 risk compared to Caucasian women.

Further Management if Diet Therapy Fails

The outcome of the neonate is directly related to the degree of glucose control in the mother, where the goal is euglycemia. If diet therapy fails, as demonstrated by the home glucose records, with fasting values consistently >90 mg/dL and 1-hr postprandial values consistently >140, then medications are required. While these values are not an indication for insulin therapy in the non-pregnant woman, they are an indication in the pregnant woman. Insulin injections can be initiated on an outpatient basis.

Oral hypoglycemic agents used to be contraindicated in pregnancy because of concerns of neonatal hypoglycemia, but glyburide crosses the placenta only minimally. Initiate outpatient insulin injections or glyburide to bring the glucose values to the target ranges.

Antenatal fetal well-being assessment in fetuses of mothers with diabetes should be managed as follows:

- **Uncomplicated GDM**

  - Fetal demise prior to 40 wks is not increased in GDM pregnancies with good glucose levels. Therefore, patients on diet therapy alone do not require NST or AFI testing prior to 40 wks. Induction of labor or delivery at 40 wks should be considered. Antepartum fetal well-being assessment in diet-controlled euglycemic gestational diabetic gravidas is only indicated if the pregnancy goes beyond 40 wks.

- **Complicated GDM or overt diabetes**

  - Fetal demise is a significant concern if risk factors are present, e.g., insulin or glyburide administration, prior unexplained stillbirth, co-existing hypertension. In these cases, NSTs and AFIs should be started 2x/weekly at 32 wks and continued until delivery (which should be planned at 39 wks).

Shoulder dystocia is increased with maternal diabetes.

- **Risk factors.** Shoulder dystocia is diagnosed when the head delivers but the remainder of the body cannot due to the fetal shoulders being wedged behind the pubic symphysis. This is commonly associated (though not necessarily) with an abnormally prolonged labor. Those at increased risk for shoulder dystocia include:

  - Diabetic patients, because of the commonly associated macrosomia; macrosomic fetuses have a disproportionate increase in fetal abdominal circumference and shoulder diameter relative to the head

  - Obese patients, with prior deliveries of babies weighing >4,000 g and prolonged gestations

- **Management.** A number of maneuvers have been described, the most common of which is the McRobert's maneuver, which entails flexing the maternal thighs and rotating the legs out laterally to increase the size of the maternal pelvis. Suprapubic pressure is also easily performed and may result in mobilizing the impacted fetal shoulder, permitting delivery of the anterior shoulder.

  - Other maneuvers include (a) delivery of the posterior shoulder, (b) rotating the fetus in utero, and (c) pushing the fetal head back into the pelvis for Cesarean delivery, essentially reversing the cardinal movements of labor

- **Prevention.** A high suspicion for shoulder dystocia should be entertained in diabetic mothers if the following intrapartum risk factors are present:

  - Prolonged second stage of labor

  - Need for oxytocin augmentation of labor

  - Use of assisted vaginal delivery with vacuum extractor or obstetrical forceps

A planned cesarean section should be offered to patients if estimated fetal weight (EFW) by obstetrical U/S suggests a high risk of shoulder dystocia. This would include EFW of >4,500 g in diabetic mothers and EFW of >5,000 g in non-diabetics.

Neonatal complications of maternal diabetes are as follows:

- Infants of diabetic mothers (IDMs) are at risk for a number of complications that are not issues for newborns of non-diabetic women. Many of these neonates will need to be observed closely in the NICU.

- IDMs should be monitored for hypoglycemia, hypocalcemia, polycythemia, hyperbili-rubinemia, and RDS. Even though the baby is large-for-gestational-age it may manifest immaturity in many organ systems.

Postpartum maternal monitoring needs to be done in cases of maternal diabetes.

- Postpartum hemorrhage (PPH) occurs much more frequently in diabetic mothers for a number of reasons. The most common cause is uterine atony, which is due to uterine overdistention resulting from a macrosomic fetus and lacerations of the perineum and vulva resulting from difficult vaginal delivery of a big neonate.

- It is important to check for elevated maternal postpartum glucose values to determine persistent need for insulin. Assessment for new onset of overt diabetes during the pregnancy can be done by performing either 2 FBS after 6 wks or by doing a 2-hour 75 gm OGTT after 6 wks.

Final Diagnosis

Gestational diabetes

CASE 10

Chief Complaint

"I woke up an hour ago to find blood all over my nightgown."

History and Physical Examination

A 30-year-old multigravida at 30 weeks gestation by dates comes to the emergency department complaining of painless vaginal bleeding. She awoke an hour ago after feeling blood trickling down her legs. She noted a pool of blood on her bedsheets and nightgown. She has minimal uterine tightening. She denies recent sexual intercourse. She states that there is good fetal movement. She has had no prenatal care. Her first pregnancy ended with an emergency low transverse cesarean section at term for breech presentation. She smokes 1 pack of cigarettes a day and admits to occasional cocaine use.

Vital signs are stable. General exam is unremarkable. The uterus is soft and non-tender. Fundal height is 28 cm. FHR by Doppler stethoscope is 135/min. Bright red blood is seen emerging from her introitus.

Differential Diagnosis

1. Placenta previa
2. Placental abruption
3. Vasa previa
4. Uterine rupture
5. Bloody show
6. Lower genital tract lesion

Initial Management

Setting: emergency department with move to inpatient

Initial Diagnostic Plan

- Abdominal obstetric U/S
- Biophysical profile with AFI/MVP
- CBC
- Type and screen

Test Results

- U/S: single live fetus with composite measurements of 30 wks gestation in transverse lie. FHR is 145/min. Complete central placenta previa.

- NST is reactive. Gross body movement, breathing movements and extension-flexion are noted. AFI is 11 cm and MVP is 2.5 cm.

- CBC: Hb 9 g/dL, Hct 27%, platelets 210,000

Assessment

The definitive diagnosis is obtained by U/S imaging showing complete placenta previa. This confirms the clinical suspicion with symptoms of painless third-trimester bleeding.

Treatment Plan

- Start IV with 16-gauge needle running isotonic fluids
- Type and cross-match for 2 units of packed RBC
- Place Foley catheter to measure urine output
- Do **not** perform a pelvic exam

Discussion

The first priority is to ensure hemodynamic stability by establishing IV access. The uterus receives approximately 20% of total cardiac output at a rate of 500 cc/minute. Young women usually do not show clinical manifestations of hypovolemic shock until they've lost 15%-20% of their total blood volume and can thus rapidly deteriorate. It is important to be vigilant regarding the possibility of acute decompensation and maintain adequate volume replacement. Several complications of excessive blood loss include hemorrhagic shock, renal-cortical necrosis, Sheehan syndrome and DIC.

It is crucial to **not perform a pelvic exam** until placenta previa is ruled out by U/S. If a pelvic exam must be done, it should occur as a double set up exam (with anesthesia present, nurses and room prepared for emergency C-section).

Further Management Plan/Results

• Kleihauer-Betke test to detect fetal RBCs in maternal circulation	• Negative for fetal RBCs
• Weigh the pads and sponges to accurately assess ongoing blood loss	• Pad-weighing shows 25 mL over past hour
• Serial CBCs to assess for blood loss	• Hgb 9 g/dL, Hct 27% (unchanged)

Further Treatment Plan

- Admit to maternity unit
- Betamethasone IM, 2 injections 24 hrs apart, to enhance fetal pulmonary surfactant
- IV $MgSO_4$ for fetal neuroprotection if delivery anticipated shortly

Discussion

Third trimester bleeding occurs in approximately 4 percent of pregnancies. RhoGAM should be administered to Rh negative gravidas. The Kleihauer-Betke test will estimate the volume of fetal blood in the maternal circulation. Each 300 mg vial of RhoGAM will neutralize 15 mL of fetal RBCs.

Abruptio placenta is the most **common** serious cause of late-pregnancy **painful** bleeding.

- The pain is often described as intense, localized and constant. The diagnosis is made **clinically**. The mechanism of bleeding in abruptio placenta is best described by the avulsion of anchoring placental villi from stretching of the lower uterine segment.

- **Risk factors** including pregnancy-induced hypertension, maternal blunt trauma (e.g., motor vehicle accident, domestic violence), cocaine use. In all these situations the placental villi lose their vascular integrity leading to hemorrhage into the decidua basalis resulting in a hematoma formation. It can be an ongoing propagation ending with complete separation of the placenta. If the hematoma does not dissect through the margin of the placenta it can remain concealed or internal, but if the blood makes its way through to the cervical os and out the vagina it becomes overt or external.

- **Management** depends on maternal and fetal status, gestational age and cervical dilation.

Placenta previa is a **common** cause of late second or third trimester **painless** vaginal bleeding.

- The diagnosis is made by OB U/S which reveals placental implantation in the lower uterine segment. The placental edge may be completely over the internal cervical os (**total** previa), partially over the os (**partial** previa) or only close to the os (**marginal** previa). The uterus is soft and nontender.

- Lower uterine segment implantation is common in early pregnancy. Atrophy of the lower placental edge combined with hypertrophy of the upper placenta gives rise to placental "migration" with advancing pregnancy.

- Fetal malpresentation is present in a third of cases (transverse lie or breech presentation). Sexual intercourse can result in significant vaginal bleeding and patients are at an increased risk if they have a history of prior placenta previa or C-sections.

- Placenta **accreta / percreta / increta** (trophoblast growing into the myometrium or deeper) is associated anterior placenta previa when the placenta is implanted over the previous C-section scar. Cesarean hysterectomy is necessary to control blood loss in these cases.

- **Management** of placenta previa depends on maternal and fetal status, gestational age, and the type of previa.

Vasa previa is a **rare** cause of **painless** vaginal bleeding but is life-threatening for the fetus.

- Prerequisites are fetal vessels running over the fetal membranes unprotected by the umbilical cord. If the vessels are over the membranes overlying the cervix, when membranes rupture the fetal vessels are torn, resulting in fetal hemorrhage and frequently exsanguination. The diagnosis is made **clinically**.

- **Risk factors** are a velamentous cord insertion or accessory placental lobe. The classic clinical triad is (1) membrane rupture followed by (2) immediate vaginal bleeding followed by (3) fetal bradycardia. Diagnosis is rare prior to the acute bleed.

- **Management** is emergency crash cesarean delivery.

Uterine rupture is a **rare** cause of **painful** late pregnancy bleeding.

- This involves full thickness disruption of the uterine wall. Massive hemorrhage is common with 50% perinatal mortality and 5% maternal mortality.

- **Risk factors** include previous uterine scar (e.g., classical uterine incision, myomectomy that entered uterine cavity), excessive oxytocin and uterine overdistention. This is a life-threatening emergency on the part of the mother and fetus.

- **Management** is emergency crash laparotomy to save the fetus if possible and repair the uterine defect if possible.

Bloody show is the passage of a small amount of blood-tinged mucus through the vagina near the end of pregnancy. It can occur just before labor or in early labor. It is evidence of cervical effacement and/or dilation. As the cervix changes shape, mucus and blood that occupied the cervical glands or cervical os is freed to pass into the vagina. Bloody show is a relatively common feature of pregnancy, and it does not signify increased risk to the mother or baby.

Lower genital tract lesion is an anatomic cause of vaginal bleeding that may come from a cervical or vaginal laceration or lesion. Possible sources of blood could be a vaginal laceration or varicosity, a cervical polyp or ulcer. Diagnosis is made by visualization of the lower genital tract using a vaginal speculum. Digital exam or speculum exam should not be done in the late second trimester or third trimester until U/S has confirmed the absence of a placenta previa.

Final Diagnosis

Complete central placenta previa

CASE 11

Chief Complaint

Elevated blood pressure

History and Physical Examination

A 16-year-old woman G1 P0 comes to the clinic for a routine return prenatal visit at 32 weeks' gestation (confirmed by 18-week U/S). She states that over the past 2 weeks she has developed swelling of her face and hands. Her prenatal course up to this point has been unremarkable, with blood pressures averaging 120/70 mm Hg. She denies any change in mental status, headaches, scotomata, blurred vision, shortness of breath, and right upper quadrant pain. She states her fetus is moving well. She has a positive family history for preeclampsia and diabetes.

On examination she appears puffy-faced and edematous with a 7-lb weight gain over the last 2 weeks. Blood pressure is 160/90 mm Hg. Retinal examination shows vasoconstriction but no exudates or neovascularization. She has a benign abdominal exam without tenderness, but deep tendon reflexes are brisk. Fundal height of the uterus is 29 cm and fetal heart tones 130/min in the left lower quadrant. Pelvic exam reveals cervix long and closed with membranes intact, and there is no vaginal discharge.

Differential Diagnosis

1. **Gestational hypertension**
   - Can be ruled out if proteinuria is present
2. **Preeclampsia without severe features**
   - No end-organ involvement – managed conservatively
3. **Preeclampsia with severe features**
   - End-organ involvement managed aggressively
4. **Eclampsia**
   - Requires unexplained generalized seizures
5. **Chronic hypertension**
   - Hypertension precedes pregnancy or <20 wks
6. **Chronic hypertension with superimposed preeclampsia**
7. **HELLP syndrome**

Initial Management

Setting: outpatient office

Diagnostic/Therapeutic Plan

- Repeat BP in 15 minutes
- Urinalysis for proteinuria
- Hemoglobin, hematocrit

- Platelet count
- BUN, creatinine, uric acid
- ALT, AST
- Urine drug screen for toxicology

Test Results

- Repeat BP: 155/95 mm Hg
- Urinalysis: 2+ protein
- Hemoglobin, hematocrit: 15 g/dL and 42% (elevated for pregnancy)
- Platelet count: 230,000/mm³ (normal)
- BUN, creatinine, uric acid: 18 mg/dL, 1.0 mg/dL, 7.5 mg/dL (all elevated for pregnancy)
- ALT, AST: 25 U/L, 35 U/L (both normal)
- Urine toxicology: negative

Assessment of Mother

Preeclampsia without severe features, mother is stable

Discussion

This patient has the classic findings of preeclampsia without severe features: sustained mild hypertension and proteinuria developing **after** 20 wks' gestation in a woman with previously normal blood pressure. There are no symptoms: headache, epigastric pain, or visual disturbances. Edema may or may not be present, but it is not a criterion for preeclampsia. The increased hemoglobin, hematocrit, BUN, and uric acid are consistent with the hemoconcentration seen with preeclampsia but are not criteria for preeclampsia.

Note that the term "mild preeclampsia" is no longer used. The preferred term is "**preeclampsia without severe features**." It is diagnosed with sustained mild hypertension in the presence of proteinuria without end-organ effects. It is typically managed conservatively until 37 wks gestation.

Similarly, the term "severe preeclampsia" is no longer used. The preferred term is "**preeclampsia with severe features**." It is diagnosed in the presence of any ONE of the following findings with or without proteinuria:

- **BP**: systolic BP >160 mm Hg or diastolic BP >110 mm Hg on 2 occasions, at least 4 hrs apart, while patient is on bed rest
- **Platelets**: thrombocytopenia <100,000/μL
- **Impaired liver function**: elevated AST or ALT to twice the normal concentrations, severe persistent unexplained RUQ or epigastric pain
- **Progressive renal insufficiency**: elevated serum creatinine >1.1 mg/dL or doubling of previous creatinine
- **Pulmonary edema**
- **Symptoms**: new onset cerebral or visual disturbances.

CLINICAL PEARL

A diagnosis of **hypertension** requires BP elevation ≥140/90 mm Hg on 2 occasions, at least 4 hrs apart at bed rest.

- Mild hypertension = ↑ BP 140/90–160/110 mm Hg
- Severe hypertension = ↑ BP >160/110 mm Hg

CLINICAL PEARL

A diagnosis of **proteinuria** requires 24-hour urine >300 mg OR protein/creatinine ratio >0.3 OR urine dipstick reading 1+ (used only if the 2 quantitative methods are not available).

CLINICAL PEARL

Preeclampsia is 8x more common in the first pregnancy, especially in women at the extremes of reproductive life. This 16-year-old is a prime candidate.

Further Management Plan/Results

• Obstetric U/S for fetal growth assessment	• Single live fetus with composite measurements of 31 wks' gestation in cephalic presentation • Fetal HR 145/min
• Biophysical profile with AFI for fetal oxygenation assessment	• Non-stress test is reactive • Gross body movement, breathing movements, and extension-flexion noted • Amniotic fluid MVP 4 cm

Assessment of Fetus

Fetal growth is appropriate for dates and fetal oxygenation and placental function is good.

Initial Management

In the presence of preeclampsia without severe features <37 wks, with maternal and fetal well-being confirmed, the management is inpatient conservative observation to allow fetal maturation to take place. No IV MgSO$_4$ is started, but serial parameters of maternal and fetal status are followed to identify if severe features develop. Two doses of IM betamethasone 12 hrs apart are given to enhance fetal lung maturity at <34 wks' gestation. At 37 0/7 wks' gestation or greater, the patient will be delivered with induction of labor or cesarean if obstetrically indicated.

The vasoconstriction of preeclampsia will not be ultimately reversed until after the pregnancy is over. However, the decision for delivery requires a judicious balance between the hazard to the mother of waiting and the hazard to the fetus of delivery early. The presence or absence of severe features will tip the scale to either conservative or aggressive inpatient management. With a gestational age in this case of only 32 wks, the risk of prematurity is significant and the risk to the mother of waiting until 37 wks is minimal. Serial assessment of maternal and fetal status will take place.

One Week Later on the Maternity Unit

At 33 wks' gestation the patient is complaining of persistent headache and epigastric pain. Her BP has been creeping up and is now persistently 165/115 mm Hg. A 24-hour urine protein collection revealed 7.5 g of protein. AST is 250 U/L, and ALT 270 U/L. Platelet count is now 85,000/mm^3. Non-stress test is reactive. Fetus is cephalic presentation. Cervical examination is 1 cm dilated, 50% effaced, soft, −2 station.

Further Assessment/Treatment

The worsening clinical findings have unequivocally moved the patient from preeclampsia **without** severe features to preeclampsia **with** severe features.

- Start IV magnesium sulfate infusion to prevent eclampsia

- Lower blood pressure with IV hydralazine or IV labetalol

- Start IV oxytocin to induce labor

Even though the fetus is only 33 wks' gestation, the hazard to the mother outweighs the risk of prematurity to her baby. The management goals of severe preeclampsia include:

- IV MgSO$_4$ to prevent convulsions

- Control blood pressure with IV hydralazine or labetalol to keep diastolic values 90–100 mm Hg and ensure adequate placental blood flow

- Prompt delivery

Vaginal delivery is a reasonable goal as long as mother and fetus are stable.

Two Hours Later on the Maternity Unit

An hour ago the patient received a 5-g IV loading dose of MgSO$_4$ over 20 minutes followed by an IV infusion of 2 g/hour. Her urine output has been 15 mL over the past hour. Her respirations, which were 20/min, are now 5/min. Continuous fetal monitor shows a baseline fetal HR of 140/min with minimal variability. There are no accelerations, but also no decelerations. Deep tendon reflexes are not obtainable.

Further Assessment/Treatment

This is probable magnesium toxicity.

- Discontinue IV magnesium sulfate infusion.

- Administer supplemental oxygen 8 to 10 liters by mask.

- Place mother on oxygen saturation monitor.

- Administer IV calcium gluconate

Magnesium is excreted through the kidney. If renal function is impaired, as it may be with preeclampsia, magnesium levels can rise and cause Mg toxicity and respiratory depression. MgSO$_4$ is contraindicated in women with myasthenia gravis since it can precipitate a severe crisis. If renal function is good, magnesium toxicity is rare. At serum Mg concentrations of 9.6–12 mg/dL, loss of deep tendon reflexes occurs; at 12–18 mg/dL respiratory paralysis takes place, and at 24–30 mg/dL cardiac arrest can develop. Calcium gluconate 1-gram IV over 5–10 min should be given to reverse life-threatening symptoms of magnesium toxicity.

Basic Science Correlate

The pathogenesis of preeclampsia involves a loss of the normal refractory state of pregnancy against the pressure effects of renin and angiotensin. There is an altered balance between the vasoactive prostaglandins: the vasodilating effect of prostacyclin is overbalanced by the vasoconstricting effect of thromboxane. This results in diffuse vasospasm, reducing systemic perfusion to vital organs and causing capillary endothelial damage. Preeclampsia is associated with a decreased intravascular volume.

CCS NOTE

When you order "magnesium sulfate" or "MgSO$_4$" in the ORDER INPUT form, a drop-down menu will appear in the ORDER QUALIFIER form to ask you to specify the route of administration (i.e., intramuscular, IV, or oral). You will then be asked to select the dosing frequency (one-time bolus or continuous).

CLINICAL PEARL

If you overtreat hypertension, lowering BP to normal range, uteroplacental perfusion may be jeopardized and thus risk fetal well-being. Keep diastolic values between 90–100 mm Hg.

Differential Diagnosis Summary

- **Gestational hypertension.** Symptoms (headache, epigastric pain, visual changes) are absent. Signs are sustained mild hypertension after 20 wks' gestation. Lab findings are those which are normal for pregnancy, including absence of significant proteinuria. Management is watching for development of preeclampsia and delivery at 37 wks.

- **Preeclampsia without severe features.** Symptoms are absent. Signs are sustained mild hypertension after 20 wks' gestation. Laboratory findings show proteinuria and mild hemoconcentration but no thrombocytopenia, liver enzyme elevation, creatinine elevation. Management is conservative and delivery is at 37 wks. No $MgSO_4$ is necessary peripartum.

- **Preeclampsia with severe features.** At least sustained mild hypertension and evidence of end-organ involvement symptoms may or may not be present. It is diagnosed in the presence of any ONE of the following findings with or without proteinuria; systolic BP >160 mm Hg or diastolic BP >110 on 2 occasions at least 4 hrs apart while patient is on bed rest; thrombocytopenia <100,000/μL; elevated AST or ALT to 2x normal concentrations, severe persistent unexplained RUQ or epigastric pain; elevated serum creatinine >1.1 mg/dL or doubling of previous creatinine; pulmonary edema; new onset cerebral or visual disturbances. Management is aggressive inpatient: prompt delivery, but not necessarily cesarean; IV $MgSO_4$ is intrapartum continued 24 hrs postpartum; lower BP with IV hydralazine or labetalol to keep diastolic pressure between 90–100 mm Hg.

- **Eclampsia.** This diagnosis is made in the presence of new-onset generalized tonic-clonic seizures in a woman with preeclampsia. Eclampsia can develop before, during, or after labor. Seizures are treated and prevented with IV $MgSO_4$. Management is otherwise aggressive inpatient, as with preeclampsia with severe features.

- **Chronic hypertension.** Symptoms are absent. Signs are sustained elevation of BP at least in the mild range **before** pregnancy or **prior** to 20 wks' gestation. Baseline laboratory findings may be normal or abnormal depending on duration and end-organ damage. Management is outpatient conservative with labetalol, nifedipine or methyldopa only if BP >160 mm Hg systolic and 105 mm Hg diastolic. Deliver at 38 wks.

- **Chronic hypertension with superimposed preeclampsia.** Symptoms may include those of preeclampsia with severe features. Signs are those of chronic hypertension plus rising BP and/or those of preeclampsia with severe features. Laboratory findings are those of preeclampsia with severe features. Management is aggressive inpatient same as for preeclampsia with severe features.

- **HELLP syndrome.** Symptoms may be present or absent. Signs may be absent or variable. Laboratory findings are hemolysis, elevated liver enzymes and low platelets. Management is aggressive inpatient same as for preeclampsia with severe features.

Final Diagnosis

Preeclampsia with severe features

CASE 12

Chief Complaint

Nonreassuring fetal monitor tracing

History and Physical Examination

A 31-year-old primigravida at 40 5/7 weeks gestation is on the maternity unit in active labor. Her prenatal course was unremarkable and she arrived with spontaneous uterine contractions at 4 cm dilation. She is now 7 cm dilated, 100% effaced, 0 station with the fetus in cephalic presentation. She has Ringer's lactate infusing in an IV line at 125 cc/hr. IV oxytocin augmentation of labor is being administered because of arrest of cervical dilation at 6 cm. Fetal membranes are intact. An external fetal HR monitor is in place along with an external uterine contractions monitor. The L&D nurse notifies you that the external EFM tracing which was initially normal now shows FHR baseline at 170/min with absent variability and repetitive late decelerations. Uterine contractions are occurring every 2 minutes lasting 90 seconds. There is no bleeding.

Differential Diagnosis

1. **Uterine tachysystole**
2. **Umbilical cord compression**
3. **Fetal head compression**
4. **Placental insufficiency**

Initial Management

Setting: inpatient workup and treatment

Assessment

Category III EFM tracing due to excessive oxytocin stimulation resulting in tachysystole, inadequate intervillous space perfusion, and placental insufficiency

Management Plan

- **Ensure IV access** with 16 gauge needle (to allow rapid infusion of isotonic fluids)
- **Turn off IV oxytocin infusion** (to space out uterine contractions and enhance intervillous placental blood flow)
- **Administer a 500 mL bolus of IV Ringer's** lactate (to counteract possible intravascular deficit and enhance uteroplacental infusion)
- **Administer 8–10 L of oxygen by face mask** (to enhance oxygen transfer across the placental gradient thereby increasing oxygen delivery to the fetus)

- **Change maternal position** (to decrease umbilical cord compression or inferior vena cava compression)

- Perform a digital vaginal exam (to rule out prolapsed umbilical cord)

- Perform a digital scalp stimulation (to observe for FHR accelerations, which would be reassuring of fetal status)

As a result of the interventions, FHR tracing normalizes with baseline now 140/min and moderate variability. Accelerations are noted with no decelerations.

Discussion

It is important to recognize that most "abnormal" tracings are not due to fetal hypoxia. Ask if the tracing has biological plausibility. Could there be a non-hypoxic explanation of the tracing (e.g., uterine tachysystole, maternal fever, complete fetal heart block, fetal tachyarrhythmia, maternal atropine)?

The following steps should be taken whenever the **EFM tracing** is **not reassuring**.

1. Examine the EFM strip carefully looking for: **baseline HR** (normal 110–160/min), degree of **variability** (normal 6–25 beats/min), and presence of **periodic changes** (accelerations, which are always reassuring, early decelerations [from head compression] which are benign, variable decelerations [from umbilical cord compression] which are concerning only if severe, late decelerations [from uteroplacental insufficiency], which are always concerning).

2. Confirm abnormal finding: tachycardia, bradycardia, absent or decreased variability, severe variable decelerations or any late decelerations.

3. Identify non-hypoxic causes present which could explain the abnormal findings: maternal fever, medication effect, prematurity, fetal arrhythmia.

4. Initiate the Intrauterine Resuscitation measures (described above) to enhance placental perfusion and fetal oxygenation.

5. Observe for normalization of the EFM tracing.

6. Prepare for delivery promptly if these interventions do not normalize the EFM tracing.

A 3-tiered system for the categorization of FHR patterns is the current standard of care. Recognize that FHR tracing patterns provide information only on the current acid-base status of the fetus.

- Categorization evaluates the fetus at that point in time but is not fixed.

- FHR tracing may move back and forth between the categories, depending on the clinical situation and management strategies used.

Category I: FHR tracings are normal. "GREEN light, GO!"

- Criteria include all of the following:

  - **Baseline rate:** 110–160 beats/min

  - **Baseline FHR variability:** moderate

  - **Late or variable decelerations:** absent

  - **Early decelerations:** present or absent

  - **Accelerations:** present or absent

- **Interpretation:** strongly predictive of normal fetal acid-base status at the time of observation

- **Action:** monitoring in a routine manner, with no specific action required

Category II: FHR tracings are indeterminate. "YELLOW light, CAUTION"

- Criteria include all FHR tracings **not categorized as category I or III** (may represent a significant proportion of EFM tracings seen)

- **Interpretation:** not predictive of abnormal or normal fetal acid-base status

- **Action:** close surveillance and reevaluation, taking into account the entire associated clinical circumstances.

Category III: FHR tracings are abnormal. "RED light, STOP!"

- Criteria include **absent** baseline FHR variability and any of the following:
  - Recurrent **late decelerations**
  - Recurrent **variable decelerations**
  - **Bradycardia**
  - **Sinusoidal** pattern

- **Interpretation:** associated with abnormal fetal acid-base status at the time of observation – requires prompt evaluation.

- **Action:** initiate expeditious intrauterine resuscitation to resolve the abnormal FHR pattern – if tracing does not resolve with these measures, prompt delivery should take place.

Intrauterine resuscitation interventions are used whenever the EFM strip shows characteristics of category II or III status. They are generic, non-specific measures designed to increase oxygen transfer from patient to fetus.

- **Decrease uterine contractions:** Turn off any IV oxytocin infusion or administer terbutaline 0.25 mg subcutaneously to enhance intervillous placental blood flow

- **Augment IV fluid volume:** Infuse 500 mL of normal saline rapidly to enhance uteroplacental infusion

- **Administer high-flow oxygen:** Give patient 8–10 L of oxygen by facemask to increase delivery of maternal oxygen to the placenta

- **Perform amnioinfusion:** useful for eliminating or reducing the severity of variable decelerations

- **Change position:** Removing the parturient from the supine position decreases inferior vena cava compression and enhances cardiac return, thus cardiac output to the placenta. Turning the parturient from one lateral position to the other may relieve any umbilical cord compression that is present.

- **Vaginal examination:** Perform digital vaginal examination to rule out possible prolapsed umbilical cord

- **Scalp stimulation:** Perform digital scalp stimulation observing for accelerations, which would be reassuring of fetal condition

Final Diagnosis

Category III intrapartum fetal monitor tracing due to excessive oxytocin administration

CASE 13

Chief Complaint

"I am 2 weeks past my due date."

Part I

A 26-year-old multigravida at 42 weeks gestation by dates comes to the outpatient clinic for a prenatal visit. She has occasional uterine contractions. Fetal movements are present and normal. Her prior pregnancy resulted in a vaginal delivery of a 4,100 g meconium-stained infant at 43 weeks gestation.

Vital signs are stable. Fundal height is 42 cm. FHT are 125/min in the RLQ. On pelvic exam the fetus is cephalic presentation with cervix closed, thick, high, posterior and firm.

Differential Diagnosis

1. **Post-term pregnancy**
2. **Inaccurate pregnancy dating**

Initial Management

Setting: outpatient office

Diagnostic/Therapeutic Plan

- Menstrual history reviewed
- Clinical landmarks reviewed
- U/S reviewed

Test Results

- LMP is normal and sure; pregnancy was planned
- Doppler fetal heart tones were heard at 11 wks with quickening at 16 wks
- 18-wk U/S: consistent with dates

Initial Assessment

- Post-term pregnancy
- Unfavorable cervix

Further Diagnostic Plan

- Nonstress test (NST)
- Amniotic fluid index (AFI) and MVP

CLINICAL PEARL

Fundal height 42 cm suggests a large, possibly macrosomic, fetus. The unfavorable cervical exam suggests a long induction of labor may be likely. This is not a good combination.

Further Test Results

- NST is reactive

- AFI is 4 cm (normal 9–25 cm); MVP is 1 cm (normal >2 cm)

Initial Treatment Plan

Cervical ripening and induction of labor with vaginal prostaglandin E2 gel

Discussion

The terminology for identifying term and post-term pregnancies is as follows:

- **Early term**: 37 to 38 6/7 wks

- **Full term**: 39 to 40 6/7 wks

- **Late term**: 41 to 41 6/7 wks

- **Post term**: 42 wks or more

The most common cause of true post-term cases is idiopathic (no known cause). It does occur more commonly in young primigravidas and rarely with placental sulfatase deficiency. Pregnancies with anencephalic fetuses are the longest pregnancies reported.

Morbidity and mortality. Perinatal M & M in post-term pregnancies is increased two- to three-fold largely from effects on placental functioning.

- In 20% of cases, placental function deteriorates, leading to **dysmaturity syndrome.** This results in inadequate nutrition and oxygenation in a starved, hypoxic fetus. Such a fetus is at risk for emergency cesarean delivery for fetal distress.

- In 80% of cases, placental function is maintained, leading to **macrosomic syndrome.** This provides fetal nutrition, resulting in an excessively large baby. Such a fetus is at risk for an operative or difficult delivery with potential birth trauma.

Importance of dating. The accuracy of diagnosis is predicated on precision of gestational dating. Confirmation of gestational age is based on assessment of menstrual history accuracy, documentation of early clinical parameters and early U/S.

- **LMP** tends to be reliable: (1) if the patient is sure of dates, (2) if the pregnancy was planned, and (3) if her menstrual cycle was normal in time as well as length and duration. Recent oral contraceptive use, abortion, pregnancy or lactation can delay ovulation. This would cause a discrepancy between assumed conception (presumed to occur 14 days after the onset of the LMP) and the actual conception.

- **Early clinical parameters** are helpful when documented at the earliest gestational age the parameter could be identified. Uterine size is best estimated in the first trimester. Early fetal heart tones can be heard by a Doppler stethoscope at 10–12 wks. Quickening occurs at 18–20 wks for primiparas and 16–20 wks for multiparas. FHT with fetoscope are heard at 18–20 wks.

- **Early U/S** is more accurate in pregnancy dating than a later one. A 10-wk U/S is accurate in dating to plus or minus 5 days. An 18-wk U/S is accurate in dating to plus or minus 10 days.

CLINICAL PEARL

AFI 3 cm and/or SDVP 1 cm is concerning. Amniotic fluid is largely derived from fetal urine, which is produced by the fetal kidneys. A low AFI and/or SDVP suggests possible inadequate placental perfusion of fetal kidneys, resulting in decreased urine production.

Management. Patient suspected to be post-term or post dates are triaged into one of 3 groups:

1. **Dates sure and cervix favorable** (Bishop score ≥8). There is no benefit to the mother or fetus to continue the pregnancy, so induce labor with oxytocin and amniotomy.

2. **Dates sure but cervix unfavorable** (Bishop ≤5). There is no benefit to the mother or fetus to continue the pregnancy. However, the unfavorable cervix (low Bishop score) can limit successful labor induction with oxytocin alone. Therefore, use either vaginal prostaglandin E or placement of a trans-cervical Foley bulb for cervical ripening, followed by IV oxytocin when the cervix softens and dilates.

3. **Dates unsure**. If the true gestational age is unknown, management is conservative with 2/week modified biophysical profile (NSTs and AFI). Delivery is indicated if there is suggestion of fetal deterioration: non-stress test is persistently non-reactive or oligohydramnios develops. (In actual practice, most obstetricians induce labor at 41 wks, when the risk of intrauterine fetal demise starts to increase. In this case the finding of a 4-quadrant AFI and MVP outside the normal is concerning, and suggests that delivery is indicated.)

Later on the Maternity Unit

After receiving cervical ripening with vaginal prostaglandin E2, the patient progressed into active labor. She is 7 cm dilated, 100% effaced, −1 station. External electronic FHR monitor shows baseline HR 155/min with moderate variability and irregularly occurring decelerations with rapid drops of 25 beats/min returning rapidly to baseline after 15 sec. Uterine contractions are occurring every 3 min lasting 50 sec. Amniotomy is performed, revealing minimal amniotic fluid with thick, "pea-soup" colored meconium.

Differential Diagnosis of Meconium

1. Fetal hypoxia due to placental insufficiency

2. Normal physiological fetal GI motility

Diagnostic/Therapeutic Plan/Results

• Placement of internal fetal scalp electrode	Scalp electrode confirms external FHR monitor findings
• Amnioinfusion with saline	Decelerations have disappeared

CCS NOTE

The order "amnioinfusion" does not appear in the order menu and is not recognized by the CS software.

Assessment

• Post-term pregnancy in active labor.

• Intrapartum meconium secondary to GI tract motility

• Mild variable decelerations, resolved, with reassuring fetal status

Treatment Plan

• Continue amnioinfusion until delivery

• Do **not** suction fetal nose and pharynx after delivery of the head

• Do **not** perform neonatal laryngoscopic tracheal aspiration after delivery unless baby is depressed

Discussion

The mechanisms for passage of **meconium** in-utero are either acidosis-mediated loss of anal sphincter tone or maturity-mediated intestinal peristalsis. Since the fetal monitor pattern is not suggestive of acidosis, the most likely explanation is fetal GI tract maturity.

It used to be thought that **meconium aspiration syndrome** (MAS) was an intrapartum phenomenon, so the routine advised was suctioning the neonatal nares/pharynx on the perineum and laryngoscopic neonatal visualization of the vocal cords to suck out any meconium.

We now know that MAS is not an intrapartum event but rather occurs well before delivery. Therefore, the current recommendations are **not to suction** the nares/pharynx on the perineum and **only to visualize** the vocal cords if the neonate is depressed.

Since the FHR **decelerations** are unrelated to contractions, they are neither **early** decelerations (from head compression) nor **late** decelerations (from myocardial depression). The rapid drop and rapid return of the FHR rate suggests a vagally mediated event. Umbilical cord compressions are the most likely explanation for these **variable** decelerations, particularly with the membranes being ruptured resulting in decreased amniotic fluid.

If we assume that decreased amniotic fluid volume is a causative factor in the variable decelerations, a reasonable intervention would be to replace fluid into the uterine cavity. This is achieved through a procedure known as **amnioinfusion**. Amnioinfusion is performed by placing an intrauterine catheter into the uterus and allowing gravity drainage of room-temperature normal saline into the amniotic cavity. The replaced fluid volume presumably allows space for the umbilical cord to float without being compressed.

Final Diagnosis

Post-term pregnancy

CASE 14

Chief Complaint

"I am not going into labor."

History and Physical Examination

A 30-year-old primigravid woman comes to the labor ward at 42 weeks gestation confirmed by an 18 week U/S examination. She had an elevated 1-hour 50 g glucose screening test but underwent a 3-hour 100 g oral glucose tolerance test which was normal. She has no other medical conditions. She takes no medications other than prenatal vitamins. She denies any allergies and previous surgeries. She was offered induction of labor 1 week ago at 41 weeks gestation but she deferred wanting to experience spontaneous onset of labor. At that time the modified biophysical profile showed a reactive NST and AFI 12 cm and MVP 4 cm.

She comes in today with irregular contractions every 8–10 minutes. Her vital signs are stable. The tocometer shows she is having irregular mild contractions coming every 8–10 minutes, lasting 25 seconds. Fetal heart tones with a Doppler stethoscope are 135/min. The uterus is soft between contractions but can be indented with a finger even during contractions.

Differential Diagnosis (questions that need to be answered)

1. **Post-term pregnancy**
   - Gestational age is ≥42 wks
2. **Is the patient in labor?**
   - Is there cervical dilation and effacement?
3. **What is fetal status?**
   - How is fetus doing on modified biophysical profile?

Initial Management

Setting: labor triage

Diagnostic/Therapeutic Plan

- Sterile vaginal digital examination for cervical status
- Modified biophysical profile (NST and AFI/MVP)
- Bedside U/S for fetal presentation

Test Results

- Cervix is closed without any effacement
- NST is reactive but AFI is only 3 cm (normal 9–25 cm) and MVP 1 cm
- Fetus in cephalic presentation

Assessment

Patient has a post-term pregnancy (now at 42 wks gestation), not in labor (cervix is closed and uneffaced). Fetal status is concerning with oligohydramnios.

Further Management Plan

- The patient has a Foley balloon placed and 5 hrs later it comes out.
- Oxytocin is started and the patient has regular contractions reaching >200 Montevideo units. She experienced spontaneous rupture of membranes and reaches a cervical dilation of 7 cm.
- However, despite regular contractions every 2–3 minutes, she does not dilate any further over the next 4 hrs.

Basic Science Correlate

Given that the patient now has a post-term pregnancy, management is induction of labor. An induction of labor can be recommended in late- or post-term pregnancy to reduce the risk of stillbirth without increasing the risk of cesarean section. Labor induction typically involves 2 phases: **cervical ripening** and **uterine contractions**:

- **Cervical ripening.** Before the cervix can dilate, it needs to soften and efface. This involves breaking the disulfide cross-linkages between the cervical collagen fibers. Prostaglandins (e.g., misoprostol and dinoprostone) are pharmacologic agents used for this ripening. Another method is mechanical, and utilizes a Foley balloon placed through the cervix, then inflated with water in the lower uterine segment and placed on tension.
- **Uterine contractions.** Once the cervical ripening has occurred, regular uterine contractions are induced utilizing oxytocin. This is a very potent drug and must be used with caution. When used excessively in an uncontrolled fashion, oxytocin can produce titanic contractions, jeopardizing both mother and fetus. A low infusion rate is initially used, titrating slowly until adequate labor is achieved.

Further Assessment

- Stage 1 of labor
- Arrest of active phase

Management of this is urgent primary cesarean section.

Discussion

The stages of **normal labor** are as follows:

- **Stage 1:** starts onset of regular contractions and ends with complete dilation
  - **Latent phase:** main task is cervical effacement; ends at 6 cm dilation
  - **Active phase:** main task is cervical dilation; ends at 10 cm dilation
- **Stage 2:** starts with complete cervical dilation; ends with expulsion of fetus
- **Stage 3:** starts with expulsion of neonate; ends with delivery of placenta

The stages of **abnormal or dysfunctional labor** are as follows:

- **Stage 1: criteria for arrest of DILATION**
  - No cervical change after ≥4 hrs of adequate contractions (≥200 Montevideo units) OR
  - No cervical change after ≥6 hrs of inadequate contractions (≤200 Montevideo units).
- **Stage 2: criteria for arrest of DESCENT**
  - No change in station with >2 hrs of pushing in a multiparous woman.
  - No change in station with >3 hrs of pushing in a nulliparous woman.
  - Longer durations may be allowed additionally if epidural anesthesia is used.

Follow-up Management

Transition the patient to routine postoperative care, with attention turned to assisting with breastfeeding and maternal infant bonding, prevention of postoperative complications, and safe discharge from the hospital.

Final Diagnosis

- Post-term pregnancy with failed induction of labor
- Active phase arrest of stage 1 of labor

CASE 15

Chief Complaint

"I am bleeding heavily after having my baby."

History and Physical Examination

A 24-year-old G2, now P2, woman has had her pregnancy complicated by gestational diabetes. She tried to follow the American Diabetes Association diet and carefully check blood glucose levels regularly. However she was unable to maintain her glucose values in the target range. When she was put on glyburide, her glucose values normalized. However, serial obstetric sonograms showed her male fetus growing at 90 percentile. She desperately wanted a vaginal delivery so labor induction was begun at 40 weeks gestation even though her cervix was not favorable. Her labor induction was prolonged with 15 hours of IV oxytocin. She underwent a 3-hour second stage of labor and finally delivered a 4,300 gram boy via outlet forceps-assisted vaginal delivery. There was no shoulder dystocia but she sustained a second-degree laceration during delivery. She has passed a significant volume of blood clots that weighed 800 grams. Estimated total blood loss until now is 1500 mL of blood.

On exam today she appears pale. You notice a large amount of blood in the bed. Pulse is 125/min and BP 80/40 mm Hg.

Differential Diagnosis

1. **Uterine atony**
   - Most common etiology of postpartum hemorrhage
2. **Genital lacerations**
   - Can involve the vagina, perineum, or cervix
3. **Retained placenta**
   - Incomplete separation of the placenta can leave fragments in the uterus
4. **Uterine inversion**
   - Rare finding; involves the uterus turning inside out
5. **Disseminated intravascular coagulation**
   - Rare finding; produces a consumptive coagulopathy

Initial Management

Setting: inpatient workup and treatment

Diagnostic/Therapeutic Plan

- Focused exam to determine the cause of bleeding.
  - Palpate uterus to assess for uterine atony (most common cause of PPH)
  - Perform vaginal exam to assess for vaginal or cervical lacerations
  - Examine both fetal and maternal surfaces of the placenta to identify retained fragments

- Simultaneously, with assistance of other personnel, stabilize the patient's vital signs
  - Two IV lines with large bore needles to ensure adequate IV access
  - Isotonic fluid bolus of normal saline or Ringer's lactate
  - Foley catheter to monitor urine output
- Appropriate laboratory tests
  - CBC, type and cross for at least 2 units of packed RBCs
  - DIC panel (as clinically indicated)

Test Results

- Uterine fundus: soft and doughy feeling above the umbilicus
- Vaginal exam: blood coming through cervical os; no cervical laceration; second-degree vaginal laceration well-approximated with no bleeding
- Placenta examined: noted to be complete
- 1 liter IV fluid bolus administered: BP increases to 100/50 mm Hg
- Foley catheter: 400 cc of clear urine returned
- CBC: results pending
- Type and cross 2 units: ordered

Further Management Plan

1. Vigorous bimanual uterine massage (can be initiated immediately and should be the first step in management)
2. Administer IV oxytocin as first drug of choice; if no response, proceed to intramuscular methylergonovine; if still no response, give intramuscular 15 methyl-F2α prostaglandin

Discussion

Postpartum hemorrhage is a true obstetrical emergency. It is defined as blood loss >500 mL with a vaginal delivery or >1000 mL with a cesarean delivery. Careful monitoring and quantification of bleeding is imperative by measuring actual blood loss and weighing pads, lap sponges and gauzes.

The most critical initial steps in management are to stabilize the patient's vital signs and ensure adequate perfusion of vital organs. Establishing IV access with a large bore needle and rapid administration of isotonic fluids as a bolus are essential.

Uterine atony. Hemostasis postpartum is dependent on uterine contractions that close the venous sinuses of the placental attachment site. Twenty percent of maternal cardiac output goes through these vessels. Inadequate uterine contractions are by far the most common cause of postpartum hemorrhage. Risk factors include:

- Prolonged oxytocin infusion
- Infected uterus (e.g., chorioamnionitis)
- Overdistended uterus (e.g., macrosomic fetus or polyhydramnios)
- Use of tocolytic agents (e.g., $MgSO_4$, terbutaline, nifedipine, indomethacin)

CCS NOTE

When you order "prostaglandin" in the ORDER INPUT form, the ORDER VERIFICATION drop-down menu will ask you to specify prostaglandin E1 or E2. Prostaglandin E1 can be administered only via the IV route. Prostaglandin E2 can be administered only via the vaginal route. Specify a one-time bolus rather than continuous administration.

Clinical findings include a soft, boggy uterus palpable above the umbilicus.

Genital lacerations. Risk factors include uncontrolled vaginal delivery (most common), difficult delivery, and operative vaginal delivery. Genital lacerations must be ruled out after every delivery with a cervico-vaginal exam. If lacerations are found they must be surgically repaired.

Retained placenta. Risk factors include accessory placental lobe (most common) and abnormal trophoblastic invasion (i.e., placenta accreta, increta, percreta). The maternal and fetal surfaces of the placenta should be inspected after every delivery to ensure there are no missing cotyledons, which may be in utero. If retained placental fragments are suspected, the treatment is removal of retained fragments by manual uterine exploration followed, if needed, by U/S-guided uterine curettage.

Uterine inversion. This is a rare finding and involves the uterus turning inside out. The uterus cannot be palpated on abdominal exam. On pelvic exam you will see a beefy-appearing bleeding mass in the vagina. Management involves immediate replacement of the uterus back into the abdomen by placing the hand in the vagina followed by IV oxytocin to ensure uterine contraction.

Disseminated intravascular coagulation (DIC). This is a rare finding and produces a consumptive coagulopathy. Risk factors include abruptio placenta (most common), severe preeclampsia, amniotic fluid embolism, prolonged fetal demise, history of excessive bleeding. Clinical findings would include generalized bleeding in presence of a contracted uterus. Treatment is removal of any products of conception, ICU support, and selective blood product replacement.

Unexplained bleeding. This is defined as persistent ongoing blood loss, after all the above causes are ruled out. It is a diagnosis of exclusion and may require vessel ligation (uterine artery or internal iliac) or, rarely, hysterectomy.

Final Diagnosis

Post-partum hemorrhage due to uterine atony

CASE 16

Adolescents

Case: A 16-year-old primigravid adolescent girl comes to Labor and Delivery with regular uterine contractions. She is accompanied by her 35-year-old mother and 10-year-old sister. She has been seen for prenatal care since 20 wks gestation and her pregnancy has progressed unremarkably. Membranes are intact and cervical exam reveals cervical exam with 4 cm dilation, 50% effacement, minus 2 station. Bedside U/S shows the fetus to be in footling breech presentation. An emergency primary cesarean is recommended. Who will sign the surgical consent?

Discussion: In matters involving pregnancy and contraception, teenagers are often legally considered emancipated minors and do not require parental consent for pregnancy care, abortion, or contraception. In most states adolescents may seek reproductive health care without parental consent. The rationale is that it is preferable for adolescents to have access to such care rather than to forego it because they are reluctant or unable to obtain parental approval. With respect to abortion, many states require no parental consent while others require the consent of one parent. However, in such cases, a judge can waive that requirement, especially if the pregnancy is the result of a rape or assault.

Married or Single Women

Case: A 35-year-old multiparous woman comes to the family planning clinic requesting an elective sterilization. She has been diagnosed with chronic hypertension and type 2 DM. She has had 4 term vaginal deliveries and has 4 living children, all of whom were fathered by her husband who is her only current and lifetime sexual partner. She describes her marriage as emotionally but not physically abusive. She does not want her husband to know about her sterilization procedure. Who needs to sign the surgical consent? Will you notify the patient's husband?

Discussion: In the past, spouses were often required to provide consent for their partner to be sterilized. Currently women do not require husband's consent for procedures including sterilization. They do not require consent for abortion from male who fathered the pregnancy.

Adult Women With Intellectual Disabilities

Case: A 24-year-old woman who has never been pregnant is brought to the family planning clinic by her parents who request a sterilization. The patient has a moderate intellectual disability. She was born with brain damage and epilepsy. She is the youngest of 5 children and has an IQ in low 50s; she cannot read, write, tell time, or care for herself. Can the sterilization be performed?

Discussion: The right of women with intellectual disabilities to sexuality and contraception is protected by law. People with intellectual disabilities have the same basic rights as other citizens. Among these rights are the rights—in conformance with state and local law—to marry, to engage in sexual activity, to have children and to control one's own fertility by any legal means available. Since sterilization is a method of contraception available to most adults, this option should be open to most intellectually disabled citizens as well. However, in order to perform a sterilization procedure without their consent will require the consent of a court-appointed conservator, not just the parents. A person who has been legally declared incompetent by a judge can be sterilized without his or her consent.

Fetal Rights

Case: A 27-year-old G3 P2 woman comes to the maternity unit with regular uterine contractions at 37 wks gestation. Her pregnancy has been complicated by chronic hypertension requiring antihypertensive medications. Her BMI is 40. Serial OB U/S has shown fetal growth is at the 5th percentile. Twice weekly antepartum fetal testing has demonstrated reactive NSTs and normal amniotic fluid. On exam today the fetus is cephalic presentation. The patient is 6 cm dilated and membranes are ruptured. A fetal scalp electrode is placed due to inadequate fetal tracing on external monitoring as a result of maternal obesity. The internal fetal monitor tracing shows absent variability and repetitive late decelerations that have not improved in spite of IV fluid bolus, oxygen by face mask at 8 L, and scalp stimulation. Because of a category III fetal monitor strip, you recommend an emergent cesarean section. The patient refuses to sign the operative consent in spite of urgent appeals by both you and her nurse. What is your next step in management? Should you get a court order for a cesarean?

Discussion: The fetus is not considered a "person" in the eyes of the law so has no legal "rights." An emergency cesarean section for fetal jeopardy can only be performed with mother's consent. In situations involving refusal of a medically advised procedure leading to issues of maternal-fetal conflict, it is important that (instead of seeking legal intervention) the physician and patient work together in establishing a plan that respects the voice and autonomy of the patient and the concerns of the physician. According to the American Congress of Obstetricians and Gynecologists, efforts to protect a fetus by restricting a woman's autonomy are not ethically or legally justified, and ultimately recommends that pregnant women's decisions must be respected.

The Newborn

Case: A 31-year-old primigravida comes to the maternity unit at 23 4/7 wks gestation with regular painful contractions that started 4 hrs ago. She has been on vaginal progesterone suppositories because of a finding of cervical length of 10 mm on an OB U/S examination at 19 wks gestation. Cervical exam now shows she is 8 cm dilated and membranes are bulging. You inform the patient that delivery is imminent and the fetus is at threshold of viability. The patient and her husband are both pediatricians and understand very well the morbidity of extreme preterm neonates. They request that no resuscitative efforts be used on the newborn and that they be allowed to hold the baby until it dies. Are you obligated to follow their request?

Discussion: After delivery, the neonate is a "person" in the eyes of the law and is afforded legal protection. Even though the mother/parents, as the child's primary caregivers, are asked for consent for medical treatment, they cannot withhold care from the child if deemed essential for the newborn's safety. A court order may be obtained by the health care professionals to allow that care to be given. Given the substantial, but improving, confidence interval on prenatal estimates of gestational age and fetal weight, neonatologists generally reserve the final decision about delivery room resuscitation for a fetus at the threshold of viability until the infant has been delivered and can be assessed. The ethical justification of this practice has been the independent moral obligation of the clinician to act in the "best interests" of the infant. When the right decision is unclear, the wishes of the parents become determinative.

Respect for Autonomy

Case: A 31-year-old G2 now P2 woman is in the operating room after just undergoing an emergency total abdominal hysterectomy for uterine atony unresponsive to vigorous and prolonged uterine massage as well as multiple uterotonic agents. She was 42 wks gestation when she underwent a spontaneous vaginal delivery of a 4,400 g male neonate. The delivery was complicated by shoulder dystocia and there were vaginal and perineal lacerations that needed suturing. Estimated blood loss is 3,000 mL. Preoperative hemoglobin was 5 g/dL and she continues to bleed. She has been advised she should have a blood transfusion but she refuses any blood products. During her prenatal care her position has been consistent and she made it clear she would choose to die before receiving blood transfusion. Will you get a court order to give life-saving blood?

Discussion: The informed consent and request of a patient with a "sound mind" must be respected even in life-death decisions where the patient refuses therapy or treatment (e.g., blood transfusion). The duty of a physician is to support patients even when their views are different from his or her own. The woman here should be kept fully informed about what is happening in a professional way, ideally by someone she knows and trusts. If standard treatment is not controlling the bleeding, she should be advised that blood transfusion is strongly recommended.

Any patient is entitled to change her mind about a previously agreed treatment plan. The doctor must be satisfied that the woman is not being subjected to pressure from others. It is reasonable to ask the accompanying persons to leave the room for a while so that she can be asked whether she is making her decision of her own free will. If she maintains her refusal to accept blood or blood products, her wishes should be respected. The legal position is that any adult patient who has the necessary mental capacity to do so is entitled to refuse treatment, even if it is likely that refusal will result in the patient's death.

CASE 1

Chief Complaint

"My vagina has a bad odor."

History and Physical Exam

A 42-year-old G3 P3 woman presents to the office with complaint of a malodorous vaginal discharge. She reports that she noticed the odor a few days ago after her period. She denies any abnormal vaginal bleeding, fever or pain. Her medical history is significant for systemic lupus erythematosus for 8 years for which she has been on hydroxychloroquine and prednisone intermittently. Her past surgical history is significant for a tubal ligation 10 years ago. She reports regular menstrual cycles every 30 days. She states that she has been married for the past 20 years and is sexually active in a monogamous relationship with her husband.

On exam she is conversational and in no acute distress. Vital signs are WNL. The abdomen is soft, non-tender with no rebound or guarding. On pelvic exam there are no vulvar or perianal lesions. On speculum exam the vagina is not erythematous but an effusive, watery-gray discharge is noted with a noticeably 'fishy' odor. On bimanual exam there is no vaginal tenderness, no cervical motion tenderness and no palpable adnexal masses.

Differential Diagnosis

1. Bacterial vaginosis (BV)
2. Trichomoniasis vaginitis
3. *Candida* vaginitis

Initial Management

Setting: outpatient workup and treatment

Initial Diagnostic Plan

- Whiff test
- Wet/saline prep
- KOH/wet prep
- Vaginal pH

Test Results

- Whiff test: positive with fishy odor
- Wet/saline prep: clue cells present
- KOH prep: no pseudohyphae
- Vaginal pH: 6.0

Assessment

Bacterial vaginosis

Treatment Plan

- Metronidazole 500 mg, orally bid for 7 days
- No need to treat sexual partner

CLINICAL PEARL

The diagnosis with vaginal discharge is based on lab results, not a clinical diagnosis. It is essential to obtain the proper tests to sort among the differential diagnoses.

Discussion. Vaginal discharge is a common gynecologic complaint. A uniform approach should be undertaken for these complaints to determine their etiology, including a detailed history and physical with a speculum exam with sampling of the vaginal discharge for testing including the whiff test, KOH/wet prep and pH.

Laboratory testing. The wet prep involves placing a smear of the vaginal discharge on a glass microscope slide. On half of the slide, a drop of saline ('wet') is placed and covered with a cover slip. On the other half, a drop of KOH is placed and covered with a cover slip. The KOH prep dissolves cellular material so that the pseudohyphae of *candida* become visible. The saline prep looks for clue cells (vaginal epithelial cells covered with bacteria) which indicate altered vaginal flora typical of BV. Lactobacilli decrease in number with marked overgrowth with anaerobes and facultative aerobes.

The whiff test involves placing a drop of KOH on the vaginal discharge. A positive test is abnormal and consists of a characteristic fishy odor.

Vaginal microbiome. The dynamics of a normal vaginal ecosystem involve a homeostasis involving a low pH (3.8–4.2) maintained by lactic acid produced by high concentrations of lactobacilli. Lactobacilli protect against bacterial and candidal infections by interfering with adherence to epithelial cells. Broad-spectrum antibiotics alter the normally high lactobacillus concentrations, resulting in overgrowth of pathogenic organisms. Any factor that increases vaginal pH can predispose to BV because of a predominance of BV pathogens, including *Bacteroides* species, *Peptostreptococcus*, and *Gardnerella vaginalis*. As lactobacilli decrease in concentration, the vaginal pH rises.

BV. This entity is not a true infection but rather a reflection of altered vaginal bacterial flora as noted above. Physical exam reveals an absence of an inflammatory response: no swelling, redness, pain. Vaginal pH is elevated, clue cells are present on the saline prep, and the whiff test is positive. Treatment is metronidazole as described above. Although associated with sexual activity, BV is not a sexually transmitted disease; thus, sexual partners of patients do not require treatment.

Trichomoniasis. Unlike BV, this is a sexually transmitted disease, caused by the flagellated protozoan *Trichomonas vaginalis*. Women may present with a purulent, malodorous vaginal discharge, often described as green-yellow in color and "frothy." On examination women may have punctate hemorrhages on the cervix ("strawberry cervix") but this occurs only in a minority of women and is not necessary to make the diagnosis. The diagnosis is based primarily on the wet prep, on which motile trichomonads are seen. Vaginal pH is elevated and whiff test is negative. Treatment is metronidazole for both patient and sexual partner(s).

Candidiasis. A majority of cases are caused by *Candida albicans*. Risk factors include: diabetes, antibiotic use, immunosuppression. Women with vulvovaginal candidiasis often present with pruritis, as well as burning and irritation. Physical exam shows erythema and a white, thick, clumpy discharge. Vaginal pH is normal, whiff test is negative, but KOH prep shows pseudohyphae. Initial treatment for symptomatic women is an oral or intra-vaginal antifungal including either single oral dose of fluconazole or multiple-day treatment with azole creams. Sexual partners do not need to be treated.

Final Diagnosis

Bacterial vaginosis

CASE 2

Chief Complaint

Abnormal Pap smear

History and Physical Exam

A 25-year-old woman presents for follow-up after an "abnormal" Pap smear. The cervical cancer screening was performed at a routine well-woman visit last week. She denies any gynecologic complaints. Her past medical history is unremarkable. She had a laparoscopic appendectomy when she was age 11. Her menses are regular, every 28 days on oral contraceptive pills. She works as a waitress. She smokes half a pack of cigarettes per day. She is in a monogamous relationship with her boyfriend.

Vital signs are stable. General exam is unremarkable with a non-tender abdomen without masses. On pelvic exam you visualize normal external female genitalia without lesions or tenderness. On speculum examination she has well-estrogenized vaginal mucosa, a grossly normal appearing cervix, without any bleeding or exophytic lesions. On bimanual exam there is no cervical motion tenderness, the uterus is normal sized, symmetrical, mobile and non-tender with no palpable adnexal masses. Her Pap smear showed high-grade squamous intraepithelial lesion (HSIL).

Differential Diagnosis

1. Cervical infection or inflammation
2. Pre-malignant cervical lesion
3. Malignant cervical lesion

Initial Management

Setting: outpatient/clinic

Diagnostic/Therapeutic Plan

- Colposcopy of cervix

Test Results

- Colposcopy of cervix: transformation zone is visualized; there are areas of "acetowhite" epithelium on anterior lip of the cervix; and mosaicism is seen at 3 and 9 o'clock positions

Assessment

HSIL Pap with areas suspicious for dysplasia on colposcopy. Since a Pap is only a screening test, any abnormality will require further evaluation using a diagnostic test.

CCS NOTE

When you order a colposcopy, an ob/gyn consult is required. You will need to provide your indication for the colposcopy in ≤10 words. Enter "Pap smear shows HSIL" where HSIL is high-grade squamous intraepithelial lesion.

Further Management Plan

• Colposcopic visually-directed biopsies	Biopsies consistent with cervical intraepithelial neoplasia 3 (CIN 3)

Treatment Plan

- Loop electrosurgical excision procedure (LEEP) **or**
- Cold knife cone (CKC)

Discussion

Current Pap guidelines. Recommendations for Pap screening for 'average risk' women, i.e., immunocompetent and/or with no recent cervical dysplasia are as follows:

- **Age <21:** do not perform Pap smear

- **Age 21–29:** Pap smear every 3 years without HPV screening

- **Age 30–65:** Pap smear every 3 years if only cytology is performed **or** every 5 years if both cytology and HPV screening are performed

- **Age ≥65:** no annual Pap screening exams or HPV testing needed

Cytology versus histology. While a Pap smear specimen represents cytologic screening only, a tissue biopsy represents histology and a definite diagnosis. The histologic diagnosis and its concordance with cytology will dictate further treatment and follow-up. The Pap is a screening test for cervical dysplasia. It involves scraping cells from the ectocervix and endocervix and then examining them under the microscope.

The purpose of a Pap smear is to detect abnormal pre-cancer cells from the transformation zone of the cervix, caused by human papillomavirus (HPV), before they progress to cancer.

Pathophysiology. Dysplasia represents premalignant changes and is caused by HPV infection. The majority of women will clear HPV on their own without any intervention and not develop dysplasia. Thus, a majority of all Pap smears will be normal, i.e., negative for intraepithelial neoplasia (NIL).

Classification. A Pap smear may be interpreted as:

- Negative for intraepithelial lesion or malignancy (**NIL**)
- Atypical squamous cells (**ASC**)
  - Of undetermined significance (**ASC-US**)
  - Cannot exclude HSIL (**ASC-H**)
- Low grade squamous intraepithelial lesion (**LSIL**)
- High grade squamous intraepithelial lesion (**HSIL**)
- Atypical glandular cells (AGS)
  - Atypical
  - Atypical, favor neoplastic
- Other (endometrial cells)

CCS NOTE

The CCS clerk does not recognize the order "exocervical biopsy." Enter: "Biopsy, cervix uteri." An ob/gyn consult will be required, and you will need to provide your indication in ≤10 words. Enter: "Colposcopy shows cervical mosaicism with Pap smear showing HSIL." This can be done on a routine basis rather than stat basis. When you order an endocervical curettage, ob/gyn consult is not required.

Role of HPV DNA typing. The mildest abnormal Pap (e.g., ASC-US) has cells that appear abnormal, but it is undetermined if that is because they are *precancerous* or only *inflamed and reactive*. To determine if the cells are dysplastic from HPV infection, perform reflex testing for high-risk HPV types on a liquid-based Pap specimen. High-risk HPV types are those that are oncogenic, meaning they can result in cancer development, and include types 16 and 18.

A majority of all cervical cancers are caused by HPV types 16 and 18. If the Pap is HPV-negative, then routine screening per age-specific guidelines can be continued. If the specimen demonstrates high-risk HPV types, then colposcopy is warranted.

Colposcopic findings. Colposcopy is a magnification of the cervix, which uses acetic acid to visualize the cervical pathology. An endocervical curettage (ECC) is a part of the colposcopic evaluation except in the pregnant state.

Preinvasive cervical lesions (dysplasias to carcinoma in situ) have no gross cervical abnormality seen on the cervix, and must, therefore, be magnified to visualize the abnormality. The abnormalities are usually caused by dysplasia-induced thickened keratin layers (e.g., white epithelium) or abnormal vascular patterns (e.g., punctation, mosaicism). Once the abnormal-appearing epithelium has been visualized colposcopically, the areas need to be biopsied. Colposcopy with visually directed biopsies should be the modality to guide treatment decisions.

Management of abnormal cytology. A Pap smear result worse than ASC-US (ASC-H, LSIL, HSIL, AGUS [AGS]) will warrant colposcopy with biopsy.

- **ASC-US**: HPV testing is preferred but repeat Pap in 1 year is acceptable
- **ASC-H or HSIL**: all patients should undergo colposcopy, regardless of HPV status
- **LSIL**: management will be dictated by HPV testing. In women age >30 who had co-testing as part of their routine screening, if HPV negative, they can repeat co-testing in 12 months.
- **LSIL Pap** and no HPV typing or high-risk HPV positive testing: women should undergo colposcopy
- **AGS** Pap: colposcopy with endocervical and endometrial sampling is needed

Abnormal Pap smears **during pregnancy** are evaluated as in the non-pregnant state, but an endocervical curettage is not done. Pregnancy has no effect on the progression of pre-invasive cervical lesions. In fact, after delivery, 75% of mild dysplasia spontaneously regresses.

Cervical intraepithelial neoplasia (CIN). If the cervical biopsy shows the basement membrane is intact, then the specimen is labeled as cervical intraepithelial neoplasia (CIN). Metastasis is not possible if the lesion is intraepithelial because the epithelium has no lymphatics or blood vessels in it. CIN is graded as:

- **CIN1** (mild dysplasia)
- **CIN2** (moderate dysplasia)
- **CIN3** (severe dysplasia or carcinoma in situ)

If the cervical biopsy demonstrates invasion of the basement membrane, i.e., invasive cancer, then metastasis is possible. Treatment is based on FIGO stage and the presence/absence of lymph-vascular space invasion (LVSI).

Management of abnormal histology. CIN1 represents a transient lesion, most likely to regress without any intervention: recommended management is repeat cervical cytology $+/-$ HPV typing in 1 year.

CIN2 and CIN3 lesions are likely to persist or progress, so women with biopsy-confirmed CIN2 or 3 should undergo excision or ablation of the cervical transformation zone. The most common excision procedure is LEEP. The most common ablation procedure is cryotherapy.

Young women (age 21–24) with CIN2 may forgo cervical excision in favor of cervical cytology and colposcopy at 6 and 12 months. When the biopsy is consistent with CIN3 or colposcopy is inadequate, treatment is preferred. After cervical excision or ablation, follow-up consists of co-testing (cytology and HPV typing) at 12 and 24 months. After 2 consecutive negative results, women may return to routine screening. If any of the initial follow-up co-testing is abnormal, colposcopy with endocervical sampling is indicated.

Final Diagnosis

Cervical intraepithelial neoplasia (CIN) 3

CASE 3

Chief Complaint

"I have a fever and pelvic pain."

History and Physical Examination

A 19-year-old nulligravida presents to the emergency department complaining of 3 days of lower abdominal/pelvic pain that is getting worse. She reports that she developed a fever today. She admits to a vaginal discharge. Her review of symptoms is positive for anorexia and generalized malaise. She has no significant medical or surgical history. She has had unprotected intercourse with several partners over the last month, with intermittent condom use. Her last menstrual period was 1 week ago.

On physical exam she is awake but appears tired and diaphoretic. Vital signs are T 39.1C (102.4F), BP 100/60 mm Hg, pulse 110/min, and respirations 20/min. On exam she has dry oral mucosa, clear breath sounds, and sinus tachycardia. On palpation of the abdomen there is generalized bilateral lower quadrant tenderness and voluntary guarding. Bowel sounds are auscultated as hypoactive. On pelvic exam she has no vulvar or perianal lesions. Speculum exam reveals mucopurulent cervical discharge. On palpation of the uterus, cervical motion tenderness (CMT) with bilateral adnexal tenderness is noted, but without palpable masses. Uterus is normal in size and mobile.

Differential Diagnosis

1. **Pelvic inflammatory disease (PID)**

   - Most likely working diagnosis in this patient who easily meets the CDC minimal criteria

2. **Appendicitis**

   - Pain is localized only to right lower quadrant

3. **Cervicitis**

   - Infection is only in lower genital tract, so there will not be adnexal or uterine tenderness

4. **Ectopic pregnancy**

   - Diagnosis can be ruled out with negative β-hCG

5. **Endometriosis**

   - Pain will be chronic, not acute, and is usually associated with infertility

6. **Ovarian cyst**

   - Sonogram would show an adnexal cystic structure

7. **Inflammatory bowel disease**

   - Unlikely, with no GI complaints

Initial Management

Setting: workup and diagnosis should start promptly in the emergency department

Diagnostic/Therapeutic Plan

- Urine or serum qualitative β-hCG
- CBC
- Chlamydia and gonorrhea specimens
- STD screening, including syphilis and HIV

Test Results

- β-hCG: negative
- CBC: hemoglobin 13 g/dL, WBC count 20,000/mL
- Gonorrhea and chlamydia cervical specimens: pending
- Syphilis serology and HIV screening tests: pending

Assessment

- Pregnancy is ruled out
- Acute PID/acute salpingo-oophoritis

Management

Inpatient treatment with IV cefotetan (for gonorrhea) and IV doxycycline (for chlamydia) until afebrile for 48 hrs and tenderness has disappeared. Then continue outpatient for a total of 14 days as follows: ceftriaxone IM x 1 plus doxycycline PO bid for 14 days with/without metronidazole.

Discussion

Acute PID is caused by an ascending infection from the lower genital tract structures (cervix, vagina) to the upper genital tract structures (uterus, fallopian tubes, ovaries). The most likely causative agents are *Neisseria gonorrhoeae* and *Chlamydia trachomatis*, but anaerobes and mycoplasma may also be involved. The dissemination and internalization of this infection result in systemic findings (i.e., fever, peritoneal signs, elevated WBC). Antibiotics are needed to treat the infection. They should be effective against *N. gonorrhoeae*, *C. trachomatis*, as well as anaerobes, *E. coli*, and group B streptococcus.

Diagnosis. The threshold for diagnosis has been lowered to only 3 minimal criteria, made on the basis of **clinical findings** as follows:

Minimal Criteria (needed to make a diagnosis)

- Sexually active young woman
- Pelvic or lower abdominal pain
- Tenderness: cervical motion or uterine or adnexal

Supportive Criteria (but not necessary to make a diagnosis)

- Oral temperature >38.3° C (>100.9° F)
- Abnormal cervical or vaginal mucopurulent discharge
- Presence of abundant WBC on vaginal fluid saline microscopy

CLINICAL PEARL

The diagnosis of acute PID is clinical, not laboratory. The CDC is so concerned about failure to treat acute PID with potential resulting chronic pain and infertility. Do not wait for lab tests to come back before initiating treatment for presumptive PID.

- Elevated ESR
- Positive lab findings of cervical *N. gonorrhoeae* or *C. trachomatis*
- Most specific criteria for diagnosis:
  - Endometrial biopsy showing endometritis
  - Vaginal sonogram or MRI imaging showing abnormal adnexa
  - Laparoscopic abnormalities consistent with PID

Sequelae. It is necessary to maintain a high clinical suspicion of PID and a low threshold to treat empirically. The sequelae of PID untreated or suboptimally treated can be devastating, including sepsis, infertility, chronic pelvic pain. The common thread of all long-term adverse sequelae is the formation of pelvic adhesions and scar tissue. Infertility risk is 15% after 1 episode of PID, 25% after 2 episodes, and 60% after 3 episodes.

Fimbrial adhesions and distal tubal occlusion are the anatomic findings. Chronic pelvic pain is the result of diffuse adhesions, which bind the pelvic organs into a "frozen pelvis," not allowing them to slide smoothly over their serosal surfaces. Dyspareunia (pain with intercourse) is a common complaint with this pathophysiology. Ectopic pregnancy can also occur.

Once PID is diagnosed, the next question is location of treatment—outpatient or inpatient. The criteria for **inpatient treatment** are:

- Presence of an abscess
- Evidence of diffuse, systemic involvement with high temperature (>39 C [102.2 F]), abdominal guarding-tenderness, and/or patient septic appearance
- Outpatient treatment failure
- IUD in place
- Uncertain diagnosis

CLINICAL PEARL

If the patient is asymptomatic but testing results come back positive, the CDC recommends treatment for both gonorrhea and chlamydia if gonorrhea is present. If testing comes back positive for only chlamydia, treat only for it.

The antimicrobial agents selected are designed to attack chlamydia, gonorrhea and anaerobes.

- Inpatient treatment for acute PID is **cefotetan** 2 g IV every 12 hrs OR **cefoxitin** 2 g IV every 6 hrs PLUS **doxycycline** 100 mg orally or IV every 12 hrs.
- Outpatient treatment for acute PID is **ceftriaxone** 250 mg IM in a single dose PLUS **clindamycin** 450 mg orally 4 times daily for 14 days WITH OR WITHOUT **metronidazole** 500 mg orally twice a day for 14 days.
- Sexual partners should also be treated if cultures are positive for gonorrhea or chlamydia.

Cervicitis. If this patient had presented prior to systemic complaints with a mucopurulent discharge, then cervicitis would be in the differential diagnosis. In general, *C. trachomatis* and *N. gonorrhoeae* are the most common causes of cervicitis. The diagnosis of cervicitis is clinical and is made on the basis of mucopurulent cervical discharge or friability of the external cervical os columnar epithelium. Definitive diagnosis includes nucleic acid amplification testing (NAAT) for chlamydia and gonorrhea. The goals of treatment are relief of symptoms and prevention of ascending infection into the upper reproductive tract with resultant acute PID. Women with cervicitis should receive empiric therapy at the time of diagnosis and evaluation. Treatment should include a single dose of azithromycin 1 gram orally (for chlamydia) and a single dose of cefixime 400 mg orally (for gonorrhea). Sexual partners should also be treated if cultures are positive.

There are other possible causes for pelvic pain.

- **Appendicitis**. Patients can present with fever, anorexia and lower abdominal pain, though the pain is usually localized to the right lower quadrant; management is surgical appendectomy

- **Ectopic pregnancy**. Patients usually present with a history of amenorrhea and pelvic pain that is unilateral; can be ruled out with a negative β-hCG

- **Endometriosis**. The presence of endometrial glands and stroma outside the uterus can result in multiple sequelae, including infertility, dyspareunia, dysmenorrhea and dyschezia. Its presentation is usually chronic, not acute. Diagnosis is confirmed by laparoscopic visualization and biopsy.

- **Ovarian cyst**. Patients usually present with unilateral pain and tenderness and a mass palpable on exam and/or visualized on imaging modalities (e.g., U/S, CT scan); sonogram would show an adnexal cystic structure

- **Inflammatory bowel disease** (e.g., Crohn's disease, ulcerative colitis). Symptoms are GI in nature and include watery diarrhea with bloody or mucoid stools, in addition to fever and abdominal pain. This patient does not have GI complaints, making this diagnosis unlikely.

Final Diagnosis

Acute salpingo-oophoritis

CASE 4

Chief Complaint

"I haven't had my period since my baby was born 15 months ago."

History and Physical Examination

A 34-year-old G2 P1 Ab1 woman has not had a menstrual period since her last delivery 15 months ago. She had a small portion of placenta retained, which required removal immediately after delivery using a large uterine curette under U/S guidance. She states she successfully breastfed her son for 6 months after delivery and electively stopped to go back to work. She has not been taking oral contraceptives or any other contraceptives. She denies any nipple discharge or secretions. General examination is unremarkable. Pelvic exam shows no vulvar, vaginal, or cervical lesions. Vaginal mucosa is pink and moist. Her uterus is asymmetrically minimally enlarged but non-tender and mobile. No adnexal masses are present.

Differential Diagnosis

1. **Pregnancy**

   - Most common cause of secondary amenorrhea; should always be ruled out (both in test situations and in the clinic); since this patient has not been utilizing contraception, it is possible she became pregnant again

2. **Hypothalamic, pituitary, ovarian axis**

   - Once pregnancy has been ruled out, nearly 90% of the causes of secondary amenorrhea will fall into this category. The most common etiologies include:

     - **Functional hypothalamic amenorrhea**: abnormal GnRH secretion due to excessive exercise, inadequate caloric intake, systemic illness, or eating disorder.

     - **Pituitary dysfunction**: due to a prolactinoma or abnormal thyroid function.

     - **Ovarian**: polycystic ovarian syndrome causing anovulation or premature ovarian failure (estrogen insufficiency).

3. **Reproductive tract outflow obstruction (about 5% of cases)**

   - In patients who have already established menses, outflow tracts such as imperforate hymen and transverse vaginal septum can be ruled out.

   - The most common cause in this category for secondary amenorrhea is uterine scarring (Asherman's syndrome).

Initial Management

Setting: outpatient workup and treatment

Diagnostic/Therapeutic Plan

- Urine β-hCG
- Serum TSH
- Serum prolactin level
- Serum FSH

CLINICAL PEARL

The criteria for secondary amenorrhea are:

- Absence of menses for 3 months with previously regular menses

- Absence of menses for 6 months with previously irregular menses

Test Results

- Urine β-hCG: negative
- Serum TSH: 1.5 uIU/mL (normal)
- Serum prolactin level: 8 ng/mL (normal)
- FSH: 4.4 mIU/mL (normal)

Initial Assessment

- Pregnancy, one of the most common causes of secondary amenorrhea, is ruled out by a negative urine β-hCG.
- Hypothyroidism and hyperprolactinemia, common correctible causes of anovulation, are ruled out by normal TSH and prolactin levels.
- Premature ovarian failure is ruled out by a normal FSH level.

Further Management Plan

Progesterone challenge test: administer medroxyprogesterone acetate (MPA) 10 mg orally for 10 days

Further Management Results

No withdrawal bleeding occurs; progesterone challenge test negative

Assessment

Secondary amenorrhea is not due to anovulation

Discussion

If the patient is chronically anovulatory, she has adequate estrogen but lacks progesterone to bring on a withdrawal bleed. In order to induce menses in the presence of adequate estrogen, a progesterone challenge test is performed by giving oral MPA. If no bleeding results when progesterone is stopped, it suggests the amenorrhea is not due to anovulation (or progesterone deficit). Thus, further testing is indicated.

At this point, the patient is either hypoestrogenic or her uterine lining is unable to respond to estrogen (most commonly due to scarring). The normal FSH indicates she is not hypoestrogenic.

The final diagnostic step is an estrogen/progesterone challenge which will differentiate the two. The test is performed by administering estrogen orally for 21 days followed by progesterone orally for 7 days. Combination estrogen/progesterone oral contraceptive pills are an alternative.

Further Management Plan/Results

- Estrogen/progesterone challenge test: negative; no withdrawal bleeding occurs

---

CLINICAL PEARL

If prolactin was elevated, this should be repeated when the patient is fasting. If persistently elevated, an MRI of the sella turcica is indicated to rule out a pituitary prolactinoma.

Given that these tests are normal, the next step is to evaluate for adequate levels of estrogen in the serum, which would cause proliferation of the lining to the extent menses could be induced with the presence of progesterone.

CCS NOTE

The CCS software does not recognize the order "progesterone challenge test." It does not appear in the drop-down menu. You will need to order "progesterone therapy" and specify PO administration for 10 days.

CCS NOTE

When ordering an estrogen-progesterone challenge test, you will need to type in "estrogen progestins combined" and specify oral route of administration and continuous dosing.

CCS NOTE

When ordering a hysterosalpingography, you will need an ob/gyn consult. You will need to provide your indication for the hysterosalpingography in ≤ 10 words. Enter "secondary amenorrhea with negative estrogen-progesterone challenge test."

Further Assessment

The secondary amenorrhea is not due to estrogen deficiency.

Discussion

The test is performed and the patient does not experience vaginal bleeding. Any woman with an anatomically normal reproductive tract should experience withdrawal bleeding after an estrogen-progesterone challenge test. The failure of bleeding suggests a structural abnormality rather than hormonal etiology. The final step is a radiographic assessment of the uterine cavity, either by hysterosalpingogram (HSG) or by saline infused sonohysterogram (SIS).

Further Management Plan/Results

- Hysterosalpingogram: obliteration of the uterine cavity due to uterine synechiae (uterine scarring)

Further Assessment

Asherman syndrome

Summary Discussion

Secondary amenorrhea is defined as absence of a menstrual period for 3 months with previously regular cycles or 6 months with previous irregular menses. There are a number of causes and a step-wise approach to the differential is important.

Pregnancy is the most common cause of secondary amenorrhea. Signs and symptoms include uterine enlargements and amenorrhea. Laboratory findings will be significant for a positive urine or serum pregnancy test. If positive, U/S should be obtained to determine if a gestation can be identified in the uterus. Management is then based upon these findings.

The remaining disorders fall into 2 categories:

Disorders of the hypothalamic, pituitary, ovarian axis (nearly 90% of cases, once pregnancy is ruled out). The most common etiologies include:

- **Functional hypothalamic amenorrhea**: abnormal GnRH secretion due to excessive exercise, inadequate caloric intake, systemic illness, or eating disorder; patients have estrogen insufficiency and thus will respond to an estrogen + progesterone challenge

- **Pituitary dysfunction**: due to a prolactinoma or abnormal thyroid function; patients will have findings on serum prolactin or serum TSH levels.

- **Ovarian**: This includes patients with polycystic ovarian syndrome causing anovulation; patients will have a positive progesterone challenge test

Reproductive tract outflow obstruction (about 5% of cases). The most common cause in this category for secondary amenorrhea is uterine scarring (Asherman syndrome). These patients will have a negative estrogen + progesterone test and will have findings on hysterosalpingogram or saline infused sonohysterogram.

This case depicts Asherman's syndrome. Intrauterine adhesions develop as the result of trauma or inflammation in the uterine cavity. Over 90% of Asherman's cases are caused by dilation and curettage procedures, most commonly those performed for obstetric indications (missed abortion, retained placental tissue). The uterine lining (endometrium) is made up of the stratum functionalis and stratum basalis. It is the damage to the basalis layer that causes adhesive disease and altered proliferation. Another cause for uterine adhesive disease is intrauterine infection, though that represents the minority.

Follow-up Management and Prevention

Treatment for uterine adhesive disease involves uterine hysteroscopy and lysis of adhesions. Post-operative care may include:

- Short-term use of estrogen to proliferate the uterine lining
- Brief use of an intrauterine balloon to allow for healing of the uterine walls and prevention of repeat adhesion formation

Final Diagnosis

Asherman syndrome (uterine adhesive disease)

CASE 5

Chief Complaint

"My stomach hurts and I've been spotting."

History and Physical Examination

A 26-year-old woman comes to the emergency department because of a sudden onset of right-sided lower abdominal pain that began 3 hours ago and has been increasing in intensity. She noticed vaginal spotting 2 hours ago. Her last menstrual period was 6 weeks ago. She has been sexually active since age 17 with multiple partners. She uses foam for contraception. She had an appendectomy in the past. She is afebrile, and vital signs are stable.

On examination she has flat abdomen with lower quadrant tenderness and rebound, right more than the left. Speculum examination reveals only minimal dark vaginal blood without cervical purulence. Bimanual examination reveals a closed, thick cervix moderately tender to motion. Her uterus is slightly enlarged and softened. Right adnexal tenderness is present, but there is no palpable mass.

Differential Diagnosis

1. **Ectopic pregnancy**
   - Whenever a patient in the reproductive years presents with amenorrhea, vaginal bleeding, and acute pelvic pain, think of ectopic pregnancy.

2. **Endometriosis**
   - When patients have chronic pelvic pain, endometriosis is always something on the differential. In this case, given the patient's LMP 6 wks ago and no prior history of pelvic pain, endometriosis becomes less likely.

3. **Pelvic inflammatory disease (PID)**
   - Given that the patient has had multiple sexual partners, she is at a higher risk for PID. However, given the lack of purulent discharge from the cervix and the fact she is afebrile, PID is less likely.

4. **Ovarian cyst**
   - The rupture of ovarian cysts can cause patients to present with pain and should be considered. They are typically associated with ovulation (hemorrhagic cysts) and this patient has not had a period for 6 wks.

5. **Appendicitis**
   - When a female presents with low abdominal/pelvic pain, it is important that non-gynecologic diagnoses remain on the differential. However, this patient has had an appendectomy and, therefore, this is lowest on the differential.

Initial Management

Setting: emergency department workup

Diagnostic/Therapeutic Plan

- Serum quantitative β-hCG: a quantitative test is imperative to help interpret U/S findings
- Blood type and Rh status: will determine whether patient requires RhoGAM
- CBC
- Transvaginal U/S: important to identify that an intrauterine gestational sac can be seen

Test Results

- Serum quantitative β-hCG: 3,500 mIU/mL
- Blood type and Rh status: O+
- CBC: hemoglobin 13.0
- Transvaginal U/S: normal uterus without an intrauterine gestational sac

Basic Science Correlate

A quantitative serum β-hCG titer of 3,500 mIU/mL exceeds the discriminatory threshold of 1,500 mIU/mL, which is the serum β-hCG titer at which a gestational sac should be seen within the uterine cavity on vaginal U/S. In an early pregnancy, the mass of chorionic villi is not large enough to produce a β-hCG titer to the discriminatory threshold. As the placental tissue grows, the serum β-hCG titer rises, doubling approximately every 48 hrs (minimum rise by 50% over 48 hrs).

Assessment

Unruptured ectopic pregnancy

Further Management Plan

Treatment will include intramuscular methotrexate therapy, as well as baseline CBC and blood chemistries. Methotrexate is metabolized by the liver and excreted by the kidneys. Subsequently, the patient will need hCG levels drawn on days 4 and 7 to ensure that a drop in hCG occurs, indicating successful treatment. Then, follow hCG levels weekly to ensure that all trophoblastic tissue has been destroyed. Levels should drop to zero.

Discussion

In a patient of reproductive age, ectopic pregnancy should be suspected in the presence of the clinical triad of amenorrhea, acute abdominal pain, and bleeding. The serum β-hCG titer has exceeded the discriminatory threshold, yet no intrauterine gestational sac is seen. This effectively diagnoses an ectopic pregnancy in this case.

Risk factors are found in only 20% of women who experience ectopic pregnancy. The site of implantation in 95% of ectopic pregnancies is in the oviduct. All risk factors are associated with congenital or acquired abnormal tubal anatomy leading to delayed or obstructed passage of the developing conceptus through the fallopian tube. These include surgical procedures on the oviduct and previous ectopic pregnancies.

CCS NOTE

The β-hCG can be ordered as qualitative (positive or negative) or quantitative (i.e., a titer is given). Urine can be ordered as qualitative, and serum either as qualitative or quantitative. In ruling out ectopic pregnancy, it is important to obtain a titer. This can only be done with a serum quantitative test.

The most significant risk factor is a **history of previous PID**, which increases risk eightfold. The other differential diagnoses (PID, appendicitis, endometriosis, ovarian cyst), although they are all associated with pelvic pain, are excluded by a positive β-hCG test.

Follow-up Management and Prevention

Whereas some ectopic pregnancies spontaneously resolve, they have significant potential for invading vascular structures leading to life-threatening hemorrhage.

- If diagnosis is uncertain (i.e., no intrauterine gestational sac on vaginal U/S with β-hCG <1,500 mIU/mL), follow serial quantitative serum β-hCGs, which should double every 2–3 days, and repeat the vaginal U/S. A slower rate of β-hCG progression or a plateau of values is suspicious for ectopic pregnancies.

- If patient is hemodynamically unstable (tachycardic and hypotensive) with findings suggestive of intraperitoneal bleeding (abdominal guarding and rebound), emergency laparotomy to stop the hemorrhage is indicated.

- Methotrexate is the treatment of choice in stable early ectopic pregnancies. Ideal candidate attributes include β-hCG titer <5,000 mIU/mL, compliant patient, and ectopic mass <3.5 cm with no cardiac activity. This cytotoxic folate antagonist destroys rapidly growing chorionic villi wherever their anatomic site. Follow-up quantitative β-hCG titers are essential to rule out persistent and/or progressive disease.

- Rh-negative patients should be administered IM RhoGAM.

- In more advanced cases, where β-hCG titer >6,000 mIU/mL, ectopic mass >3.5 cm, or cardiac activity is seen, laparoscopic surgery is the treatment of choice. If the patient has completed childbearing, a salpingectomy should be performed. Fertility-preserving procedures include a linear salpingostomy with unruptured ampullary ectopics and segmental resection with proximal isthmic ectopics.

Preventive management should involve a discussion with the patient regarding effective forms of contraception. This patient is using an ineffective form of contraception, placing her at high risk for a subsequent undesired pregnancy and, given her present condition, increased risk for a subsequent ectopic pregnancy. She should be offered effective forms of reversible contraception which can be utilized until she is ready to begin her family.

Final Diagnosis

Unruptured ectopic pregnancy

CASE 6

Chief complaint

"I have pelvic pressure."

History and Physical Examination

A 25-year-old woman, G1 P0 Ab1, comes to the office for a well-woman visit. Her only complaint is a feeling of occasional pelvic pressure. Onset of menarche was age 13 with initially irregular menses for 2 years. Since age 15 she has had regular 30-day menstrual cycles, with her LMP starting 12 days ago and lasting 4 days. She denies urgency, frequency, or burning with urination. She has been married for 2 years and her husband is her only sexual partner. They are considering trying for pregnancy in the next year. She uses a diaphragm for contraception, which was fitted 2 years ago.

Inspection of the external genitalia reveals a normal urethral meatus and vaginal introitus. There are no vulvar or perianal lesions. On speculum examination you note a pink and moist vaginal epithelium with no discharge. The cervical mucus is clear, thin, and watery. On bimanual examination the uterus is normal size, symmetrical, mobile and nontender. There is no cervical motion tenderness. However there is a 6 cm, cystic, mobile, non-tender, right adnexal mass. Rectovaginal exam confirms your finding.

Differential Diagnosis

There are 3 organ systems in the pelvis from which pelvic masses could originate.

1. **Reproductive tract**

   - Pregnancy (most common cause of a pelvic mass in reproductive years)

   - Functional ovarian cyst (most common cause of a pelvic mass if pregnancy ruled out)

   - Benign ovarian neoplasm (most common in young women is benign cystic teratoma)

   - Malignant ovarian neoplasm (most common in young women is germ cell tumor)

2. **Urinary tract**

   - Pelvic kidney (rare, usually asymptomatic)

   - Hydroureter (rare, usually from obstruction)

3. **GI tract**

   - Diverticulosis (unlikely in a young woman)

Initial Management

Setting: outpatient workup

Diagnostic/Therapeutic Plan

- Urine β-hCG

- Pelvic sonogram

Test Results

- Urine β-hCG: negative

- Pelvic sonogram: normal uterus and left adnexae. There is a right sided $5 \times 5 \times 6$ cm thin-walled, fluid filled simple cyst without septations or calcifications.

Assessment

Functional ovarian cyst, probably follicular cyst

Treatment Plan

- Conservative outpatient observation

- Follow-up exam and sonogram in 6–8 wks

Discussion

There are 2 diagnostic tests for premenopausal pelvic masses.

Pregnancy test: The most common cause of pelvic mass in the reproductive years is pregnancy. A negative urine β-hCG easily rules out pregnancy. A qualitative β-hCG that gives a simple "positive" or "negative" is cost-effective and is adequate for this case. This should be the first test with a pelvic mass of unknown etiology regardless of whether a patient admits or denies sexual activity.

Pelvic ultrasound: The next diagnostic test needed once pregnancy has been ruled out is pelvic sonogram. The value of an U/S imaging study is to identify the anatomic location of the mass and assess its sonographic characteristics. U/S appearance helps differentiate masses of ovarian origin as opposed to those arising from the urinary tract or GI tract. It is essential to know if the pelvic mass is a simple cyst, a complex mass or a solid mass.

Further Management Plan/Results

Pelvic sonogram 6 wks later finds normal uterus and bilateral adnexae with no evidence of cystic masses. Functional ovarian cyst is retrospectively confirmed. Routine follow-up is required.

Subsequent Discussion

The most common cause of a **simple cyst** of the ovary in the reproductive years is a physiological cyst. During the reproductive years the ovaries are functionally active, producing a dominant follicle in the first half of the cycle and a corpus luteum in the second half of the menstrual cycle. Either of these structures—the ovarian follicle or the corpus luteum—can be fluid-filled and enlarged, producing a functional cyst. If their size >5 cm, they are palpable on a bimanual examination of the pelvis. Other diagnoses of thin-walled, fluid-filled adnexal cystic structures could include a paratubal cyst or hydrosalpinx.

Basic Science Correlate

A functional ovarian mass is part of the physiologic changes a normal ovarian follicle undergoes throughout the menstrual cycle, in response to the rising and falling levels of FSH and LH from the anterior pituitary. A follicle cyst is seen during the pre-ovulatory period of the cycle as FSH stimulates the formation of the dominant follicle to produce estrogen. A corpus luteum cyst is seen during the post-ovulatory period of the cycle after the mid-cycle LH surge stimulates ovulation leading the formation of the corpus luteum at the site of ovulation producing progesterone.

A **functional mass** will always disappear over time. The management of a presumptive functional or physiologic ovarian cyst is conservative observation. Follow-up examination should be in 6–8 weeks, at which time the functional cyst should have spontaneously disappeared. If the cystic mass is still there after the observation time period, the assumption is the cyst is not functional and surgical evaluation and removal by laparoscopy will need to be performed.

Basic Science Correlate

If the normal hypothalamic-pituitary gonadotropins are suppressed by steroid contraceptives for ≥2 months, there should be no stimulation of ovarian follicles by FSH or LH surge, which is needed for formation of the corpus luteum. Therefore, physiologic ovarian cysts should not occur if the patient is using combination steroid contraception (e.g., OCPs, vaginal ring, transdermal contraceptive patch).

The most common benign, **complex adnexal mass** in young women is a dermoid cyst or benign cystic teratoma. They can be bilateral in 15% of cases. They are benign tumors that can contain cellular tissue from all 3 germ layers including hair, sebaceous glands, teeth and thyroid tissue. All complex masses require surgical exploration and should not be managed conservatively. Ideally, with benign conditions, a cystectomy can be performed with a laparoscope shelling out the abnormal tissue and preserving the normal ovarian tissue. The pathology report will confirm the precise diagnosis. Rarely teratomas can be malignant.

The most common malignant **solid adnexal mass** in young women is dysgerminoma, a germ cell tumor of the ovary. All dysgerminomas are considered malignant, but only one third of dysgerminomas behave aggressively. Dysgerminomas have most commonly been associated with elevations in LDH, although it is not elevated in all cases. All solid masses require surgical exploration and should not be managed conservatively. If malignancy is suspected, surgical staging is essential to plan appropriate treatment.

If the adnexal mass is large (>8 cm in diameter) and **mobile**, regardless of etiology, it can undergo **torsion** or twisting, cutting off the blood supply causing severe sudden onset of abdominal/pelvic pain. This is a surgical emergency requiring untwisting of the pedicle and cystectomy allowing revitalization if ischemic injury has not occurred. If the ovary is necrotic and non-viable, a unilateral salpingo-oophorectomy must be performed.

Final Diagnosis

Functional ovarian cyst, resolved

CASE 7

Chief Complaint

"My breasts are sore and I feel bloated and moody."

History and Physical Examination

A 31-year-old single woman comes to the clinic because of emotional lability, bloating, and breast tenderness. The symptoms are so severe in the week before her menses that she has difficulty functioning in the home and at work. She has been eating and drinking more fluids lately, especially coffee, because of fatigue, but says she has recently been under more stress at work, which makes her anxious, irritable, and often depressed when she goes home. She has a 26-day menstrual cycle and 5 days of menstrual flow. She has been diagnosed with fibromyalgia for which she takes pregabalin (Lyrica).

General physical examination is unremarkable. Diffuse minimal bilateral breast tenderness is noted, with no dominant masses.

Differential Diagnosis

1. Pregnancy

2. Premenstrual syndrome

3. Thyroid dysfunction

4. Stress/anxiety

5. Depression

Initial Management

Setting: outpatient office

Diagnostic/Therapeutic Plan

- Urine β-hCG

- Menstrual diary over 3 months

- Evaluation of medications including hormonal treatment

Test Results

- Urine β-hCG: negative

- Menstrual diary: symptoms predictably occur only in second half of menstrual cycle

- Medications: none

Assessment

Premenstrual syndrome (PMS)

Further Management Plan

Many treatments have been proposed, though none are universally effective.

- Simple physician reassurance for mild cases

- Elimination of coffee and caffeine from the diet to relieve breast pain

- Spironolactone alone to decrease edema by inhibiting aldosterone concentrations, which are usually increased in late luteal phase

- SSRIs such as fluoxetine and the combination oral contraceptive containing the progestin drospirenone have been approved by the FDA to relieve premenstrual syndrome

Discussion

PMS is a constellation of physical and behavioral symptoms that occur in the luteal phase (second half of the menstrual cycle). Mild symptoms that do not cause distress or functional impairment are considered premenstrual symptoms, not syndrome. It is **unlikely** to be premenstrual syndrome if:

- Symptoms are present throughout the cycle

- Symptoms come and go throughout the cycle

- Symptoms are present in some cycles but not others

Whereas depression can be associated with some somatic symptoms, this case presentation is typical of premenstrual syndrome, with breast tenderness/swelling and trace edema.

Diagnostic criteria. Diagnosis is based on the findings of a menstrual diary the patient keeps, tracking all the physical and behavioral symptoms quantified on a 1 to 5 rating scale and noting which day of the cycle the symptoms occur. The diary must show that symptoms have the following characteristics:

- Are associated with economic or social dysfunction

- Begin during the 5 days before the onset of menses

- End within 4 days of the onset of menses

- Are severe enough to interfere with normal activity

- Are present in at least 3 consecutive menstrual cycles

Symptom clusters. Premenstrual syndrome symptoms can be grouped under symptom clusters:

- Fluid retention (breast tenderness, edema, weight gain, bloating)

- Autonomic symptoms (heart pounding, confusion, insomnia, fatigue)

- Emotional symptoms (tension, forgetfulness, mood swings, irritability)

- Musculoskeletal symptoms (muscle aches, joint aches, cramps)

The most common affective or behavioral symptom is mood swings. The most common physical manifestation is abdominal bloating and extreme sense of fatigue.

CLINICAL PEARL

There are no specific lab tests for PMS. The diagnosis is clinical and utilizes a symptom diary for 3 months. The temporal sequence of symptoms is important to determine if a relationship to the menstrual cycle exists.

Treatment options should target the specific symptom cluster that seems to dominate a patient's complaints. Generic treatments may include lifestyle changes (relaxation methods, support group, exercise), nutritional changes (decrease caffeine, simple sugars, and salt), and medications.

Pharmacologic treatment may include SSRIs administered during the luteal phase of the menstrual cycle, effective in 60–70% of patients. However, a concerning side effect of SSRIs is decreased libido, something that occurs in 40–50% of patients. Alternatively, the oral contraceptive Yaz may be helpful if administered with a shortened pill-free interval. Yaz is given for 24 days with a 4-day hormone-free period rather than the 21–7 day sequence used with most oral contraceptive pills.

Follow-up Management

Prospective monitoring of symptom improvement with self-rating scale. The daily record of severity of problems (DRSP) form, which has been validated as a self-administered questionnaire is commonly used.

Final Diagnosis

Premenstrual syndrome

CASE 8

Chief Complaint

"I have heavy periods every few weeks or so."

History and Physical Examination

A 32-year-old G4 P4 woman comes to the office complaining of irregular bleeding in between normal menstrual cycles. She has had 2 vaginal deliveries and 2 cesarean sections. She underwent a tubal sterilization procedure 3 years ago with her last cesarean. She has been prescribed proton pump inhibitors for GI reflux. She was diagnosed with irritable bowel syndrome 6 years ago but is not taking any medications for it other than stool softeners. She denies a history of bleeding disorders and easy bruising. Vital signs are stable.

General physical exam is unremarkable. Pelvic examination reveals no vulvar, vaginal, or cervical lesions on visual inspection. Speculum exam reveals dark blood in the vaginal vault. Cervical mucus is profuse, thin, and watery. Vaginal mucosa is pink and moist. The uterus is asymmetrically minimally enlarged but non-tender and mobile. No adnexal masses are present.

Differential Diagnosis

PALM-COEIN is a mnemonic that includes all possible causes of abnormal uterine bleeding. It is endorsed by the International Federation of Gynecologists and Obstetricians (FIGO).

1. Polyp
2. Adenomyosis
3. Leiomyoma
4. Malignancy and hyperplasia
5. Coagulopathy
6. Ovulatory dysfunction
7. Endometrial
8. Iatrogenic
9. Not yet classified

Initial Management

Setting: outpatient office

Diagnostic/Therapeutic Plan

- Urine qualitative β-hCG (to rule out pregnancy-related causes of bleeding)
- CBC (to assess severity of bleeding and possible anemia)
- Menstrual history
  - Irregular, unpredictable cycles are predictive of ovulatory dysfunction
  - Regular cycles with inter-menstrual bleeding are suggestive of an anatomic lesion

- Contraceptive/medication history: certain medications and steroid contraceptives can cause breakthrough bleeding
- Physical exam (to determine source of bleeding: lower or upper genital tract, urinary tract, GI tract)

Test Results

- Urine β-hCG: negative
- CBC: Hgb 12.2 mg/dL; Hct 36
- Menstrual history: regular cyclic bleeding with inter-menstrual bleeding
- Contraceptive history: tubal ligation 10 yrs ago
- Pelvic exam: no vulvar, vaginal, or cervical lesions

Assessment

The patient is not pregnant since the negative β-hCG virtually rules out any viable trophoblastic villi. Menstrual history is suggestive but not diagnostic of an anatomic cause of bleeding but the thin, watery cervical mucus suggests anovulation.

- Bleeding has not been excessive with a normal hemoglobin/hematocrit.
- Steroid contraceptives are not a cause of the bleeding.
- Lower genital tract etiology is ruled out by the normal pelvic exam.
- Coagulopathy is unlikely with no known bleeding disorders or easy bruising.

Further Management Plan/Results

- Progestin trial (medroxyprogesterone acetate PO × 7 days): bleeding does not stop

Further Assessment

Anovulation is ruled out by the absence of bleeding response to progestin trial. If the bleeding were due to unopposed estrogen, characteristic of anovulation, it should have stopped.

Discussion

Anovulation symptoms include irregular, unpredictable vaginal bleeding without cramping. Signs include thin, watery cervical mucus and uniphasic basal body temperature. Laboratory findings include low serum progesterone levels and possible low TSH and high prolactin.

It is now important to visualize the endometrial cavity to identify either a submucous leiomyoma or endometrial polyp. A history of irregular bleeding between normal predictable menstrual cycles is classic for an anatomic lesion. This could involve the lower genital tract (evaluated by speculum exam) or upper genital tract (evaluated by hysteroscopy).

Follow-up Management

Hysteroscopy: endometrial polyps

Further Assessment

The patient has bleeding caused by endometrial polyps. These abnormal benign endometrial folds do not respond to progestins in the same way as normal endometrium. The polyps can be resected at the time of hysteroscopic visualization.

Discussion

U/S visualization of the endometrium can be performed on an outpatient basis by using a saline hystero-ultrasound. This procedure is only diagnostic because anatomic lesions are imaged but not removed.

Hysteroscopy, on the other hand, is diagnostic and therapeutic; it allows for direct visualization of the endometrial cavity. Uterine anatomic lesion symptoms include abnormal bleeding in between regular menses. Signs may be absent. Hysteroscopy or saline U/S may show an intrauterine endometrial polyp or submucous leiomyoma.

Management is hysteroscopic resection of lesion seen at time of procedure.

Final Diagnosis

Endometrial polyps

CASE 9

Chief Complaint

"I can't get pregnant."

History and Physical Examination

A 28-year-old nulligravida comes to the clinic because of an 18-month history of infertility in spite of unprotected mid-cycle intercourse. She states her menses are usually regular, lasting 4 days, but she does skip periods occasionally. She denies dysmenorrhea. She has been treated in the past for sexually transmitted diseases, whose names she does not recall. Intercourse with her husband is regular (1 to 2 times a week) with no sexual dysfunction.

General physical examination is unremarkable. Pelvic examination shows normal vulva, perianal area, vagina, and cervix without lesions. Clear, thin, watery cervical mucus is seen. Bimanual examination reveals a symmetrical, mobile, nulliparous uterus. There is mild right adnexal tenderness but no palpable masses. Rectovaginal examination is normal.

Differential Diagnosis

1. **Male factor infertility**

   - Male factor infertility due largely to altered semen parameters is causal in 25% of cases

2. **Fallopian tube disease**

   - Patient has a history of an STI, a risk factor for tubal occlusive disease. Tubal disease is causal in 15% of cases.

3. **Ovulatory dysfunction**

   - Issues related to ovulation can be determined in large part by menstrual cycle history. These are often related to thyroid disease, hyperprolactinemia, polycystic ovarian disease, or premature ovarian insufficiency. This patient has overall normal periods, making these options less likely.

4. **Endometriosis**

   - Although seen in 5–8% of patients with infertility, endometriosis is not likely when dysmenorrhea and pelvic pain are absent and there is a normal pelvic examination.

5. **Coital dysfunction**

   - Although seen in 5–8% of couples, the history solicited indicates regular coitus without dysfunction that would impair reproductive efficiency.

6. **Unexplained infertility**

   - Although it accounts for >25% of cases, unexplained infertility is a diagnosis of exclusion.

Initial Management

Setting: outpatient workup and treatment

Diagnostic/Therapeutic Plan

- Semen analysis
- Hysterosalpingogram (HSG)
- Serum TSH and prolactin levels
- Luteal phase progesterone level to assess for ovulation
- Day 3 FSH and estradiol levels to assess ovarian function

Test Results

- Semen analysis: normal
- HSG: normal uterine cavity, bilateral distal fallopian tube occlusion and hydrosalpinges
- TSH 1.5 uIU/mL; prolactin 8 ng/mL (normal)
- Luteal phase progesterone level 5 ng/mL (both normal)
- Day 3 FSH 5 mIU/mL; day 3 estradiol 35 pg/mL (both normal)

Assessment

Primary infertility due to tubal disease.

Further Management Plan/Results

- Gonorrhea and chlamydia testing should be performed in patients who have evidence of fallopian tubes such as this patient. Ascending pelvic infection is a common cause of abnormal intrinsic fallopian tube disease as revealed by this patient's HSG.
- Doxycycline 100 mg 2/day for 5 days should be given to patients found on HSG to have evidence of dilated fallopian tubes to prevent a post-procedure infection.

Follow-up Management and Prevention

Diagnostic laparoscopy is in order to assess if surgical repair of tubal disease is feasible. In the event the tubal reconstruction cannot be performed, more advanced treatment will be necessary. This treatment will require subspecialist referral to a reproductive endocrinologist and the patient will undergo in vitro fertilization (IVF).

Discussion

Infertility is diagnosed by failure to conceive with regular intercourse without contraception (a) for 12 months in women age <35 or (b) for 6 months in women age ≥35. Eighty to 90% of couples will conceive after 12 months of trying. The 3 most common causes of infertility are:

- **Male factor**. A semen analysis is an effective, inexpensive, and non-invasive diagnostic test that is performed on an outpatient basis after 2–3 days of abstinence.
- **Ovulatory function**. Assessment begins with a complete menstrual cycle history and initial serum testing to rule out thyroid disease and hyperprolactinemia. Confirmation of ovulation is achieved by observing an elevation in the luteal phase

progesterone level. Ovarian function can also be assessed utilizing day 3 FSH and estradiol testing. Elevated FSH may indicate ovarian insufficiency as a cause of infertility.

- **Fallopian tube disease.** An HSG is the test of choice for evaluating fallopian tube patency. It entails injecting radio-opaque dye through the cervix into the uterus and watching for bilateral intraperitoneal dye spillage from the tubes. A hydrosalpinx is a collection of fluid within the fallopian tube most commonly due to a distal obstruction. Patients exhibiting this finding at the time of hysterosalpingogram are at risk for infection and should be treated with antibiotics.

Basic Science Correlate

When evaluating ovarian reserve, obtain both an FSH and estradiol on **day 3**. This is because FSH levels are influenced by the feedback of estradiol on the hypothalamus and pituitary. Recall normal hormonal regulation:

- FSH influences the granulosa cells and LH theca cells. Although both are present throughout the cycle, FSH predominates in the follicular phase and LH predominates in the luteal phase.

- Similarly, estradiol is the primary sex steroid produced in the follicular phase and progesterone is the predominant sex steroid produced in the luteal phase.

- As follicles are depleted in later reproductive life, FSH rises earlier in the prior luteal phase of the menstrual cycle with a corresponding earlier rise in estradiol level. This increased estradiol feeds back on the hypothalamus and pituitary and lowers the FSH.

- Thus, you can have a falsely low day 3 FSH in older patients. An estradiol level >80 pg/mL on day 3 is suspicious for ovarian insufficiency, even with a normal FSH.

CLINICAL PEARL

If present, an elevated fasting prolactin level may represent a pituitary lactotroph adenoma. MRI imaging of the sella turcica is indicated.

Discussion

Infertility is defined as inability to achieve pregnancy after 12 months of unprotected and frequent intercourse. Both male and female factors have to be included when evaluating the causes of infertility. Around 15% of American couples suffer infertility.

Initial Noninvasive Tests

Semen analysis

- **Normal values.** Expected findings are volume >2 mL; pH 7.2–7.8; sperm density >20 million/mL; sperm motility >50%; and sperm morphology >50% normal. If values are abnormal, **repeat the semen analysis** in 4–6 wks.

- **Minimally abnormal.** If sperm density is mild to moderately lower than normal, intrauterine insemination (IUI) may be used. Washed sperm is directly injected into the uterine cavity. Idiopathic oligozoospermia is the most common male infertility factor.

- **Severely abnormal.** If semen analysis shows severe abnormalities, intracytoplasmic sperm injection (ICSI) may be used in conjunction with in vitro fertilization (IVF) and embryo transfer.

- **No viable sperm.** With azoospermia or failed ICSI, artificial insemination by donor (AID) may be used.

Ovulation assessment

- **History.** The patient typically gives a history of irregular, unpredictable menstrual bleeding, most often associated with minimal or no uterine cramping.

- **Objective data**. A basal body temperature (BBT) chart will not show the typical midcycle temperature elevation. A serum progesterone level will be low. An endometrial biopsy shows proliferative histology.

- **Correctible causes**. Hypothyroidism or hyperprolactinemia are causes of anovulation that can be treated.

- **Ovulation induction**. The agent of choice is clomiphene citrate administered orally for 5 days beginning on day 5 of the menstrual cycle. The biochemical structure of clomiphene is very similar to estrogen, and clomiphene fits into the estrogen receptors at the level of the pituitary. The pituitary does not interpret clomiphene as estrogen and perceives a low estrogen state, therefore producing high levels of gonadotropins. hMG is administered parenterally and is used to induce ovulation if clomiphene fails. Careful monitoring of ovarian size is important because ovarian hyperstimulation is a major side effect of ovulation induction. When a patient is given clomiphene, her own pituitary is being stimulated to secrete her own gonadotropins, whereas when a patient is administered hMG, the patient is being stimulated by exogenous gonadotropins.

Follow-Up Invasive Tests

Hysterosalpingogram and laparoscopy

Tubal disease. Assessment of fallopian tube abnormalities is the next step if the semen analysis is normal and ovulation is confirmed.

- **Hysterosalpingogram (HSG).** In this imaging procedure, a catheter is placed inside the uterine cavity, and contrast material is injected. The contrast material should be seen on x-ray images spilling bilaterally into the peritoneal cavity. It should be scheduled during the week after the end of menses and prophylactic antibiotics should be given to patients noted to have a hydrosalpinx (fluid filled fallopian tubes) to prevent causing a recurrent acute salpingitis. No further testing is performed if the HSG shows normal anatomy. If abnormal findings are seen, the extent and site of the pathology are noted and laparoscopy considered.

- **Chlamydia antibody.** A negative IgG antibody test for chlamydia virtually rules out infection-induced tubal adhesions.

- **Laparoscopy.** If potentially correctible tubal disease is suggested by the HSG, the next step in management is to visualize the oviducts and attempt reconstruction if possible (tuboplasty). If tubal damage is so severe surgical therapy is futile, then IVF should be planned.

Final Diagnosis

Primary infertility due to fallopian tube disease

CASE 10

Chief Complaint

"My periods are painful."

History and Physical Examination

A 21-year-old woman comes to the clinic complaining of recurrent, severe, disabling pain on the first 3 days of her menses. She describes the pain as cramping nature and located in her lower abdomen and pelvis. The pain is so severe that she has difficulty functioning. The cramping is associated with nausea, vomiting, diarrhea, tiredness, and headache. She has no pain with intercourse (she has had 2 partners in the past 6 months) or bowel movements. Her menstrual periods are regular, 28 days apart and lasting 3 days. She did not have any pain with menses initially after starting her periods at age 12. The onset of the pain was within 2 years of menarche at age 14.

Physical examination is unremarkable, except for moderate obesity. Her vulva and vagina have no lesions or discharge. Her uterus is small, anteverted, non-tender, and mobile. There are no palpable adnexal masses. Recto-vaginal examination is normal.

Differential Diagnosis

1. **Primary dysmenorrhea**

   - Can be suspected when a patient has pelvic pain that is (a) cramping in nature (from smooth muscle contractions of the uterus); (b) onset within 2 yrs of menarche (regular ovulatory cycles take 2 yrs to stabilize), and (c) absence of pathological findings on pelvic exam.

2. **Endometriosis**

   - Ectopic endometrial tissue that is responsive to hormones is a common cause of cyclic pelvic pain. The amount of endometriosis does not correlate well with the symptoms caused by the lesions.

3. **Uterine polyps**

   - Uterine polyps can cause pain but are more commonly associated with abnormal uterine bleeding. Most commonly, they manifest with inter-menstrual bleeding.

4. **Chronic PID**

   - Ascending infections of the uterus and fallopian tubes (caused most commonly by chlamydia and/or gonorrhea) can be a source of pelvic pain. In addition, the adhesive disease that can complicate these ascending infections may also contribute to pain.

5. **Uterine leiomyoma**

   - Uterine fibroids are common and will often cause abnormalities in uterine bleeding and/or pelvic pain/pressure symptoms due to compression on surrounding structures or outgrowth of their blood supply, which causes degeneration.

6. **Adenomyosis**

   - This is when endometrial glands and stroma are found in the uterine musculature; can present with abnormal bleeding and/or pelvic pain.

Initial Management

Setting: outpatient workup and treatment

Diagnostic/Therapeutic Plan

- Pelvic U/S
- Cervical cultures for gonorrhea and chlamydia

Test Results

- Pelvic U/S: normal uterine contour and size. No leiomyoma seen. Uterine lining is thin and regular. Ovaries of normal size and volume. No cysts or masses.
- Cervical cultures: negative.

Further Management Plan

1. Non-steroidal anti-inflammatory agents (NSAIDs)
2. Continuous oral contraceptive pills (OCPs)

Assessment

Primary dysmenorrhea is the most likely diagnosis. Primary dysmenorrhea is diagnosed in the presence of painful severe menstrual cramps without any evident pathology to account for them. Pathophysiology is an excessive response to prostaglandins released from the endometrium during menstruation. Intense dysrhythmic uterine contractions result in increased myometrial tone and increased intrauterine pressure reducing uterine blood flow causing ischemia and pain. Diagnosis rests on a good history with negative pelvic evaluation findings.

The first line of treatment for primary dysmenorrhea is medical therapy using prostaglandin synthetase inhibitors or NSAIDs. These agents suppress prostaglandin release and decrease the inflammatory reaction that occurs at the time of menses and contributes to the pain. Oral contraceptive pills are another helpful adjuvant. They interrupt the hypothalamic-pituitary-ovarian axis and eliminate the menses. This interrupts the inflammatory cascade involving prostaglandins thereby alleviating the pelvic pain.

Follow-up Management and Prevention

The patient should be followed up in 3 months to assess the pelvic pain. With the use of NSAIDs and OCPs (thereby eliminating menses) her pain should improve. If no improvement is seen, a discussion of additional diagnostic tools must be had. The next step would be a diagnostic laparoscopy to further assess the pelvis for anatomic pathology and evaluate the entire pelvis for evidence of endometriosis. If endometriosis is present, ablation of the lesions should be performed.

The pelvic U/S can rule out many anatomic pathologic processes that are related to pelvic pain. In this case the uterus is of normal size and contour (no adenomyosis, characterized by a large, symmetric, globular uterus) and no uterine fibroids (characterized by an asymmetric uterus) are noted. The endometrial lining is thin and regular (no polyps). Finally, her cervical cultures are negative, ruling out the most common causes for PID.

General Discussion

Chronic pelvic pain is defined as pain that is present for at least 6 months in duration, is found below the umbilicus, and is severe enough to impair daily function. The differential diagnosis for pelvic pain is broad and can include GI, urologic, gynecologic, psychologic, musculoskeletal, and neurologic causes.

When evaluating gynecologic causes, a complete history and physical are important. The history should include a detailed menstrual history as many of the causes of pelvic pain center around menstruation and/or involve the organs that regulate the process. Laboratory testing is of limited value when evaluating pelvic pain, although infectious disease testing is helpful. Limited radiologic testing is warranted and can be helpful. Ultimately, laparoscopy may be required in patients with persistent pain.

Some of the most common gynecologic causes of chronic pelvic pain include:

Secondary Dysmenorrhea

- Symptoms usually begin in the twenties and thirties and may be present pre- and/or post-menses. The pain is usually described as dull and aching but may be variable. It may be associated with dyspareunia (painful intercourse), infertility, and abnormal bleeding.
- Mechanism of secondary dysmenorrhea is often anatomic, leading to an abnormal pelvic examination.
- Management varies according to the diagnosis.

Endometriosis

Endometriosis is a benign condition in which endometrial glands and stroma are seen outside the uterus.

- Symptoms are infertility and pain with intercourse and bowel movements arising from scarring and adhesions from irritation from the bloodshed from the endometrial tissue.
- Signs include the characteristic findings of uterosacral ligament nodularity and cul-de-sac adhesions leading to a fixed, retroverted uterus.
- Diagnosis is by laparoscopic visualization and biopsy of lesions.
- Medical management involves preventing progesterone withdrawal bleeding through continuous steroid contraceptives (pseudopregnancy) or suppression of estrogen through antiestrogens, such as danazol, or GnRH agonists, such as leuprolide (pseudomenopause).

Chronic Pelvic Inflammatory Disease (PID)

Chronic PID is a benign condition in which painful pelvic adhesions remain after healing of an inadequately treated acute salpingo-oophoritis.

- Symptoms are chronic pelvic pain.
- Signs include bilateral adnexal tenderness and cervical-motion tenderness.
- Diagnosis is made by laparoscopic visualization of adhesions.
- Management may be medical (outpatient mild analgesics) or surgical (pelvic cleanout requiring total abdominal hysterectomy, bilateral salpingo-oophorectomy).

Adenomyosis

Adenomyosis is a benign condition in which endometrial glands and stroma are found within the wall of the uterus.

- Symptoms include chronic cyclic pelvic pain.

- Signs include symmetrically enlarged, soft, and tender uterus.

- Sonography may show a thickened myometrium containing cystic areas.

- Diagnosis is confirmed histologically on the hysterectomy specimen.

- Management is hysterectomy.

Leiomyomas

Leiomyomas are benign smooth muscle tumors of the uterine wall. They may enlarge with rising levels of estrogen.

- Symptoms may be absent or may include pelvic pain or bleeding between regular menses.

- Signs include asymmetrically enlarged, firm, and nontender uterus.

- Sonography may show subserosal, intramural, or submucosal locations.

- Management may be medical (leuprolide for premyomectomy shrinkage) or surgical (myomectomy or hysterectomy).

Final Diagnosis

Primary dysmenorrhea

CCS NOTE

In the event diagnostic laparoscopy is required, you will need a gynecology consult.

CASE 11

Chief Complaint

"I don't want any more children."

History and Physical Examination

A 30-year-old multipara woman comes to the clinic requesting permanent sterilization. She has 3 healthy children. She and her husband have discussed the issue at length, and they agree they have completed their family. They have discussed birth control pills but are unwilling to try them. She states she just "wants her tubes tied." Her last menstrual period was 3 weeks ago. Physical and pelvic examinations are unremarkable.

Initial Management

Setting: outpatient workup, office-based or operating room-based treatment

Diagnostic/Therapeutic Plan

- Urinary β-hCG
- Pre-operative CBC

Test Results

- Urinary β-hCG: negative
- CBC: normal

Assessment

This couple has come to discuss long-term family planning. They state that they have completed their family with 3 children. Nevertheless, she is young and a complete conversation about all available options along with their risks, benefits, and alternatives is in order. A full discussion should take place regarding all forms of contraception available including oral contraceptive pills, diaphragms, IUDs, condoms, tubal occlusion and vasectomy.

Possible options are as follows:

- **Female sterilization:** transection or occlusion of the fallopian tubes
- **Male sterilization:** vasectomy, a fast and effective form of sterilization
- **Female long-acting reversible contraception:** progesterone or copper IUDs and implantable progesterone devices; it is important to discuss these options

Further Management Plan/Results

After a complete discussion, the patient elects to have a copper IUD placed. The basis of her choice is the following:

- Can be placed in outpatient office (rather than operating room)
- Long duration of action (FDA-approved for 10 yrs)
- Easily reversed

Intrauterine Contraception

There are 2 types of medicated intrauterine contraception.

- **Copper IUD**: The ParaGard has copper as the active ingredient and does not alter bleeding patterns; in fact, bleeding may at times become slightly heavier. It needs replacement in 10 yrs.

- **Progestin IUD**: The Mirena has levonorgestrel as the active ingredient and is associated with lighter periods and at times, even amenorrhea (though patients continue to be ovulatory). Bleeding may be intermittent and unpredictable. It needs replacement in 5 yrs. A smaller version of Mirena is known as the Skyla and needs replacement in 3 yrs.

There are several factors that should be considered when deciding to use an IUD.

- **Benefits**. Effectiveness is high similar to permanent sterilization with failure rates <1%. Only one decision is needed that lasts 3–10 yrs.

  - No systemic side effects

  - Okay to use in diabetics and patients with HIV

  - Has user satisfaction with continuation rates (% of women still using a method after one year) of 80%

  - Does not cause abnormal Pap smears

- **Risks**. Expulsion rates are low with most occurring in first 6 wks. Uterine perforation is rare with most occurring at the time of placement. Risk of ectopic pregnancy is low but if pregnancy occurs with an IUD in place, it is more likely to be an ectopic pregnancy.

- **Contraindications**. Known or suspected pregnancy. Unexplained vaginal bleeding. Distorted uterine cavity. Acute PID (but not a history of PID).

Barrier-Spermicidal Methods

- These are locally active devices preventing sperm entry into the cervix. They become increasingly effective with advancing age with the associated natural decline in fertility.

- Male and female condoms do not require the individual fitting. Vaginal diaphragms need individual fitting and are used with spermicidal jelly or cream. The diaphragm can be placed an hour before intercourse and should be left in place for 6 hrs after.

- Condoms should be recommended for patients with multiple sexual partners who are at high risk for sexually transmitted disease.

- Patients using barrier contraception alone should be counseled on how to obtain and use emergency contraception. Also known as postcoital contraception, this consists of a single-dose of levonorgestrel 1.5 mg PO taken within 72 hrs of intercourse but ideally taken as soon as possible. Effectiveness is 80–90%.

Steroid Contraception

- **Estrogen-progestin modality.** This includes oral contraceptives, transdermal patch (Ortho Evra) and vaginal ring (Nuva Ring). Gonadotropins are suppressed so ovulation does not occur. Venous and arterial thrombosis risk is low but is dose-related.

CCS NOTE

When ordering tubal ligation, you will need to specify whether it will be performed by laparotomy or laparoscopy. In an uncomplicated patient, order laparoscopy. An ob/gyn consult will be required, and you will need to provide your indication in ≤10 words. Enter: "Elective female sterilization."

Non-contraceptive benefits include: improved pain with primary and secondary dysmenorrhea, treatment of anovulatory bleeding, decreased functional ovarian cysts and iron deficiency anemia, 50% decrease in ovarian and endometrial carcinoma. Assessing for thromboembolic risk (smoking history, history to assess for migraines, measurement of blood pressure, etc.) are important before initiating combined estrogen-progestin contraception.

- **Progestin-only modality.** Daily oral pill ("Minipill"), monthly IM injection (DMPA), good for 3 yrs subcutaneous implant (Nexplanon), one dose Emergency Contraception (Plan B), levonorgestrel IUD (Mirena). No effect on venous or arterial thrombosis.

- **Contraindications.** Known or suspected pregnancy, acute liver disease, hormonally-dependent cancer, smoker age >35 (only for EP modality).

Female Sterilization

- This procedure can be done using **laparoscopy** (transaction or occlusion with cautery or occluding devices) or using **hysteroscopy** (inserting occlusive devices through the cervix into the uterus and finally into the oviduct).

- Risk factors for regret (wishing they had not been sterilized) include: age <30, pressure from family, ambivalence about decision, decision after a fetal or neonatal death.

- Procedure should be considered permanent and irreversible with a failure rate of 1 in 200.

Final Diagnosis

Multiparity desiring long-term contraception with IUD

CASE 12

Chief Complaint

"I can't control my bladder."

History and Physical Examination

A 58-year-old woman, G3 P3, comes to the outpatient clinic with involuntary loss of urine. The symptoms began 4 years ago after she experienced menopause, but have been gradually getting more noticeable. She takes no hormone therapy. She denies burning on urination and loss of urine at night, though she loses urine in small spurts when coughing and sneezing. Ten years ago she was diagnosed with type 2 DM, for which she is being treated with metformin. She does home glucose checking irregularly and her blood glucose control is suboptimal. Five years ago she also was diagnosed with chronic hypertension, for which she is being treated with thiazide diuretics. BP is 155/95 mm Hg, HR 80/min, and respirations 15/min.

General exam is unremarkable with the exception of obesity. On pelvic examination as you are inspecting the vulva you note normal labia minora, labia majora and perianal area without lesions. Visualization of the perineum reveals a protrusion of the upper anterior vaginal wall to the level of the introitus. Speculum exam shows mildly atrophic vaginal epithelium and cervix without lesions or bleeding. On bimanual examination the uterus is midline, small, symmetrical, mobile and nontender. No ovaries or adnexal masses are palpable.

Differential Diagnosis

1. **Irritative incontinence**

   - Look for abnormal urinalysis

2. **Genuine stress incontinence**

   - Look for no urine lost at night

3. **Hypertonic urge incontinence**

   - Look for involuntary detrusor contractions

4. **Hypotonic overflow incontinence**

   - Look for overdistended bladder

5. **Fistula or bypass incontinence**

   - Look for continuous urine loss

Initial Management

Setting: outpatient workup

Diagnostic/Therapeutic Plan

- Urinalysis (U/A)
- Urine culture
- Voiding diary for 3 days
- Q-tip test
- Cystometric studies

Test Results

- UA: no RBC, WBC or bacteria
- Urine culture: negative
- Voiding diary: urine is lost intermittently during daytime hours but never at night; urine is lost in small spurts and is more common when coughing or sneezing
- Q-tip test: urethral angle changes >45 degrees
- Cystometric studies
  - Residual volume 60 cc
  - Sensation of fullness volume 250 cc
  - Urge-to-void volume 400 cc
  - No involuntary detrusor contractions are seen

Assessment

Genuine stress urinary incontinence. This is based on the negative U/A, classic history of loss in small spurts, absence of night symptoms and normal cystometric studies.

Management Plan

Medical therapy is used for mild symptoms and includes Kegel exercises and pelvic floor exercises; first line of treatment; local or systemic estrogen has not been shown to improve symptoms

When medical therapy fails or there are severe symptoms, surgical therapy is used; the goal is to elevate the urethral sphincter—which has lost its anatomic support—with a urethropexy procedure so proximal urethra is again supported.

Discussion

The prevalence of involuntary loss of urine steadily increases with advancing age, with up to 50% of older women experiencing problems. The history and physical exam are the first and most important steps in evaluation.

- A prospectively collected 3-day voiding diary is a practical and reliable method of obtaining information on voiding behavior because patient recall by history taking may be unreliable.
- A clean-catch urinalysis should be obtained to rule out a lower UTI (WBCs and bacteria) and bladder irritation sources (RBCs)
- Office-based simple cystometry is a test of detrusor function and can assess bladder sensation, capacity and compliance as well as identify involuntary detrusor contractions.

Irritative Incontinence

- **Pathophysiology**: bladder pathology: infection, stone, tumor or foreign body
- **Laboratory findings**: abnormal urinalysis (either WBCs and bacteria or RBCs)
- **Diagnosis**: urine culture (causing infection) or cystoscopic visualization of the lesions (causing microscopic hematuria)
- **Management**: varies according to diagnosis

Genuine Stress Incontinence

- Most common form of true urinary incontinence.
- **Pathophysiology**: rises in bladder pressure caused by intra-abdominal pressure increases (e.g., coughing and sneezing) are transmitted to the bladder but are not transmitted to the proximal urethra due to urethral hypermobility and loss of support.
- **Symptoms**: absence of urine loss at night (this is a **unique** finding for stress incontinence).
- **Exam**: cystocele may or may not be present. Neurologic findings are normal. Q-tip test shows a change in the urethral angle of ≥30 degrees.
- **Cystometric studies**: normal residual volume, normal sensation of fullness volume, normal urge to void volume, and absence of spontaneous detrusor muscle contractions.
- **Management**: **medical** (Kegel exercises and pelvic floor exercises) or **surgical** (elevate the urethral sphincter with a urethropexy or sling procedure so that the proximal urethra is again in an intra-abdominal location).

Hypertonic, Urge Incontinence

- **Pathophysiology**: involuntary rises in bladder pressure from idiopathic detrusor contractions that cannot be voluntarily suppressed.
- **Symptoms**: loss of urine in large amounts often without warning day and night. The most common symptom is urgency. Signs include normal pelvic examination and normal neurological examination.
- **Exam**: normal pelvic and neurologic findings.
- **Cystometric studies**: normal residual volume, reduced sensation of fullness volume and reduced urge to void volume. Presence of spontaneous detrusor muscle contractions is a **unique** finding.
- **Management** is medical: bladder training (timed voiding exercises) and anticholinergic medications (e.g., oxybutynin, tolterodine) or NSAIDs to inhibit detrusor contractions.

Mixed Incontinence

- Up to 1/3 of patients can have mixed incontinence, i.e., both genuine stress incontinence and hypertonic, urge incontinence.
- It is crucial that a correct diagnosis be made because the treatments vary significantly.
- Stress incontinence can be managed either medically or surgically, whereas hypertonic incontinence is only managed medically.

Hypotonic, Overflow Incontinence

- **Pathophysiology**: rises in bladder pressure occurring gradually from an overdistended, hypotonic bladder. Involuntary urine loss occurs but only until the bladder pressure exceeds urethral pressure; however, the bladder never empties. Then the process begins all over again. Systemic medication or chronic neurologic disease may be underlying causes.

- **Symptoms**: intermittent urine loss occurs continually day and night.

- **Signs**: normal pelvic anatomy. However, an enlarged, overdistended bladder is a **unique** finding. Neurologic examination shows decreased pudendal nerve sensation (S 2,3,4)

- **Cystometric studies**: markedly increased residual volume, but involuntary detrusor contractions do not occur.

- **Management**: intermittent self-catheterization or discontinuance of the offending systemic medications. Cholinergic medications can stimulate bladder contractions, and alpha adrenergic agonists can relax the bladder neck.

Fistula, Bypass Incontinence

- **Pathophysiology**: ischemic devascularization of pelvic structures from either radical pelvic surgery or pelvic radiation therapy. Vesico-vaginal fistula is most common finding.

- **Symptoms**: loss of urine continually in small amounts day and night is a **unique** finding.

- **Diagnostic studies**: IV pyelogram demonstrates dye leakage from a urinary tract fistula. With a urinary tract-vaginal fistula, IV indigo carmine dye leaks onto a vaginal tampon and turns it blue.

- **Management** is surgical repair of the fistula.

Final Diagnosis

Genuine stress incontinence

CASE 13

Chief Complaint

"I am bleeding from my vagina."

History and Physical Examination

A 60-year-old obese woman presents to the clinic with complaint of vaginal bleeding. She reports that she has been having vaginal bleeding intermittently for the last 2 months. She states that this is her first episode since she went through menopause at age 52. Her medical history is significant for obesity (BMI = 44 kg/m^2), non-insulin dependent diabetes and osteoarthritis. Her past surgical history is significant for a laparoscopic cholecystectomy and a remote history of a dilation and curettage for heavy, irregular vaginal bleeding. Her most recent Pap smear 2 years ago was normal. She has never been pregnant despite her and her husband not using any contraception.

Vital signs are WNL except BP 155/90 mm Hg. Physical exam reveals a heavy-set woman in no acute distress. She has a large pannus. Pelvic exam shows a normal appearing vulva, well estrogenized vaginal mucosa with normal rugae and no cervical lesions. There is some dark blood visible in the cervical os. On bimanual exam the uterus is midline, symmetrical, mobile and normal sized. No adnexal masses are palpable.

Differential Diagnosis

1. **Endometrial cancer**
   - Needs to be first on the differential diagnosis even though only 15% of women with postmenopausal bleeding have endometrial cancer

2. **Endometrial hyperplasia**
   - Can be with or without atypia; the former is a premalignant condition

3. **Endometrial polyps** (overgrowths of localized endometrial tissue that can be malignant)

4. **Vaginal atrophy**
   - Unlikely, considering speculum exam demonstrated an estrogen effect

5. **Cervical cancer**
   - Unlikely, considering normal-appearing cervix and normal Pap 2 yrs ago

Initial Management

Setting: outpatient workup

Diagnostic/Therapeutic Plan

- Endometrial sampling via endometrial pipelle (performed in office) or dilation and curettage (D&C) (performed as an outpatient surgical procedure) **OR**
- Vaginal probe U/S to evaluate endometrial lining thickness (a thin endometrial stripe can rule out pathology)

CLINICAL PEARL

Postmenopausal bleeding should never be considered normal or physiologic and should always be evaluated. An endometrial tissue sample is imperative for definitive diagnosis.

CCS NOTE

When you order an endometrial biopsy, an ob/gyn consult will be required, and you will need to provide your indication in 10 words or less. Enter "postmenopausal bleeding."

CCS NOTE

When ordering total abdominal hysterectomy with bilateral salpingo-oophorectomy, you can enter simply "TAH BSO." You will need to specify that the procedure will be done by laparotomy. The order converts to "laparotomy," and an ob/gyn consult is not required. If you order the procedure unnecessarily, a PATIENT UPDATE screen will appear, stating, "After discussion of potential benefits and risks with the patient, appropriate family member(s), or guardian, the procedure is declined at this time."

Test Results

- Endometrial biopsy: endometrioid adenocarcinoma (Grade 1) in a background of endometrial hyperplasia

Assessment

Endometrial cancer

Further Management

Staging laparotomy, including total abdominal hysterectomy with bilateral salpingo-oophorectomy (TAH-BSO) and lymphadenectomy.

Discussion

This patient has endometrial cancer, the most common gynecologic malignancy in the United States. While only a minority of women with post-menopausal bleeding have endometrial cancer, it represents the most serious diagnosis and thus must be diagnosed promptly and treated appropriately. Any bleeding or spotting that occurs after menopause must be evaluated by endometrial biopsy to rule out endometrial cancer.

Most women present with post-menopausal bleeding and are diagnosed at an early stage, often cured with hysterectomy. Endometrial cancer is surgically staged and treated with TAH-BSO and lymphadenectomy. The most common stage is stage I. There is no screening test for endometrial cancer.

Women at **highest risk** for endometrial hyperplasia and cancer have unopposed estrogen: high estrogen levels without any progesterone to mature the endometrium. These include:

- Exogenous unopposed estrogen replacement therapy
- Obese women who aromatize androstenedione to estrone in their peripheral adipose
- Women with an estrogen-producing tumor

Women on tamoxifen (a selective estrogen-receptor modulator) have an increased risk of endometrial cancer. Tamoxifen, used to treat estrogen-receptor positive breast cancer, has an estrogen-antagonist effect on the breast, but an estrogen-agonist effect on the endometrium.

Hyperplasia. Endometrial hyperplasia is an abnormal proliferation of endometrial glands and stroma. It represents a premalignant state. Hyperplasia with complex structure and atypical cells on microscopic examination may be an indicator of an underlying endometrial cancer and should be treated with a hysterectomy and BSO. A high-dose progestin is an alternative to hysterectomy in patients who are a poor operative risk and in those whose hyperplasia does not contain atypical cells.

Workup. Endometrial cancer and endometrial hyperplasia are histologic diagnoses that require tissue sampling. They both result from excess estrogen stimulation and present with vaginal bleeding. They are associated with a thick endometrial lining so as an alternative to endometrial sampling, women can have a vaginal probe U/S and if the endometrial lining is thin (<5 mm) endometrial cancer can be ruled out.

Final Diagnosis

Endometrial adenocarcinoma

CASE 14

Chief Complaint

"My periods have stopped, and my moods are unpredictable."

History and Physical Examination

A 50-year-old woman whose last menstrual period was 12 months ago comes to the outpatient clinic stating that she has been depressed, angry, easily agitated, and having difficulty concentrating. She has frequent hot flashes that can come at both day and night and result in trouble sleeping. Her vagina feels dry, resulting in painful sexual intercourse. She also has urinary frequency and dysuria. On examination she has flushed features and is somewhat irritable. Pelvic examination reveals normal external genitalia with dry vaginal mucosa. The remainder of the examination is normal.

Differential Diagnosis

1. **Pregnancy**

   - Although unlikely here, pregnancy must always be considered when a patient presents with secondary amenorrhea.

2. **Menopause**

   - The patient meets criteria for menopause, which requires 12 months without menses in the absence of a pathophysiologic cause. The average age for menopause is age 51. The presenting and most troublesome features are vasomotor symptoms, which this patient exhibits. Obese patients are less likely to have these symptoms because of persistent estrogen levels from peripheral conversion of adrenal androgens in the adipose tissues.

3. **Oligomenorrhea**

   - Although possible here, this is unlikely in light of patient's other symptoms such as vaginal dryness, hot flushes, and dyspareunia.

Initial Management

Setting: outpatient workup and treatment

Diagnostic/Therapeutic Plan

- Urinary β-hCG test

Test Results

- Urinary β-hCG test negative

Assessment

The patient appears to be menopausal. Although pregnancy is very unlikely, it should still be ruled out in the setting of amenorrhea without a history of irregular menses. In menopause, FSH, LH, and GnRH are all elevated. FSH is a sensitive marker and the most cost-effective; however, it is not required to make the diagnosis.

Further Management Plan/Results

Serum FSH elevated

Discussion

Menopause is defined as 12 months without menses in the absence of pathophysiologic causes. The transition is marked by irregular menstrual cycles and is often accompanied by vasomotor complaints, sleep disturbances, and changes in sexual function. As menopause progresses, genitourinary atrophy symptoms including vaginal dryness, dyspareunia, and sometimes sexual dysfunction arise. These symptoms occur when insufficient ovarian follicles result in inadequate estrogen levels to maintain estrogen-dependent tissues. When endometrial proliferation is inadequate to yield menstruation, then menses cease.

Age 51 is the mean age at which menopause occurs; it is unaffected by race, socioeconomic status, education, age of menarche, parity, oral contraceptive use, and alcohol use. Cigarette smoking is the only thing to have been shown to hasten follicular exhaustion. Obesity, hypertension, and diabetes do not affect the age of menopause.

Endocrine changes: With no functional ovarian follicles left, estrogen, progesterone, and inhibin levels are decreased. With estrogen levels low, there is minimal feedback to the hypothalamus/pituitary. Thus, GnRH levels are high, which stimulates increased levels of pituitary gonadotropins. Thus, FSH and LH are increased.

Follow-up Management and Prevention

The patient should be counseled about her diagnosis and given expectation for the menopausal transition. In addition, the option of HRT should be discussed.

The patient elects to proceed with HRT for her vaginal dryness, dyspareunia, and hot flush symptoms. In patients with a uterus (i.e., they have not had a hysterectomy) it is important to prescribe combination (both estrogen and progesterone) therapy. Estrogen-only therapy will treat her symptoms but unopposed estrogen puts her at risk for endometrial hyperplasia and cancer. Thus, her prescription should include: conjugated estrogen 0.3 mg PO daily and medroxyprogesterone acetate 1.5 mg PO for 1 wk per month.

The patient should return in 3 months to assess symptoms. The treatment goal should be to utilize the lowest dose of hormones for the shortest period possible to alleviate symptoms.

Discussion

Estrogen receptors are ubiquitous in a woman's body. Organ systems with estrogen receptors include the lower and upper reproductive tract, the urinary tract, the musculoskeletal system, the cardiovascular system, and the liver, brain, and breasts. The most pronounced clinical evidences of estrogen deficiency are noted in the genital and urinary tract. The vaginal epithelium undergoes atrophy, the vaginal diameter narrows, and the vaginal pH increases, making the vagina more susceptible to infections.

Osteoporosis complications occur in 1 out of 3 postmenopausal American women. It involves loss of trabecular, not cortical, bone. Whether or not it develops depends on a combination of estrogen levels, calcium intake, and weight-bearing exercise. Osteoclastic resorption of bone exceeds osteoblastic deposition of bone.

- The most common site of osteoporotic fractures in postmenopausal women is the vertebra, with a female-to-male ratio of 10:1.

- The second most common site is the hip, with a female-to-male ratio of 4:1.

- The third most common site is the wrist.

Although the Women's Health Initiative (WHI) study (2002) showed that estrogen and progestin hormone replacement therapy (EP-HRT) was found to decrease the risk of osteoporosis, it should not be used solely for osteoporosis prevention; that is because there are other medications that can prevent osteoporosis/fractures and appear to carry lower risks for breast cancer and heart disease.

Cardiovascular disease is the main cause of mortality in postmenopausal women, causing twice as many deaths as cancer. Estrogen deficiency results in increased levels of LDL cholesterol and decreased levels of HDL cholesterol. Vaginal pH increases. Estrogen replacement as a prevention of heart disease is not indicated. On the basis of the WHI study, EP-HRT is no longer recommended to prevent heart disease in healthy women (primary prevention) or to protect women with pre-existing heart disease (secondary prevention). The WHI data suggest that not only does EP-HRT not work, it may also actually increase the risk of heart attack and stroke.

Contraindications to estrogen-replacement include breast/endometrial cancer, active thrombophlebitis, undiagnosed vaginal bleeding, and active liver disease.

Although the WHI showed a significantly decreased risk of colon cancer and bone fractures in EP-HRT users, it also showed a small but significant increase in breast cancer, as well as thrombotic and cardiovascular events. This difference was enough to stop the EP-HRT arm of the study. It is significant that the estrogen-only arm of the WHI did not show any increase in breast cancer or cardiovascular disease.

The WHI conclusions are valid for women in their sixties without vasomotor symptoms. However, there are significant limitations in the WHI study that raise questions regarding the application of its conclusions to the average woman entering menopause in their fifties. The limitations include the following:

- Subjects with significant vasomotor symptoms (the most common indication for hormone therapy) were excluded from the study groups

- Mean age of study subjects at enrollment was age 63, 12 yrs past the mean age of menopause

- All subjects received the same dose of hormones, regardless of age

Hormone replacement therapy is the most effective treatment for the relief of vasomotor symptoms, such as hot flashes and sleep disturbances, which can affect both physical and mental health. It's also effective in treating genitourinary symptoms, such as vaginal dryness. If hormone replacement therapy is used, it should be administered at the lowest possible effective dose for up to 4 yrs and subject to annual review with the physician.

All women given hormone replacement therapy should receive continuous estrogen replacement. Women with a uterus need continuous or intermittent (at least 4 times a year) progestin to prevent unopposed estrogen stimulation of endometrial hyperplasia and carcinoma.

Final Diagnosis

Menopause

CASE 15

Chief Complaint

"My abdomen feels bloated and full."

History and physical exam

A 63-year-old woman presents to the clinic complaining of the sensation of increasing abdominal bloating. She reports an increasing abdominal girth, with her pants fitting tighter. She admits to early satiety and urinary frequency without dysuria. Her medical history is significant for hyperlipidemia. Prior to her current presentation, she states that she was healthy. She went through menopause at age 50 and denies any subsequent episodes of vaginal bleeding. Her family history is significant for an aunt who was diagnosed with breast cancer at age 42.

On physical exam she is alert and oriented. Her lungs are clear to auscultation. No tachycardia. Her abdomen is distended with fluid. There is no palpable hepatomegaly. A fluid wave is present. On bimanual pelvic exam a large, firm, fixed right-sided pelvic mass is palpated.

Differential Diagnosis

1. Epithelial ovarian cancer
2. Uterine mass/fibroid uterus
3. Metastatic tumor to ovary
4. Old tubo-ovarian abscess (TOA)

Initial Management

Setting: outpatient workup

Initial Diagnostic Plan

- Pelvic U/S
- CA-125 level
- CBC, metabolic panel

Test Results

- U/S: multicystic, complex right ovarian mass measuring 8 × 12 cm
- Free fluid in pelvis
- CA-125 level 650 U/mL (normal <35 U/mL)
- Hgb 10.2 gm/dL, WBC 6,000, creatinine 0.7, liver enzymes normal

Initial Discussion

Ascites and/or an ovarian mass in a post-menopausal woman is never normal and should always be evaluated for its etiology. A post-menopausal woman does not have functional ovarian follicles and therefore cannot have a functional ovarian cyst. A renal or hepatic etiology of the ascites can be ruled out with a normal creatinine and liver function tests. U/S characteristics that make an ovarian mass suspicious for malignancy include: large size, solid components and irregular contours.

CA-125 is a nonspecific tumor biomarker. While it is elevated in a majority of women with advanced stage epithelial ovarian cancer, it is not used for screening for ovarian malignancy. Any condition resulting in peritoneal inflammation or irritation can cause it to be elevated, e.g., peritonitis, diverticulitis, endometriosis. However, in the setting of ascites and a pelvic mass, a markedly elevated CA-125 is highly suspicious and predictive of malignancy.

Further Diagnostic Plan

Cytoreductive surgery. This includes total hysterectomy, bilateral salpingo-oophorectomy, omentectomy, and removal of ascitic fluid.

Further Results

The pathology report shows both ovaries and fallopian tubes with serous adenocarcinoma. Omentum is noted to have "caking" secondary to tumor involvement. There was diffuse peritoneal "studding" with tumor implants. The ascitic fluid is positive for carcinoma.

Further Treatment

Chemotherapy

Discussion

Epidemiology. Ovarian cancer is the second most common gynecologic malignancy, with over 20,000 cases diagnosed each year in the United States. A woman's lifetime risk of developing ovarian cancer is 1 in 70. A majority of cases are sporadic. However, women with a family history and/or an inherited genetic predisposition (e.g., BRCA1, BRCA2) are at increased risk of developing ovarian cancer. Secondary to a lack of effective screening, a majority of cases are diagnosed at an advanced stage (i.e., stage III or IV).

Symptoms. They are often non-specific, including bloating, early satiety and urinary complaints. Women with findings suspicious for ovarian cancer (e.g., ovarian mass, ascites, worrisome symptoms) should undergo a workup for ovarian cancer, including imaging and CA-125 level. The exact etiology of ovarian cancer is unknown. Protective factors include those that decrease the number of ovulatory cycles in a woman's lifetime (e.g., oral contraceptive use, pregnancy, breast feeding). There is no screening test for ovarian cancer.

Method of spread. The disease first spreads to the abdomen by exfoliation of malignant cells into the peritoneal fluid and direct extension. Metastatic disease can involve the liver parenchyma, lungs, and pleural space. Stage I disease is confined to one or both ovaries. Stage II is disease confined to pelvis. Stage III is cancer that has spread to the abdomen (often the omentum resulting in thickening with tumor "caking"). Stage IV describes metastatic disease, often pleural fluid and/or liver parenchyma involvement.

Management. The initial management involves surgical resection, with the goal of removing all grossly visible disease. The purpose of surgery is fourfold:

1. Obtain a tissue diagnosis
2. Assess extent and spread of disease
3. Remove symptomatic disease burden
4. Increase efficacy of chemotherapy

Women with advanced stage disease and those with early stage disease with risk factors (poorly differentiated and/or aggressive histologic subtypes) warrant chemotherapy. Recommended chemotherapy is a platinum-based combination of 2 agents, e.g., carboplatin and paclitaxel. Women with advanced stage disease should be considered for intraperitoneal administration of chemotherapy, as it has proven to result in improved progression-free and overall survival when compared with IV administration. A majority of patients respond to initial chemotherapy. Ultimately, though, most patients will relapse and eventually succumb to their disease.

Final Diagnosis

Metastatic serous ovarian carcinoma, stage III

CLINICAL PEARL

Treatment of advanced ovarian cancer is primarily surgical debulking and chemotherapy. Even though the seeding of the peritoneal cavity is often diffuse, external beam radiation therapy is contraindicated because of severe morbidity and mortality.

CASE 16

Chief Complaint

"I have vulvar itching."

History and Physical Examination

A 64-year-old woman comes to the outpatient office with complaints of vulvar itching. She has a 30 pack-year history of tobacco use and she drinks wine with her dinner daily. She was diagnosed with chronic hypertension 15 years ago and BP is controlled on hydrochlorothiazide daily. She states she has hyperlipidemia for which she has been prescribed statins. She reports that she first noticed the vulvar itching 6 months ago. She gets some relief from scratching. She reports having been treated for the same complaint with a steroid cream without relief. More recently she felt a "bump" on her labia. She reports that the palpable lesion and itching are confined to her left labia. Inspection of external genitalia reveals a hyperemic, raised, excoriated 1 × 2 cm left vulvar lesion.

Differential Diagnosis

1. Squamous hyperplasia
2. Lichen sclerosis
3. Vulvar intraepithelial neoplasia (VIN)
4. Vulvar cancer
5. Paget's disease

Initial Management

Setting: outpatient workup

Diagnostic Plan

Vulvar biopsy

Results

Vulvar biopsy: Well-differentiated squamous cell carcinoma, keratinizing type; depth of invasion 3 mm

Assessment

Vulvar carcinoma

Treatment

Radical vulvectomy with ipsilateral inguinofemoral lymphadenectomy

CLINICAL PEARL

The most common symptom of both benign and malignant lesions is vulvar itching resulting in scratching. All vulvar lesions of uncertain etiology should be biopsied. Patients with vulvar pruritus should be considered for the possibility of preinvasive or invasive vulvar carcinomas if there is a vulvar lesion.

CLINICAL PEARL

With vulvar cancer, look for the 3 P's: **p**ersistent, **p**ostmenopausal **p**ruritis.

Discussion

Epidemiology. In the United States, there are nearly 4,000 new cases of vulvar cancer diagnosed each year. This is primarily a disease of post-menopausal women; however, there is a trend toward an earlier age at presentation. Risk factors include:

- Vulvar dystrophy
- HPV infection
- Cigarette smoking
- Cervical dysplasia and/or cancer
- Immunocompromised state

The variety of risk factors highlights the existence of 2 distinct pathways for the development of vulvar cancer. One pathway involves chronic inflammation while the other is related to an infectious etiology, specifically human papillomavirus. There is no screening test for vulvar cancer.

Squamous cell carcinoma (SCC) is the most common type of vulvar cancer. Pruritus and the presence of a mass are the most common presenting symptoms. Vulvar cancer is surgically staged. The standard initial management of SCC of vulva involves surgical resection. The extent of surgery is dependent upon the size of the lesion, its location, depth of invasion and risk for lymph node metastasis.

- Patients with lesions with ≤1 mm stromal invasion have a negligible risk of lymph node metastases and therefore do not require a lymphadenectomy and can be cured with wide local excision (WLE) with the goal of a 1.5 cm tumor-free margin.

- For patients with stromal invasion >1 mm, the risk of lymph node metastasis is great enough to warrant an inguinofemoral lymphadenectomy. Unilateral lymph node dissection is appropriate for unilateral involvement with bilateral procedures reserved for bilateral lesions. A vulvar tumor-free margin of at least 1.5 cm should be obtained.

Melanoma is the second most common malignant tumor of the vulva. It constitutes 5–10% of all vulvar malignancies. This tumor frequently affects post-menopausal white women. Presenting symptoms for vulvar melanoma include pruritis, bleeding, and ulceration.

Paget's disease is a rare slow-growing malignancy. It presents with vulvar pruritis and a red, excoriated appearing lesion. There may be an invasive component beneath the surface and surgical excision is needed to rule this out and for symptom relief. Women with Paget's should be evaluated for possible synchronous neoplasms, as they are at risk for noncontiguous cancers, e.g., breast, rectum.

Vulvar dystrophies, including lichen sclerosis and squamous hyperplasia, also present with pruritis and a vulvar lesion. Diagnosis is confirmed with biopsy.

- Lichen sclerosis is classically described as "parchment-like" appearance. On histology, epidermal thinning and loss of rete ridges are seen. Treatment is clobetasol cream.

- In contrast, squamous hyperplasia will show hyperplasia of the epithelium with overlying hyperkeratosis. Treatment is fluorinated corticosteroid cream.

Final Diagnosis

Vulvar squamous cell carcinoma

PART III

SURGERY

CASE 1

Chief Complaint

Right-sided abdominal pain

History and Physical Examination

A 24-year-old man comes to the emergency department complaining of right-sided abdominal pain. He was well until the pain began in the periumbilical area 24 hours ago, followed by some episodes of nausea and vomiting. It has now moved to the right lower quadrant and remains there. The patient is anorexic. He denies any significant medical history. He states that he has not had any episodes like this prior to this one. He denies blood, mucus, constipation, diarrhea, dysuria, or blood in urine. He is a well-appearing male in mild distress, lying still. Vital signs are temperature 37.8 C (100.0 F), pulse 96/min, and BP 130/75 mm Hg.

On physical examination the abdomen is soft and non-distended, and there is right lower quadrant tenderness with rebound and guarding. There are no masses, hernias, or costovertebral angle tenderness. Psoas and obturator signs are positive. Rectal examination shows right-sided tenderness but no palpable masses. The remainder of the physical examination is unremarkable.

Differential Diagnosis

1. Appendicitis

   - Consistent with history and physical examination findings

2. Renal colic

   - Can present with similar history and physical examination findings, but typically has more back pain and costovertebral tenderness to palpation; low grade fever may be present due to imminent UTI

3. Peptic ulcer

   - Often presents initially with periumbilical region, but typically radiates to epigastrium or right upper quadrant.

4. Gallstones/cholecystitis

   - Can present as periumbilical pain which then radiates to the right upper quadrant, but can also present as right lower quadrant pain; often presents with low-grade fever

CLINICAL PEARL

Acute appendicitis should always be considered in the differential diagnosis of abdominal pain even if physical examination findings are negative.

5. Diverticulitis

   • Periumbilical pain, low grade fever, and rectal exam findings are all consistent with this diagnosis, although the patient is not in the typical age group

6. Inflammatory bowel disease (IBD)

   • More consistent with this patient's age, should be strongly considered in the differential; pain and tenderness are usually not as focal as presented in this scenario; no family history is given but this should be considered in assessing the likelihood of this diagnosis.

Initial Management

Setting: emergency department

Diagnostic/Therapeutic Plan

• CBC

• Comprehensive metabolic panel

• Abdominal x-ray

• Chest x-ray

• Urinalysis

Test Results

CLINICAL PEARL

It is not uncommon to have WBCs in the urine secondary to bladder irritation from appendicitis. This is not due to a primary UTI.

• CBC: WBC count 15,000/mm^3

• Comprehensive metabolic panel: normal

• Abdominal x-ray: fecalith identified in right lower quadrant

• Chest x-ray: no pleural effusion or pneumoperitoneum

• Urinalysis: 5 WBC, no RBCs or bacteria

Assessment

This patient has acute appendicitis based on the history, physical examination, laboratory results, and the presence of a fecalith on x-ray.

• Renal colic is generally associated with RBCs in the urine and a migrating colicky pain.

• A perforated peptic ulcer is usually associated with free air on chest x-ray, or a leak may be demonstrated with an upper GI series using water-soluble contrast; there is usually a history of dyspepsia.

• Diverticulitis is rare in this age group, and other types of IBD (e.g., Crohn's disease, UC) are associated with mucus or blood in diarrhea and a history of chronic GI symptoms.

• Cholecystitis is associated with a positive Murphy sign in the right upper quadrant, and gallstones may be seen on x-ray 15% of the time.

Additionally, a comprehensive metabolic panel includes hepatic function tests, which would be at least slightly abnormal. Appendicitis is a clinical diagnosis, and a fecalith is seen on x-ray in only 15–20% of cases. Be sure to rule out mild menstrual pain, ovarian cysts, and torsion in women.

Further Management Plan

- NPO (nothing by mouth)

- IV antibiotics

- Appendectomy

Discussion

Appendicitis is the most common cause of abdominal pain requiring surgery. The incidence is 10% worldwide. The lumen of the appendix becomes obstructed by a fecalith, lymphoid hyperplasia, a foreign body (e.g., popcorn), a tumor (e.g., carcinoid, pancreatic rests), or strictures. The bacteriology typically associated with appendicitis is *E. coli, B. fragilis*, and *Pseudomonas*.

The diagnosis is clinical in 80% of cases, with the pain starting in the periumbilical region (visceral) and later moving to the right lower quadrant, where it is more sharp and localized (somatic). Seventy-five percent of cases have anorexia or vomiting associated with pain. Laboratory studies often show mild-to-moderate leukocytosis (12,000–16,000/mm^3), with a left-sided shift and low-grade fever, all suggesting acute inflammation. However, WBC count may be normal, even in the presence of perforation.

Referred tenderness in the right lower quadrant when palpated in the left lower quadrant is called Rovsing's sign and when present is pathognomonic for acute appendicitis. The psoas sign (pain in right lower quadrant with hyperextension of right hip joint) and the obturator sign (pain in right lower quadrant on flexion and internal rotation of right hip joint) may be positive in acute appendicitis. However, the most constant signs of acute appendicitis are pain and tenderness localized to right lower quadrant.

Basic Science Correlate

With acute appendicitis, to understand why the pain "moves" from periumbilical to right lower quadrant requires an understanding of the embryology, anatomy, natural history, and clinical presentation of the disease.

- Embryologically, the intestines are divided into the foregut, midgut, and hindgut.

- The visceral peritoneal innervation of the regions of the gut tube is provided by the ANS.

  - Parasympathetic nerves (vagus; CN X and pelvic splanchnics) provide the functional innervation of the gut, controlling peristalsis and glandular secretions.

  - Sympathetic innervation of the gut is largely inhibitory, but is important because sympathetic nerves carry visceral pain fibers from the region of the gut that they innervate.

When there is an inflammation of the visceral peritoneum of the gut tube, the sensation conveyed by visceral pain fibers will be REFERRED to a specific area based on its embryologic origin and the cord segments that receive the visceral pain fibers.

- Foregut visceral peritoneal inflammation refers pain to the epigastrium, because foregut visceral pain enters the cord from about T5- T9.

- The midgut refers pain to the periumbilical area T9- T11, and the hindgut refers pain to the suprapubic area (T10- L1). Visceral pain referred to the body wall is not a terribly "sharp" pain, but rather a kind of "dull ache and discomfort."

The somatic nervous system innervates the body wall and the parietal peritoneum that covers it. If an inflamed gut structure directly involves the body wall, it is—in contrast to visceral pain—very sharp and "localized." Therefore, the clinical presentation of appendicitis, periumbilical referred pain that "moves" to right lower quadrant of the body wall reflects progression of the natural history of the disease: visceral peritoneal involvement of a structure derived from the midgut to direct involvement of body wall (parietal peritoneum) adjacent to the actual location of the appendix.

Remember that it is **parietal** peritoneal involvement which produces on physical exam the "acute abdomen"—involuntary guarding, rigidity, and rebound. However, a retrocecal appendix that is inflamed may present with atypical pain and a less impressive abdominal exam.

Even though the diagnosis is usually established clinically, image studies are sometimes useful.

- Abdominal x-rays can infrequently show a fecalith.
- Sonogram is most useful in children and occasionally in women of childbearing age.
- CT scan is indicated only in cases where the history and physical examination are suspicious for acute appendicitis, but tests are inconclusive and sigmoid diverticulitis, cecal neoplasm, or tuboovarian pathology cannot be excluded. CT findings consistent with appendicitis include a distended, thick-walled appendix with inflammatory streaks of fat, a pericecal phlegmon or abscess, or a fecalith.

The appropriate management is to keep the patient NPO, begin IV antibiotic therapy with a third-generation cephalosporin, and prepare the patient for immediate appendectomy. A ruptured appendix is much more serious than an acute appendicitis. Always err on the side of caution; it is safer to remove a normal appendix than to miss a ruptured appendix.

There are several complications of appendicitis:

Wound infection (most common complication)

To prevent this, prophylactic antibiotics are generally given at the time of induction. In cases where the appendix has already perforated and there has been gross spillage, the surgical incision site should not be closed but instead packed with wet gauze until it heals with granulation tissue. Alternatively, laparoscopic approach helps avoid larger wounds and hence less chances for a wound infection.

Intra-abdominal infection

Pelvic abscesses present with rising fevers, leukocytosis, and diarrhea with tenesmus. (Rectal examination can reveal a boggy, painful mass.) CT scan can typically establish the diagnosis, and treatment can be performed with CT-guided percutaneous draining of the abscess. Open drainage can be performed transabdominally or transrectally (if abscess is adjacent to the rectum). In the current surgical practice, laparotomy to drain the appendicular abscess is rare, as CT-guided drainage is now an established practice. However, in cases of abscess rupturing and generalized peritonitis, open surgical lavage is an appropriate option.

Enterocutaneous fistula

This may develop from a nonhealing appendicular stump; a right hemicolectomy may be required. This is also called a "fecal fistula."

Small bowel obstruction, secondary to adhesions

If a patient presents 5–7 days after the onset of pain, an appendiceal mass develops, and this is referred to as a "missed appendicitis." Historically, this was managed with antibiotics and interval appendectomy at 6–8 weeks to prevent recurrence of appendicitis, which occurs in 5–10% of patients. Currently, this is more controversial, with many advocating no surgery unless recurrent appendicitis occurs because the risk is so low.

Final Diagnosis

Acute appendicitis

CASE 2

Chief Complaint

"I'm having trouble breathing."

History and Physical Examination

A 23-year-old man is brought in by paramedics to the emergency department after being involved in a motor vehicle accident. The patient was the driver of an automobile traveling at 40 mph. He lost control and struck a telephone pole. He denies any loss of consciousness. He was not wearing his seatbelt at the time and recalls striking the steering wheel. He complains of chest pain and shortness of breath. He admits that he had been out drinking. Past medical history is otherwise negative. He appears to be a healthy man in moderate distress. Vital signs are BP 110/70 mm Hg, pulse 115/min, and respirations 30/min. Airway is patent, and he is moving air without difficulty. He is awake and responsive. Nasogastric aspirate is bilious. Further examination reveals:

Head: no traumatic injuries; no oral or nasal blood; no ecchymoses or raccoon eyes

Neck: in a cervical collar; no point tenderness, jugular distension, hematoma, or crepitus

Lungs: clear bilaterally; mild sternal tenderness to palpation but no deformity

Chest: small abrasions are visible on skin, no ecchymosis

Heart: regular rhythm but tachycardic; no muffling or murmur

Abdomen: nondistended, soft, mild mid-epigastric tenderness to palpation

Pelvis: stable, tender anteriorly; no blood at urethral meatus

Extremities: no musculoskeletal deformities; palpable distal pulses

Rectal: no gross blood, guaiac negative; prostate not palpable

Neurologic: answers appropriately, cranial nerves intact, no focal deficits

Differential Diagnosis

1. Blunt trauma to the abdomen or pelvis: visceral injury, hemorrhage, pelvic fracture

2. Blunt trauma to chest: aortic dissection, pulmonary contusion, cardiac contusion, sterna or rib fractures

   - A pulmonary laceration resulting in pneumothorax or hemothorax is less likely given the presence of bilateral breath sounds.

Basic Science Correlate

Deceleration injuries such as motor vehicle accidents or falls from significant heights can result in a descending aortic dissection due to the aorta's relative mobility except at the distal aortic arch. This is where it is fixed at the ligamentum arteriosum, the remnant of the ductus arteriosus which connected the distal aortic arch to the pulmonary artery in utero. Significant blunt force will result in a tear at this fixed point, which propagates down the aorta in the form of a dissection.

Initial Management

- Transfer to trauma evaluation room
- Continuous monitoring of heart rate and oxygen saturation; serial blood pressure monitoring
- Chest x-ray, pelvis x-ray
- Focused abdominal sonography for trauma (FAST)
- Blood work: type and cross match, serum electrolytes, CBC, coagulation profile, amylase, blood alcohol level
- 12-lead EKG
- Foley catheter insertion
- Nasogastric tube placement and aspiration

Test Results

- Continuous monitoring of heart rate and oxygen saturation; serial blood pressure monitoring: HR consistently sinus rhythm 100–120 bpm, O_2 saturation 96–98% on 2L nasal cannula; BP 90–120/40–60 mmHg.
- Chest x-ray: no pneumothorax, hemothorax, widened mediastinum, sternal or rib fractures
- Pelvis x-ray: non-displaced right superior ramus fracture
- Focused abdominal sonography for trauma (FAST): no intra-abdominal free fluid, no pericardial fluid
- Blood work: type and cross match, serum electrolytes, CBC, coagulation profile, lipase, blood alcohol level: pending
- 12-lead EKG: no dysrhythmia
- Foley catheter insertion: clear urine
- Nasogastric tube placement and aspiration: bilious drainage, no blood

Assessment

This patient is hemodynamically stable following blunt trauma in the setting of alcohol intoxication, with the only finding on initial assessment being a non-displaced minor pelvic fracture. Although a major thoracic injury is unlikely given the findings, he is still at risk for significant intracranial, spinal, and abdominal or pelvic injuries.

CLINICAL PEARL

Radiographic signs of an aortic injury include a widened mediastinum, pleural effusion, apical cap (due to extrapleural blood), left main stem bronchus displacement (downward), and nasogastric tube displacement (lateral).

Alcohol intoxication and other distracting injuries make neurological and abdominal exams unreliable. Although the FAST exam is reassuring for no intra-abdominal injury, it is user-dependent and only evaluates the intra-abdominal compartment, not the entire pelvis and any retroperitoneal structures. Accordingly, CT scan of the head, cervical spine, and abdomen and pelvis with IV contrast is indicated. A hemodynamically unstable patient with a pelvic fracture belongs in the interventional radiology suite for angiographic embolization of the internal iliac arteries.

Further Management Plan

- CT head: no intracranial injury

- CT c-spine: no cervical fracture or dislocation

- CT abdomen/pelvis: no intra-abdominal fluid, no retroperitoneal injury, no solid organ injury; 2×2 cm hematoma around the right superior pelvic ramus, which is fractured but non-displaced

- Admit patient to monitored setting

- Pain control

- Serial hemoglobin checks

- Orthopedic consultation

Discussion

The primary survey of trauma involves **a**irway and cervical spinal cord; **b**reathing; **c**irculation; **d**isability; and **e**xposure/environment control (ABCDE).

Airway: Loss of airway function can lead to irreversible brain damage within minutes. Cervical spine control must be maintained during airway assessment and management. Possible methods are:

- Clear oropharynx of secretions: blood, mucus, and vomitus can be removed by suction

- Do jaw thrust to prevent tongue obstruction

- Remove dentures or loose teeth (potential obstructors of the airway in unconscious and semiconscious patients)

If the patient's condition as assessed by the Glasgow Coma Scale (GCS) is <8, the airway control of choice is endotracheal intubation.

- If endotracheal intubation is not possible (i.e., patient has a midface fracture), an immediate airway is achieved by cricothyroidotomy.

- If long-term airway management is required, then a tracheostomy can be placed subsequently to cricothyroidotomy.

- In a child age <12, cricothyroidotomy is contraindicated because of the risk of subglottic stenosis.

- In a child with a midface fracture, emergent airway control is achieved with needle cricothyroidotomy with pulse oxygen therapy, which allows brain oxygenation for 20–40 min but is inadequate for ventilation (carbon dioxide accumulation). However, it allows more time for a more definitive surgical tracheostomy.

Breathing: Assess for oxygen saturation, bilateral symmetric chest rise, and auscultate for breath sounds. Palpate the trachea for deviation and also the chest wall to check for fracture or emphysema (crepitus).

Tension pneumothorax is characterized by profound hypotension, distended neck veins, tachycardia, decreased breath sounds, and tracheal deviation to the opposite side. Fractured ribs or a penetrating injury to the chest are often the cause. (Rib fractures can also lead to a flail chest and hemothorax.) Air becomes trapped in pleural space; this results in a progressive buildup of tension on the affected hemithorax. Treatment is with needle thoracostomy in the midclavicular line at the second intercostal space or with tube thoracostomy in the midaxillary line at the fifth intercostal space.

Flail chest occurs with multiple rib fractures that allow a segment of the chest wall to cave in during inspiration and bulge out during expiration (paradoxical breathing). The real problem is the underlying pulmonary contusion. A contused lung is very sensitive to fluid overload, thus treatment includes fluid restriction, use of colloids, plasma or albumin, rather than crystalloids (regular IV fluids) and diuretics. Pulmonary dysfunction may develop, so arterial blood gases have to be monitored. Pulmonary contusion can be secondary to rib fracture or from penetrating or blunt chest injury. A contused lung is perfused but hypoventilated (ventilation–perfusion mismatch), leading to hypoxemia and to acute respiratory distress syndrome. If the patient desaturates in spite of supplemental oxygen and undergoes clinical respiratory embarrassment, intubation may become necessary. Always drain pleural spaces prophylactically even with no pneumothorax, before placing the flail chest cases on ventilators lest tension pneumothorax develops.

Hemothorax occurs when there is blood in the pleural space secondary to a rib fracture or a penetrating injury. A "white out" on a chest x-ray is diagnostic. The affected side will be dull to percussion. Treatment is urgent thoracostomy drainage. When bleeding is from a systemic vessel (typically an intercostal artery), thoracotomy is needed. Delayed treatment may cause complications such as empyema or fibrothorax. Factors which dictate the need for surgery include:

- Recovery of ≥1,500 mL of blood when chest tube is inserted into pleural space
- Discovery of ≥250 mL/h of blood in tube drainage over ensuing 4 hrs or 2.5 liter blood loss over 24 hrs

Circulation: Shock occurs in trauma by one of the following mechanisms:

- Cardiogenic: tension pneumothorax, cardiac tamponade, and air embolism
- Hypovolemic: hemorrhage, dehydration
- Neurogenic: spinal cord injury

Cardiac tamponade can result from blunt or penetrating chest trauma. It is characterized by Beck's triad: elevated jugular venous pressure, decreased BP, and muffled heart sounds. As little as 20 mL of blood in pericardial space can be hemodynamically significant. Treatment is with pericardiocentesis or open drainage.

Air embolism presents similarly with elevated jugular venous pressure and decreased BP, but there is sloshing—not muffled—heart sounds. It can be caused by iatrogenic injury (e.g., central line insertion), neck wound, or a pulmonary parenchymal laceration. Treatment includes placing the patient in the Trendelenburg position with the right side up, and performing thoracotomy with air aspiration.

CLINICAL PEARL

Needle thoracostomy is a one-way valve in which pleural pressure is greater than atmospheric pressure. This converts a tension pneumothorax to a simple pneumothorax. A chest tube is still required.

Hypovolemic shock is characterized by decreased BP, increased heart rate, cold and clammy skin, weak pulse, and oliguria. Treat with volume replacement, not pressors.

Neurogenic shock is characterized by decreased BP, decreased heart rate (inappropriate bradycardia), warm skin, loss of rectal tone, and loss of sweating. Treat with alpha-agonists (phenylephrine drip leads to pharmacologic restoration of sympathetic tone) and volume replacement.

All shock patients are monitored by good end-organ perfusion, as measured by adequate urine output and improvement of metabolic acidosis on arterial blood gas.

Disability: Neurologic evaluation including mental status as assessed by GCS and any focal neurologic deficits.

Exposure: Completely examine patient from head to toe; be sure to keep patient warm as trauma patients tend to be hypothermic and this can propagate coagulopathy and bleeding.

Secondary survey then ensues incorporating chest x-ray, pelvic x-ray, and FAST when indicated. CT scan may be necessary as outlined above. Should there be any deterioration in his clinical status, the appropriate interventions would be necessary based on the organ system involved. If respiratory deterioration develops, then repeat chest x-ray is indicated to exclude delayed pneumothorax or aspiration pneumonitis. The most commonly injured abdominal organs are the spleen and liver.

Management Blunt Trauma: Trauma evaluations, both in real life and on examinations, are standardized to take into account the variety of mechanisms of injury. Always stick with the ABCDE evaluation, followed by a secondary survey including proper imaging modalities.

- Blunt head trauma with loss of consciousness or retrograde amnesia or neurologic signs is an indication for head CT.

- Blunt abdominal trauma should raise alarms as to the operative ability as well as patient selection. After the initial volume replacement and FAST, if the patient appears STABLE, the best way to evaluate blunt abdominal trauma is CT scan of the abdomen and pelvis.

- Blunt chest trauma can be more easily evaluated based on examination and chest x-ray.

Final Diagnosis

Blunt trauma, nondisplaced pelvic fracture

CASE 3

Chief Complaint

"My foot hurts."

History and Physical Examination

A 67-year-old man comes to the emergency department complaining of an acute onset of left foot pain that began one hour ago. He denies any history of trauma or previous episodes such as this one. He still has feeling in the foot and is able to move it. The patient has a history of a myocardial infarction and atrial fibrillation. He stopped taking his warfarin 2 weeks ago for unclear reasons. He does not smoke. His only current medication is a beta-blocker.

Vital signs are temperature 37.0 C (98.6 F), BP 120/70 mm Hg, and pulse 70/min. His chest is clear to auscultation, heart rhythm is irregular, but without murmurs, and his abdomen is soft, nontender, and without any palpable masses. Examination of the extremities shows bilaterally strong femoral pulses. Right popliteal and pedal pulses are normal. Left popliteal and pedal pulses are absent. There is no evidence of chronic ischemic disease in either extremity. The left foot is pale and cool to the touch to the ankle. Sensation is intact, and there is voluntary motion. Thigh and calf muscles are soft and not tender to palpation.

Differential Diagnosis

1. Arterial embolus

   - Most likely diagnosis given history of atrial fibrillation without anticoagulation

2. Arterial thrombosis

   - Less likely, as this is due to chronic atherosclerotic disease and leads to long standing signs and symptoms of ischemia, which are not present

3. Gout

   - Can present as acute onset foot pain, but is typically localized to the first digit and not associated with loss of pulses

Initial Management

Setting: emergency department

Diagnostic/Therapeutic Plan

- Blood work
- CBC
- Comprehensive metabolic panel
- Creatinine phosphokinase (CPK)
- Coagulation profile
- Type and cross match
- EKG
- Chest x-ray

CLINICAL PEARL

Suspicion of ischemia should prompt concern for **compartment syndrome**. Edema of the lower extremity muscle compartments, which are fixed by their fascial investments, results in ischemia. This can cause an elevated CPK, which can result in acute kidney injury, but there is a delay in elevation of serum creatinine. An early rise in CPK or serum potassium is a sign of potential ischemia and should prompt urgent intervention.

Test Results

- Blood work: unremarkable other than INR 1.4
- CPK: normal
- EKG: atrial fibrillation at 70/min; no ST or T changes
- Chest x-ray: unremarkable

Assessment

The acute onset of pain in a lower extremity, associated with loss of pulses, is characteristic of an embolic event. Atrial fibrillation predisposes the patient to systemic emboli.

Further Management Plan

- Systemic heparinization
- Angiogram: sharp cutoff at level of the left popliteal artery with no filling of distal vessels
- Surgical embolectomy: fresh clot removed from distal arterial tree with good back bleeding and restoration of popliteal and pedal pulses; if evidence of limb ischemia or prolonged delay from onset of symptoms to intervention (>6 hours), perform a lower extremity fasciotomy

Discussion

In 70% of cases, acute embolic occlusion occurs as a result of embolic material originating in the heart. This is typically due to stagnant flow due to one of the following:

- Atrial fibrillation
- Post-myocardial infarction
- Endocarditis
- Aortic dissection
- Ulcerated plaque in the aorta
- Arterial trauma
- Iatrogenic injury

Classic presentation is the "5 P's":

- Pallor
- Pain
- Paralysis
- Pulselessness
- Poikilothermia

The time interval between onset of pain and presentation is critical, as irreversible ischemia can develop after 6 hours of occlusion.

- All patients should be heparinized and immediate angiogram performed.

- If angiogram confirms diagnosis of embolism, emergent embolectomy is indicated.

- If the patient presents late (4–6 hours) after the onset of pain, perform an emergent embolectomy with an on-table angiogram because there is no time for a preoperative workup.

Basic Science Correlate

The "Ps" of acute arterial embolism primarily involve the sensory nerves, which are quite sensitive to ischemia: paresthesia, pain, and poikilothermia. Motor nerves are much more resilient than sensory nerves and can generally withstand ischemia better; therefore, when a patient has paralysis, this reflects very severe ischemia and should prompt a higher level of concern.

Ongoing ischemia, as well as post-embolectomy reperfusion injury, can lead to swelling and ultimately, compartment syndrome. The resultant myoglobinuria can lead to nephropathy, hyperkalemia, malignant arrhythmia, and death. Compartment pressures should be evaluated either by physical exam or direct invasive pressure monitoring.

- Elevated compartment pressures consistent with compartment syndrome should be treated with fasciotomy to relieve the edema.

- Elevated potassium and serum creatinine should be treated with aggressive fluid resuscitation, sodium bicarbonate to alkalinize the urine and increase clearance, and hemodialysis if necessary.

Follow-up Management and Prevention

After recovery from this acute event, the patient should be restarted on systemic anticoagulation. Management of atrial fibrillation can include rate control with a beta-blocker or another class of anti-arrhythmics and potentially electrical cardioversion.

Final Diagnosis

Arterial embolization

NOTE

On the exam, vignettes may include a patient who has a stiff and painful compartment with normal vascular exam and capillary refill. These normal findings can make the diagnosis of compartment syndrome difficult and can delay decompressive fasciotomy.

- If one waits for absent pulses to diagnose compartment syndrome, it's already too late and ischemia has progressed to necrosis. Ischemia is reversible, but necrosis is not. The only option left will be amputation.

- Be sure to keep a low threshold for diagnosis of compartment syndrome and err toward fasciotomy when in doubt. That is the safest answer for the Step 3 exam.

CASE 4

Chief Complaint

"My belly hurts."

History and Physical Examination

A 33-year-old woman comes to the emergency department complaining of increasing RUQ pain that began earlier in the day. She has a fever and chills, and had an episode of emesis this evening. She has had similar type pain in the past but never this severe. It is typically associated with bloating after eating fatty foods and is sometimes accompanied by anorexia. The attacks usually last a few hours to 1 day. She denies jaundice or a change in color of stool or urine.

She is a well-appearing female in mild distress. Vital signs are temperature 38.3 C (101 F), BP 130/70 mm Hg, and pulse 105/min. Her skin is not jaundiced and sclera are nonicteric. Heart and lung examinations are normal. Abdominal examination shows marked RUQ and midepigastric tenderness with rebound tenderness and some mild guarding. No discreet masses are palpable. The peritoneal signs seem to be localized to the RUQ. Rectal examination is unremarkable. Pelvic examination is unremarkable with no bleeding or adnexal masses.

Differential Diagnosis

1. Acute cholecystitis

   - Most likely diagnosis given the patient's demographics and history

2. Acute cholangitis

   - Possible based on physical exam, fever, and tachycardia; however, patient is non-icteric and would be expected to be in more acute distress

3. Pancreatitis

   - Possible given history and physical

4. Ulcer disease

   - History is compatible but physical exam makes this less likely and fever unexplained without frank perforation, which would result in a more acute presentation

5. Viral hepatitis

   - Typically has more indolent symptoms with less acuity

6. Appendicitis

   - Possible given history and physical, and can result in RUQ and not RLQ tenderness

7. Ruptured ovarian cyst

   - Must be considered in any woman of childbearing age, but is less likely to present with upper abdominal symptoms; a negative pelvic exam makes this less likely

8. Ectopic pregnancy

   - Must be ruled out in any woman of childbearing age, but typically presents with lower abdominal pain and evidence of hemorrhage

9. Renal colic

   - Can present as upper abdominal pain, but less likely given post-prandial symptoms and patient demographics

---

CCS NOTE

Be sure to select a HEENT exam to check for scleral icterus.

Initial Management

Setting: emergency department

Diagnostic/Therapeutic Plan

- CBC with differential
- Serum electrolytes with lipase
- Abdominal x-ray
- Urinalysis, urine HCG

Test Results

- CBC: WBC count 15,000/mm^3
- Serum electrolytes with lipase: normal
- Abdominal x-ray: RUQ calcification; normal bowel gas pattern; no pneumoperitoneum
- Urinalysis, urine HCG: urinalysis without blood cells, HCG negative for pregnancy

Assessment

A 33-year-old woman with recurrent post-prandial RUQ pain, fever, tachycardia, and RUQ tenderness on physical exam has acute cholecystitis until proven otherwise. Additional evaluation will help confirm this diagnosis.

Further Management Plan

1. RUQ U/S: gallstones present in gallbladder with a mildly thickened wall; the common bile duct is normal in size
2. HIDA scan: nonvisualization of gallbladder after 4 hrs, with emptying into the duodenum indicative of cystic duct obstruction; this test is indicated only if U/S fails to definitively diagnose cholecystitis
3. NPO
4. IV antibiotics
5. Cholecystectomy

Discussion

Cholecystitis is a complication of gallstones. Most gallstones are asymptomatic; however, they can cause biliary colic, which is characterized by RUQ pain radiating to the back along with nausea and vomiting. Pain is colicky and builds up to a crescendo. It is usually associated with fatty foods and results from intermittent obstruction of a cystic duct with stones.

In acute cholecystitis, the stone gets impacted in the cystic duct and causes continuous, unyielding, RUQ pain with signs of localized peritonitis (Murphy's sign), leukocytosis, and fever. If not treated, acute cholecystitis can progress to gangrenous cholecystitis and perforation of the gallbladder, which could lead to biliary peritonitis.

Cholecystitis must be differentiated from cholangitis, another dangerous complication of gallstones. With cholangitis, the gallbladder is not obstructed but the escaped stones have obstructed the common bile duct (choledocholithiasis). This biliary stasis can lead to infection with *E. coli* (90% of cases) or less commonly, *Klebsiella*.

CLINICAL PEARL

Murphy's sign is often erroneously documented as pain upon palpation of the right upper quadrant; it is actually defined as cessation of inspiration during palpation of the abdomen and is due to the downward motion of the inflamed gallbladder against the anterior abdominal wall and the examiner's hand as the diaphragm descends during inspiration.

Cholangitis is characterized by Charcot's triad of RUQ pain, fever, and jaundice. If untreated, it can progress to Reynold's pentad, which is Charcot's triad plus hypotension and mental status changes. This is a perimoribund condition requiring immediate decompression of the biliary tree, either by percutaneous transhepatic cholangiography (PTC), endoscopic retrograde cholangiopancreatography (ERCP), or operative exploration and decompression. Operative exploration is reserved as a last resort as PTC or ERCP are associated with a decreased morbidity.

Calculous cholecystitis is the most common type of cholecystitis, but acalculous cholecystitis (diagnosed with HIDA scan) and biliary dyskinesia (diagnosed with CCK-HIDA scan) are sometimes seen as well. The CCK-HIDA exploits the function of the endogenous hormone that contracts the gallbladder and relaxes the sphincter of Oddi, which is normally released in response to fats and amino acids into the duodenum.

CLINICAL PEARL

Always check the coagulation profile in cases of obstructed bile duct, as bile is needed for vitamin K absorption (as well as Vitamins A, D, and E).

Final Diagnosis

Acute cholecystitis

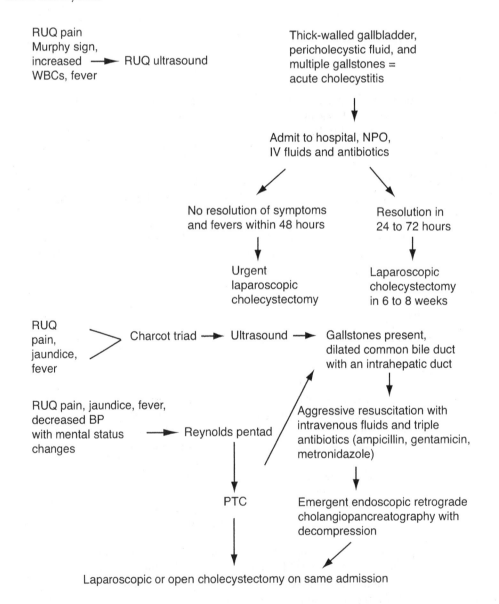

Follow-up Management and Prevention

In cases of acute cholecystitis, the established practice for decades has been urgent cholecystectomy done laparoscopically. When laparoscopy was first introduced, the practice was to first stabilize the patient with antibiotics and then do an elective laparoscopic cholecystectomy. That is no longer the case, as there has been extensive research studying this approach.

Furthermore, if a patient has gallstones complicated by acute pancreatitis, one should first rest the pancreas by keeping the patient NPO, and consider surgical removal of the gallbladder only once the pain and lipase levels stabilize. One should try to perform the surgery during the same admission period to decrease the chances of further attacks of pancreatitis if the patient is allowed to go home without cholecystectomy.

The same principles apply to cholangitis, which require biliary decompression with ERCP followed by laparoscopic cholecystectomy on the same admission.

After cholecystectomy, fatty foods will be more difficult to digest as the GI tract relies on active biliary secretion by the liver and there is no reservoir to store excess bile. Accordingly, patients should be counseled to avoid eating large amounts of fatty foods, or the malabsorption will result in symptoms of diarrhea.

CASE 5

Chief Complaint

Abdominal distention

History and Physical Examination

A 65-year-old man comes to the emergency department complaining of abdominal distention. He has been in his usual state of health, but in the last 2 weeks has had a sense of fullness in the lower abdomen. Yesterday he stopped passing gas, did not have any bowel movement, and became markedly more distended over the course of the night. He has vomited once and is somewhat nauseated since then. He also notes a 10-lb weight loss over the last 3 months. He has recently noted that he is having more constipation with occasional diarrhea and stringier-looking bowel movements. He denies gross blood but notices mucus and occasional dark stool. He denies dysuria. He has no significant past medical history.

The patient is a somewhat thin, pale-appearing male in no apparent distress. Vital signs are temperature 37.0 C (98.6 F), BP 100/70 mm Hg, and pulse 110/min. Physical examination shows a non-tender, distended abdomen with hypoactive bowel sounds and tympany on percussion. There are no surgical scars, hernias, or palpable masses. There is no hepatomegaly. Rectal examination shows that the vault is empty with no stool available for guaiac-staining.

Differential Diagnosis

1. Large bowel obstruction secondary to a mass

   - Tympany and distention are consistent with an air-filled hollow viscus such as the bowel; the lack of upper GI symptoms such as vomiting and lack of stool in the rectal vault support a large bowel obstruction

2. Diverticulitis

   - Can present with abdominal distention but typically have fever and tenderness as well

3. Pseudo-obstruction (Ogilvie's syndrome)

   - Will present with same symptoms as a true large bowel obstruction and should be considered, but this patient does not have the typical risk factors

4. Sigmoid volvulus

   - Can present with same symptoms as large bowel obstruction and should be considered, but is more common in the elderly, sedentary patient, often with chronic constipation. It also presents more acutely than the patient described in this vignette.

Initial Management

- CBC

- Serum electrolytes

- Abdominal x-ray

Test Results

- CBC: hemoglobin 10 g/dL

- Serum electrolytes: BUN 28 mg/dL, creatinine 1.4 mg/dL

- Abdominal x-ray: dilated small bowel with air-fluid levels and air in right colon; no air visualized in left colon or pelvis

Assessment

This patient has a large bowel obstruction. Tympany on percussion indicates large amounts of air in the abdomen. The lack of tenderness and fever on the clinical exam goes against the diagnosis of an inflammatory process such as diverticulitis. Although diverticulosis without diverticulitis could explain the low hemoglobin, it typically presents with active rectal bleeding, not dark stool associated with a slow bleeding process.

The abdominal x-ray excludes volvulus and pseudo obstruction. Overall, the lack of tenderness, the obstruction, stool changes, and slowly developing anemia point to a mass that is likely a neoplasm.

Further Management Plan

- Inpatient admission

- NPO

- IV hydration

- Nasogastric tube placement (for proximal decompression)

- Rigid sigmoidoscopy: negative for any lesions up to 20 cm

- Contrast enema study: filling of the colon from the rectum to the mid-descending colon then an abrupt cutoff with no passage of contrast in the rest of the colon.

- After resuscitation, exploratory laparotomy, possible bowel resection and colostomy creation.

Basic Science Correlate

Obstruction results in bowel edema and decreased oral intake, which leads to dehydration, which results in electrolyte disturbances. Specifically, potassium and magnesium are vital for bowel motility, and therefore hypokalemia and hypomagnesemia worsen the obstruction, causing a vicious cycle. These electrolytes must be aggressively repleted during resuscitation.

Discussion

Ten percent of left-sided colon cancers present as acute colonic obstruction with abdominal distension, constipation, pain, and vomiting. Plain abdominal x-ray may reveal a massively dilated colon to the point of obstruction with a sudden cutoff point and with no gas in the distal colon and rectum. The patient should be resuscitated with IV fluids. Diagnosis is confirmed by water-soluble contrast enema and colonoscopy, followed by emergent surgery.

CLINICAL PEARL

In small bowel obstruction, use oral water-soluble or barium contrast (eg, upper GI study with small bowel follow-through) judiciously, as the study is proximal to the obstruction and reflux of contrast can cause vomiting. The osmotic gradient from hypertonic water-soluble oral contrast may help resolve partial obstruction. Contrast may be safely used in an enema study, as it is distal to the obstruction.

CLINICAL PEARL

Hartmann's procedure refers to sigmoid resection with end colostomy and closure of the distal rectum. Reversal of this operation at a later time refers to closure of the colostomy and reconnection of the bowel ends. Although this strategy was first described in reference to the management of sigmoid carcinoma (now typically done in a single stage), it is now primarily used to refer to the management of acute sigmoid diverticulitis.

Abdominoperineal resection refers to resection of the rectum all the way to the anus with surgical closure of the anus and a permanent end colostomy. This is done in cases where the rectal carcinoma has invaded the anal muscles or when the cancer originates within the anus.

Preoperative colonoscopy may help differentiate between mechanical obstruction of the colon due to tumor and functional obstruction without a mass, i.e., Ogilvie's syndrome; however, extreme care must be taken to not insufflate the bowel too much as extremely dilated bowel is at risk for perforation and peritonitis. Whereas obstructing colon carcinoma is treated surgically, treatment of Ogilvie's syndrome is primarily medical. The operative options are either one stage or two:

- Primary resection with anastomosis if bowel is not too dilated and patient is stable
- Proximal diverting loop colostomy followed by resection of the tumor and anastomosis at a later time

In the elective setting, colon cancer presents with a history of altered bowel habits, weight loss, anorexia, anemia, and in some cases, altered or fresh bleeding from the rectum. Most right-sided causes present with weight loss, anorexia, and anemia. Most left-sided causes present with obstructive symptoms (cecal diameter is larger than left colon diameter, and obstruction is seen in very advanced cases of cecal cancer only). For the same reason, left colon cancer is symptomatic earlier in its course and hence has a better prognosis compared with right colon lesions. Right-sided-colon cancers, in addition to presenting with anemia, can present with "slimy" diarrhea-due to the mucinous nature of these right colon cancers

Diagnosis of colon cancer is with a colonoscopy and biopsy (gold standard). The entire colon must be evaluated even if a lesion is found in order to rule out a synchronous lesion. If this is discovered, treatment of choice is a total abdominal colectomy, and not two or more segmental resections.

To determine the stage of the disease, use chest x-ray and CT scan. Bowel preparation is with polyethylene glycol 3350/electrolytes oral solution and antibiotics, and radical resection is indicated for a tumor and its draining lymph nodes. If a left-sided tumor is identified, either on colonoscopy or contrast study, a complete colonoscopy must be performed to rule out synchronous tumors in the right or transverse colon.

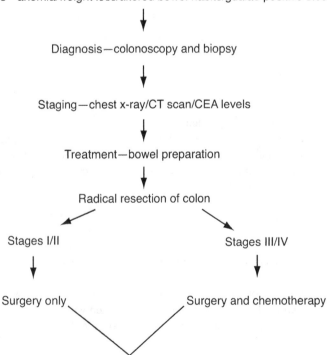

Carcinoma of Colon

Symptoms—anemia/weight loss/altered bowel habits/guaiac-positive stools

↓

Diagnosis—colonoscopy and biopsy

↓

Staging—chest x-ray/CT scan/CEA levels

↓

Treatment—bowel preparation

↓

Radical resection of colon

Stages I/II   Stages III/IV

Surgery only   Surgery and chemotherapy

Follow-up—chest x-ray/CEA/CT scan, colonoscopy/PET scan

Postoperative Staging

Dukes A Stage I	• Muscularis is free of invasion 90% • 5-year survival
Dukes B Stage II	• Penetrates muscularis 60–80% • 5-year survival
Dukes C Stage III	• Lymph nodes positive 20–50% • 5-year survival
Dukes D Stage IV	• Distant metastasis <5% • 5-year survival

Adjuvant Treatment

Stages I and II	Colon carcinoma: surgery and close follow-up
Stages II and III	Colon carcinoma: surgery and chemotherapy; 5-fluorouracil plus levamisole or leucovorin

Radiotherapy has no standard role in advanced colon cancer.

Follow-Up

Year 1	Every 3 months CEA and LFTs every 3 months
Year 2	Every 6 months Colonoscopy and chest x-ray yearly
Year 3+	PET scan and CT scan if CEA levels rise

For rectal cancer, surgery should be performed in stage I, or surgery and radiotherapy in stages II and III.

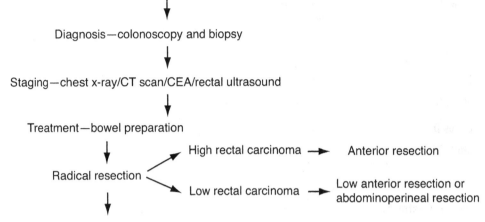

Rectal Cancer

Symptoms—bright-red blood per rectum/altered bowel habits/mass on digital rectal examination

Diagnosis—colonoscopy and biopsy

Staging—chest x-ray/CT scan/CEA/rectal ultrasound

Treatment—bowel preparation

Radical resection

High rectal carcinoma → Anterior resection

Low rectal carcinoma → Low anterior resection or abdominoperineal resection

Stage I: surgery only
Stages II and III: chemotherapy and radiation, with surgery to follow

Follow-up as for colon cancer

Follow-up Management and Prevention

Ideally, colon cancer is managed electively and a metastatic workup is performed. However, when patients present in extremis, e.g., with large bowel obstruction, they must be managed immediately and evaluated later for the possibility of distant disease.

In this patient, chest x-ray can be performed at admission to evaluate for pulmonary nodules, and post-operatively serum LFTs and CT scan of the abdomen to evaluate for liver metastasis.

- If neurologic symptoms suggestive of brain metastases are present, MRI of the brain is indicated.

- If distant disease is present, post-operative chemo- and radiotherapy are indicated.

- Depending on the pathological stage of the tumor, systemic chemotherapy may be indicated for this patient.

Screening for colon cancer in patients with no risk factors begins at age 50 with a colonoscopy. Historically, flexible sigmoidoscopy and serial fecal occult blood testing were utilized, but in the current era—and on the exam—colonoscopy has a higher sensitivity and an acceptably low morbidity.

Risk factors that determine an earlier screening age include:

- Strong family history

- History of familial cancer syndromes

- IBD

Appropriate screening allows for earlier diagnosis and intervention and thereby a lower mortality from colon cancer.

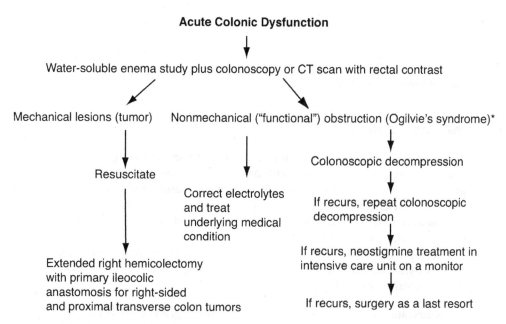

Acute Colonic Dysfunction

Water-soluble enema study plus colonoscopy or CT scan with rectal contrast

Mechanical lesions (tumor)

Nonmechanical ("functional") obstruction (Ogilvie's syndrome)*

Resuscitate

Correct electrolytes and treat underlying medical condition

Colonoscopic decompression

If recurs, repeat colonoscopic decompression

Extended right hemicolectomy with primary ileocolic anastomosis for right-sided and proximal transverse colon tumors

If recurs, neostigmine treatment in intensive care unit on a monitor

If recurs, surgery as a last resort

*Ogilvie's syndrome is associated with hypertonic colonic segment (usually splenic flexure), which fails to relax secondary to imbalance between colonic sympathetic and parasympathetic. It is associated with electrolyte imbalance (potassium), vertebral fractures, traumatic retroperitoneal bleeds, and pneumonias. Sometimes, obstructed sigmoid colon cancer can present like acute diverticulitis. CT scan will not differentiate between the two entities.

Final Diagnosis
Large bowel obstruction secondary to colon cancer

CASE 6

Chief Complaint

Abdominal pain with nausea and vomiting

History and Physical Examination

A 67-year-old woman comes to the emergency department complaining of diffuse, crampy, abdominal pain with nausea and vomiting. The pain began gradually in the epigastrium 2 days ago, is crampy in nature, and in the last 24 hours has worsened. She reports some current nausea and vomiting. The pain is somewhat relieved after vomiting. The patient's last bowel movement, or passage of flatus, was last night. She was well and on no medications prior to this episode. Her past medical history is significant for a hysterectomy for fibroids 2 years ago. She denies any recent change in bowel or bladder habits or any groin, vulvar, or thigh pain.

Her temperature is 37.0 C (98.6 F), BP is 120/70 mm Hg, and pulse is 110/min. Her abdomen is distended and tympanitic with hyperactive bowel sounds. It is non-tender with no peritoneal signs. There is a lower midline scar extending from the umbilicus to the suprapubic region. No incisional hernias are palpated. There are no inguinal masses or vulvar masses identified. Rectal examination shows a minimal amount of guaiac-negative stool. Pelvic examination is negative for masses and tenderness. The remainder of the physical examination is unremarkable.

Differential Diagnosis

1. SBO secondary to adhesions
2. SBO secondary to incarcerated hernia
3. Biliary tract disease with pancreatitis
4. Gastric outlet obstruction secondary to ulcer disease
5. Gastroenteritis

Initial Management

- CBC
- Serum electrolytes, LFTs, and amylase/lipase
- Abdominal x-ray

Test Results

- CBC: significant for WBC 10,000/mm³ and hemoglobin 14 mg/dL
- Serum electrolytes, LFTs, amylase/lipase: significant for BUN 28 mg/dL, creatinine 1.3 mg/dL, and amylase 40 U/L
- Abdominal x-ray: dilated small bowel with multiple air-fluid levels and air in the colon

CLINICAL PEARL

Never use barium for an antegrade study because its viscous nature can worsen an obstruction. Use water-soluble contrast judiciously, as it can injure the pulmonary epithelium and result in aspiration pneumonitis if vomited.

Assessment

The history, physical, laboratory, and radiologic studies are all consistent with a small bowel obstruction. These are most commonly due to adhesions from prior surgery, hernias, or intra-abdominal malignancies.

Pancreatitis is unlikely with amylase 40 U/L and abdominal x-rays showing obstruction rather than an ileus.

Further Management Plan

- Nasogastric tube placement: will decompress the GI tract and hopefully allow the obstruction to self-resolve. At the very least the patient will feel better and prevent vomiting.

- IV fluid administration: bowel edema leads to intravascular hypovolemia and dehydration, as evidenced by this patient's BUN and creatinine.

- Foley catheter placement: vital signs and urine output are the best indicators of adequate resuscitation.

- Admit to surgical ward for serial physical exams; if abdominal exam worsens or patient shows evidence of peritonitis consistent with bowel ischemia or perforation, immediate operative exploration is warranted. Operation at the minimum is a lysis of adhesions, and could potentially require a bowel resection if the intestine is too ischemic or frankly gangrenous.

Basic Science Correlate

The most common electrolyte disturbance seen with a SBO is hypochloremic metabolic alkalosis with hypokalemia from loss of gastric contents. Potassium must be aggressively repleted to prevent dysrhythmias as well as to improve bowel motility.

Discussion

The primary features of SBO are crampy abdominal pain, vomiting, and constipation or obstipation (no bowel movement or flatus). The most common causes of SBOs are post-operative adhesions, hernias, and tumors. It is crucial to distinguish small bowel obstruction as mechanical/functional and complete/incomplete.

A **mechanical** obstruction is due to a physical blockage, such as scar tissue (adhesions), a fascial defect (hernia), or a mass. This should be differentiated from a paralytic ileus, which occurs secondary to surgery in the immediate postoperative period and is a **functional** problem.

An **incomplete** small bowel obstruction typically presents with intermittent, colicky abdominal pain (crescendo–decrescendo pattern). Patients are able to pass flatus, and an abdominal radiograph shows multiple air-fluid levels with gas in the rectum. Patients have a soft, nontender abdomen, with no leukocytosis or fever. The following treatment will resolve 75% of cases:

- Making the patient NPO
- Administration of IV fluids
- Placement of nasogastric tube
- Serial radiographs (kidney, ureter, bladder)
- Physical examinations

If the patient's pain worsens, if leukocytosis progresses, if radiographs show persistent small-bowel dilatation, or if the patient does not move the bowels by 12 hours of nonoperative management, surgery is essential.

Complete obstruction typically presents with absolute constipation; constant, unyielding pain with signs of peritonitis; leukocytosis; increased fever; and increased heart rate. Radiographs may show multiple air-fluid levels with no gas in the rectum. Aggressive management with isotonic fluids is required, along with surgical exploration before gangrene of the bowel sets in.

Prognosis of small bowel obstruction is as follows:

- Complete: 8% mortality
- Gangrene: 25% mortality
- Incomplete: 2% mortality

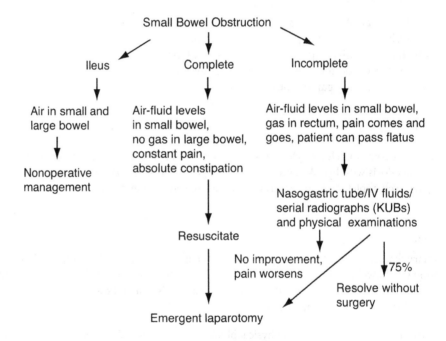

Follow-up Management and Prevention

Unfortunately, managing patients with bowel obstructions surgically continues the vicious cycle: more scar tissue develops, putting the patient at risk for future obstruction from adhesions.

There is some evidence that laparoscopic surgery decreases the amount of intra-abdominal inflammation and therefore scar tissue, so the long-term risk of small bowel obstruction is lower. Intra- and post-operative hemorrhage is also a risk factor for future adhesions, so meticulous hemostasis must be obtained at every single operation.

CT scan is critical to diagnosing the obstruction and identifying the transition point. This is augmented by oral contrast, though care must be taken when administering to avoid vomiting and even worsening the obstruction. IV contrast can define the bowel wall and identify areas of ischemia, but should be used judiciously as it can be nephrotoxic, especially in a patient who already has an acute kidney injury from dehydration.

If the patient is not in extremis, a reasonable strategy is to resuscitate with IV fluids for several hours, place a nasogastric tube to decompress the proximal GI tract, and then perform CT scan with oral and IV contrast.

Patients should be adequately screened for age- and gender-appropriate malignancies, including colon, rectal, cervical, and prostate. Successful screening could prevent late diagnosis when a mass has already invaded other structures resulting in an obstruction.

Final Diagnosis

Small bowel obstruction

CLINICAL PEARL

The Step 3 exam vignettes can help direct the management of the patient when read carefully. All SBO cases fall into operative versus non-operative management. The key is in the patient's history.

- If the patient has **intermittent pain** with periods of no pain, it is likely a partial obstruction and hope for a non-operative resolution remains valid.

- If the patient has **persistent pain** with no relief, it is likely an early sign of ischemia of an obstructed bowel loop; one need not wait for fever, leucocytosis or even worse, frank peritonitis, to take surgical action.

Good surgical management of SBO entails intervention when the bowel is ischemic and not necrotic.

CASE 7

Chief Complaint

Irregular heartbeat and severe abdominal pain

History and Physical Examination

A 74-year-old woman with a history of atrial fibrillation is brought to the emergency department because of a sudden onset of severe, diffuse abdominal pain. There is no nausea, vomiting, or recent change in bowel habits. There are no urinary symptoms. She stopped taking her warfarin 3 weeks ago due to insurance problems. She is very uncomfortable and writhing in pain. Her temperature is 37.0 C (98.6 F), blood pressure 140/90 mm Hg, pulse 105/min, and respirations 30/min.

Upon physical examination the heartbeat is irregular with variable S1. The lungs are clear. The abdomen is slightly distended with hypoactive bowel sounds. She is diffusely tender without guarding, rigidity, or rebound; there are no pulsatile masses. Rectal examination shows brown stool that is trace guaiac-positive; there are no rectal masses.

Differential Diagnosis

1. Mesenteric ischemia
2. Perforated viscus
3. Pancreatitis
4. Appendicitis
5. Diverticulitis

Initial Management

Setting: emergency department

Diagnostic/Therapeutic Plan

- Blood work: CBC with differential, serum electrolytes, lactic acid, LFTs, lipase, and arterial blood gas
- Abdominal x-ray
- Chest x-ray

Test Results

- WBC 13,000/mm^3; potassium 5.3 mM; amylase 54 U/L; pH 7.26; lactic acid 2.6 mg/dL
- X-rays: slightly distended small bowel, no evidence of obstruction, no pneumoperitoneum, no infiltrate

Assessment

Any of the diagnoses in the differential could cause abdominal pain. Diverticulitis and appendicitis are less likely because of the sudden onset of symptoms. They are often associated with fever, though this is an unreliable sign in an elderly patient who can be afebrile in the presence of sepsis. Diffuse tenderness indicates peritonitis, but the lack of free air on x-ray helps exclude perforated viscus.

The lack of guarding or rebound tenderness, guaiac-positive stools, sudden onset, and atrial fibrillation point to a diagnosis of mesenteric ischemia. Mesenteric ischemia is classically associated with "pain out of proportion to physical findings."

Further Management Plan

1. Emergency mesenteric angiography: sharp cutoff several centimeters from the origin of the superior mesenteric artery

2. Systemic heparinization

3. Surgical exploration for embolectomy and possible bowel resection if gangrenous changes are found.

Discussion

Atrial fibrillation predisposes this patient to systemic embolization of cardiac thrombus, which may travel to the mesenteric artery. Warfarin anticoagulation prevents cardiac thrombus, which is the source of these emboli, and the patient has stopped taking hers. Also, because she is not currently anticoagulated, the guaiac-positive stool also suggests mucosal damage secondary to ischemia.

Mesenteric vascular disease is classified as acute vs. chronic and arterial vs. venous. In this case, the patient has acute arterial mesenteric vascular disease.

Acute mesenteric occlusion is most commonly seen in the superior mesenteric artery. Most often, it involves:

- Cardiac patient with history of atrial fibrillation on warfarin and is noncompliant

- Patient recently admitted to cardiac care unit after an acute myocardial infarction who has developed arrhythmia

- Usually followed by "severe" abdominal pain; however, on clinical examination the abdomen is soft and nontender (typically referred to as "pain out of proportion to physical findings")

- Increased WBC, increased potassium, and persistent metabolic acidosis may also be seen

- Diagnosis is based on a high index of suspicion

- Gold standard test is mesenteric angiogram

- Treatment is emergent embolectomy and resection of the obviously necrotic bowel segment with anastomosis

The bowel may not always be well-demarcated between grossly ischemic and grossly necrotic segment. In these cases, a 'second-look operation' 24-48 hours later is done to reassess whether a bowel that looked suspiciously nonviable in the first operation is truly necrotic. This approach helps to preserve bowel length and avoid short gut syndrome.

CLINICAL PEARL

Although all of the differential diagnoses must be considered, think mesenteric ischemia when there are no significant findings on physical exam.

Chronic mesenteric ischemia is seen in elderly patients with atherosclerosis and is caused by atherosclerotic stenosis of the superior mesenteric artery and collateral blood flow to intestines. The classic presentation is "abdominal angina" (post-prandial pain). This leads to "food fear," an avoidance of food, and eventual malnutrition and weight loss. Diagnosis is established with a mesenteric angiogram. Some patients have mild atherosclerotic disease that is exacerbated with dehydration, and can be managed with IV hydration and anticoagulation alone; more severe cases require surgical bypass of the affected area using an autologous vein or a synthetic vascular graft.

The most common cause of venous occlusion of the portal vein is typically seen in hypercoagulable patients, i.e., protein C and S deficiency, antithrombin III deficiency, factor V Leiden, and homocysteinemia. It often presents with abdominal pain, distension, diarrhea, or an incidental finding on laparotomy. CT scan confirms the diagnosis. Treatment is nonsurgical when attempting to correct hypercoagulation with long-term anticoagulation with warfarin. Surgery is needed only if gangrene of the bowel is suspected. No attempt should be made to thrombectomize the portal vein.

Follow-up Management and Prevention

Atrial fibrillation must be managed to avoid the development of thrombus in the left atrial appendage that is at risk for embolization. Management includes anti-arrhythmic medications and systemic anticoagulation, and possibly electrical cardioversion if no current thrombus is visualized on echocardiography.

Final Diagnosis

Ischemic bowel disease

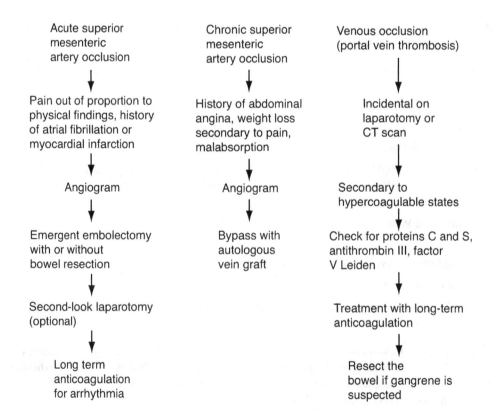

CASE 8

Chief Complaint

Sudden onset of pain in the groin and lower abdomen

History and Physical Examination

A 16-year-old boy comes to the emergency department complaining of sudden onset groin and lower-abdominal pain. He experienced severe lower-abdominal and scrotal pain causing him to double over during football practice. He denies any trauma to the groin, hematuria, or dysuria. He is not sexually active. He is currently nauseous.

His temperature is 37.0 C (98.6 F). He is a healthy-appearing male in moderate to severe distress. The examination is all WNL, except for a swollen, mildly erythematous, right-sided scrotal sac with extreme testicular tenderness, slight elevation, and a horizontal orientation of the right testicle as compared with the left. There is no adenopathy. There is no prostatic tenderness or mass on rectal examination. No groin hernia is palpable, but it is difficult to assess the right side.

Differential Diagnosis

1. Testicular torsion

2. Incarcerated inguinal hernia

3. Tumor hemorrhage

4. Epididymitis

5. Orchitis

Initial Management

Setting: emergency department

Diagnostic/Therapeutic Plan

- CBC

- Urinalysis

- Abdominal x-ray

Test Results

- CBC: normal

- Urinalysis: no WBCs

- X-ray: no dilated bowel

CLINICAL PEARL

Order an abdominal x-ray to look for signs of a hernia (e.g., dilated small bowel, air below inguinal ligament).

Assessment

The sudden onset of groin pain and the lack of white cells in the urine or blood go against an infectious process such as epididymitis or orchitis. In addition, the patient is not sexually active, making him less likely to have these infections. Although his history is consistent with a possible incarcerated hernia, the physical examination did not show a hernia mass. Because his exam was difficult, the abdominal x-ray also helps exclude this diagnosis, as no bowel loop is visibly trapped below the level of the inguinal ligament. The sudden, extreme pain, the horizontal orientation, and elevation of the testicle are classic for torsion. Cancer cannot be absolutely excluded by clinical examination and is dependent on tissue diagnosis.

Further Management Plan

- Immediate surgical detorsion (untwisting) and bilateral orchiopexy

Discussion

This patient needs to undergo immediate surgical exploration to physically correct (untwist) the testicular torsion and affix the testicle (orchiopexy) to the surrounding soft tissue to prevent recurrent torsion. A bilateral orchiopexy should be performed to prevent future contralateral torsion. This must be treated as a surgical emergency, as the only hope of salvaging the testicle is to restore blood flow within a few hours.

Testicular torsion results from a congenital defect in fixation. The problem is due to a high insertion of the tunica vaginalis, which allows for 360° torsion of poorly fixated testicles. This defect is by definition bilateral, so one should always fix both sides.

Also, if the testicle is obviously necrotic (delay in treatment beyond 4 hrs), it must be removed before an auto-immune reaction attacks the sperm, rendering the child sterile for life.

Testicular necrosis can occur within 6 hours. This patient's clinical history and the horizontal orientation of the testicle on examination are pathognomonic for torsion. A nuclear-medicine scan to evaluate the testicle for blood flow (decreased in torsion, increased in inflammation) would delay time in getting to the operating room and could result in testicular loss. If unusual findings, such as a tumor, are noted in operating room, biopsy and resection would be undertaken as indicated.

CLINICAL PEARL

When a presentation is atypical, U/S or nuclear scan is very helpful in the diagnosis. Viability can be determined visually and, if necessary, by biopsy.

Follow-up Management and Prevention

Post-operatively, follow-up with urology should be at around 1 week to assess scrotal wound healing and evaluate for hematoma. No long-term sequelae should develop from this problem.

Bilateral orchiopexy is performed at the time of operation to prevent torsion of the contralateral testis.

Final Diagnosis

Testicular torsion

CASE 9

Chief Complaint

"He's been stabbed!"

History and Physical Examination

An 18-year-old man is brought to the emergency department with a stab wound to the mid-abdomen. He was stabbed approximately 20 minutes earlier with a 6-inch butcher knife while backing away from his attacker. He has been awake and alert and is brought to the emergency department by paramedics who report stable vital signs in transit. Past medical history is negative. Tetanus immunization is up to date. The patient is awake and alert with an adequate airway; he is breathing without difficulty. His BP is 120/70 mm Hg and pulse is 90/min.

Upon physical examination the head is without trauma, neck is without tenderness, and chest is clear bilaterally. The abdomen is soft and non-tender. There is a 1-inch stab wound to the right abdominal wall below the umbilicus, but there is no active bleeding or large hematoma. There is no peritonitis on examination, and he is mildly tender only at the stab site. Rectal examination is unremarkable, and the prostate is in normal position. Extremities are without injury.

Differential Diagnosis

1. Superficial skin laceration
2. Rectus laceration
3. Intra-abdominal injury

Initial Management

Setting: emergency department

Diagnostic/Therapeutic Plan

- Blood work: CBC, electrolytes, type and cross match
- Foley catheter placement
- Chest and abdominal x-rays

Test Results

- Blood work normal
- Foley catheter: no blood
- X-rays: no pneumoperitoneum, no pleural effusion

Assessment

The patient was "moving away" while stabbed, making severe injury less likely. The central issue in evaluating a stab wound is to determine the **depth of penetration** and **exclude possible organ injury**. The fact that the abdominal exam is benign does not completely rule out injury, because blood in the abdominal cavity may not produce tenderness on examination.

CLINICAL PEARL

You must assume peritoneal penetration until proven otherwise.

Further Management Plan/Results

- Local wound exploration: penetration of the anterior rectus sheath

- CT scan of the abdomen and pelvis with IV contrast: no free air or fluid

- Exploratory laparotomy: a small laceration of the small bowel serosa is identified without a full-thickness enterotomy; it is oversewn. No other intra-abdominal injuries are found after careful exploration. The laparotomy incision is closed in a standard fascia, including skin. The fascia at the stab wound site is debrided and closed and the skin is left open and packed to avoid infection.

CLINICAL PEARL

There is a 25% chance of visceral injury with violation of the anterior fascia.

Abdominal Trauma

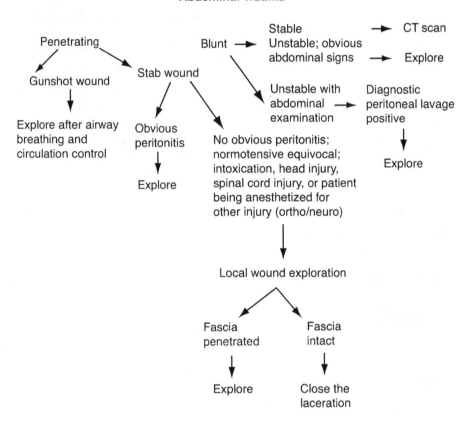

Discussion

Historically, operative exploration was mandatory for all penetrating abdominal trauma. Currently, admission and abdominal examination every 3–4 hours is justified in a patient with intact mental status and no evidence of fascial penetration on local wound exploration.

When abdominal wall fascia is penetrated, exploration is warranted to rule out organ injury, and the fascial hernia must be closed. Laparoscopic examination in a stable patient has been well documented, but it is too early in the experience and is associated with a high percentage of missed injuries, therefore should be avoided on the exam. It is always safer to do a negative laparotomy than to miss an intra-abdominal injury.

At operative exploration for penetrating trauma, vascular injuries resulting in hemorrhage should be controlled first, followed by GI injuries to control spillage and contamination. If necessary, resuscitation should be done after all bleeding is controlled before moving ahead to definitive management of injuries.

Liver laceration

- CT scan shows hematoma: observe
- Active bleeding: angiographic embolization
- Bile leak: stents/drains

Splenic laceration

- Stable hematoma: observe
- Uncontrolled bleed: splenectomy

Follow-up Management and Prevention

If splenectomy is performed, vaccination against capsulated organisms must be performed prior to discharge from hospital. No long-term follow-up is necessary.

Unfortunately, many population-based studies have demonstrated a high recidivism rate despite social programs aimed at decreasing violence and the incidence of penetrating trauma.

Final Diagnosis

Penetrating abdominal trauma

CASE 10

Chief Complaint

Distended abdomen

History and Physical Examination

An 85-year-old nursing-home patient is transferred to the emergency department because of a distended abdomen. The patient suffers from Alzheimer's disease and also has difficulty walking because of osteoarthritis. The patient is brought in by her aide, who tells you that the patient was in her usual health until 24 hours earlier, when her abdomen became bloated and no passage of flatus or stool was noted since that time. The patient had one episode like this about a week and a half ago, and it seemed to go away on its own. She has not been nauseous or vomiting. She denies any history of surgery or any intestinal problems. She has had no change in bowel habits, although she has had a long-term history of constipation. Her temperature is 37.0 C (98.6 F) and BP is 108/75 mm Hg.

Upon physical examination you find a slightly confused elderly woman in no apparent distress. Heart and lung examinations are normal. The abdomen is soft, distended, and tympanitic with hypoactive bowel sounds. There are no discrete masses, hernias, or scars. Rectal examination shows no stool in the vault and no masses.

Differential Diagnosis

1. Large bowel obstruction secondary to a mass, fecal impaction, or volvulus

   - Most likely diagnosis given the history and physical

2. Ogilvie's syndrome (i.e., pseudo-obstruction of the colon)

   - Possible and fits the patient's demographic, but should be a diagnosis of exclusion once a true mechanical obstruction has been ruled out.

3. Small bowel obstruction due to occult incarcerated hernia

   - Would expect more nausea and vomiting, but would also produce abdominal distention

4. Mesenteric ischemia (less likely)

   - Typically presents as "pain out of proportion to exam," whereas this patient has physical exam findings and is not in particular distress; nonetheless, must be considered for its significant potential sequelae

Initial Management

Setting: emergency department

Diagnostic/Therapeutic Plan

- CBC

- Serum electrolytes, lactic acid

- Abdominal x-ray

Test Results

- CBC: normal

- BUN 22 mg/dL; creatinine 1.2 mg/dL; lactic acid normal

- X-ray: dilated loop of large bowel, emanating from the pelvis up into the RUQ, shaped somewhat like the letter omega ("bent inner tube")

Assessment

This patient has a sigmoid colonic volvulus. Her advanced age and inactivity predispose her to colonic volvulus, with the pathognomonic omega loop on x-ray. In addition, the history of a transient episode of similar symptoms—which remitted spontaneously—suggests volvulus. Obstruction from a mass or hernia does not usually remit.

In Ogilvie's syndrome, there might be a similar presentation, but abdominal x-ray will show megacolon (i.e., widely dilated throughout), not just an omega loop.

CLINICAL PEARL

Sigmoid colonic volvulus is the second most common cause of large bowel obstruction.

Further Management Plan

- Rigid sigmoidoscopy: normal, healthy-appearing mucosa to about 18 cm, then a clear collapse of the bowel, consistent with a twist

- Rectal tube placement: gush of air and colonic contents are obtained as the bowel untwists; further inspection of the mucosa above the area of the twist shows the bowel to be viable with no evidence of necrosis

- Inpatient admission

- NPO/IV hydration

- Monitoring of vital signs, including urine output, and serial abdominal examinations to evaluate for ischemia

Discussion

The rectal tube can be left in situ but should not remain in >48 hrs due to risk of erosion of rectal or colonic mucosa. After resuscitation and stabilization for a couple of days, the patient should undergo bowel preparation and barium enema or colonoscopy to rule out an underlying lesion. An elective resection of the sigmoid colon should be performed, as these types of patients have a propensity for recurrent volvulus.

The rigid sigmoidoscope reaches in only 20 cm. A soft rubber rectal tube is used to reach the twist causing obstruction when it is beyond the reach of the sigmoidoscope. The gush of air and stool indicates successful untwisting.

Sigmoid volvulus accounts for 80–90% of all volvulus seen in elderly, institutionalized individuals with neurologic impairment.

- Presents with abdominal pain, constipation, and distension

- Abdominal x-ray shows "bent inner-tube" and "coffee-bean" shapes

- Water-soluble enema shows "bird's beak"–type deformity

- Treatment is first with sigmoidoscopy and rectal tube placement; perform sigmoid resection during same hospital admission

- Emergent sigmoidectomy is necessary if peritonitis is present.

CLINICAL PEARL

CT scan with rectal contrast will also show this characteristic deformity.

Basic Science Correlate

Neostigmine is an acetylcholinesterase inhibitor that acts as a parasympathomimetic by decreasing degradation of acetylcholine. Although the exact mechanism of Ogilvie's syndrome is unclear, it can resolve the condition by stimulating the parasympathetic nervous system and increasing bowel motility.

Patient Safety Note

Neostigmine induces a systemic parasympathetic response, not just in the GI tract. The effect on the heart is bradycardia and potentially life-threatening bradyarrhythmias; the effect on the airway is bronchospasm. Accordingly, a patient undergoing treatment for Ogilvie's with neostigmine should be transferred to the ICU for continuous heart rate and airway monitoring.

Follow-up Management and Prevention

After appropriate recovery from surgery, the patient should be transferred back to her nursing facility with routine follow-up about 2 weeks after surgery to assess incisional healing and bowel habits. No interventions have been demonstrated to prevent this problem in the elderly, although high fiber diets may improve bowel motility and potentially be helpful.

Final Diagnosis

Colonic volvulus

CASE 11

Chief Complaint

Left-sided chest pain

History and Physical Examination

A 29-year-old man comes to the emergency department complaining of left-sided chest pain. He had been out drinking with friends when he began to retch and vomit up some blood specks. The left side of his chest soon started to hurt. He denies any history of cardiopulmonary disease or similar episodes in the past. He and his friends deny any illicit drug use. He is in mild distress. Vital signs are temperature 37.0 C (98.6 F), BP 100/60 mm Hg, and pulse 120/min. Physical examination shows diminished breath sounds at the left base. His heart sounds are rapid without any murmurs. Abdominal examination is negative for signs of peritonitis.

Differential Diagnosis

1. Esophageal perforation (Boerhaave's syndrome): not common but foremost in diagnosis due to severity

2. Spontaneous pneumothorax: can occur with fits of coughing, especially in younger males; would result in absent (not decreased) breath sounds, but may be partial

3. Myocardial ischemia: unlikely in this demographic, but can cause the symptoms described and can be induced by illicit drug use, especially cocaine

4. Aspiration pneumonitis: can cause vomiting; possible here given history of alcohol ingestion and depressed mental status

5. Esophageal spasm: can cause similar chest pain, but is typically retrosternal and not acute-onset

Initial Management

Setting: emergency department

Diagnostic/Therapeutic Plan

- Blood work: CBC, serum electrolytes
- EKG
- Chest x-ray
- Abdominal x-ray

Test Results

- Blood work: normal
- EKG: sinus tachycardia, no acute ischemic changes
- Chest x-ray: blunting of the left costophrenic angle with minimal amount of air in the mediastinum; no evidence of pneumothorax
- Abdominal x-ray: no pneumoperitoneum, no dilated bowel

Assessment

The history and chest x-ray findings are most consistent with esophageal perforation, with resultant pneumomediastinum and a left pleural effusion.

Pneumothorax has been ruled out on x-ray. Myocardial ischemia has been ruled out by EKG. Aspiration pneumonitis is unlikely without an infiltrate on chest x-ray. Esophageal spasm is most likely to cause pain with swallowing, and be progressive and not acute onset.

Further Management Plan/Results

- IV hydration and broad-spectrum antibiotics (based on clinical suspicion; do not delay antibiotics for final diagnostic confirmation as patient could become septic)
- Upper GI study with water soluble contrast: extravasation of contrast into left chest
- If an upper GI study is not available or non-diagnostic, perform CT scan with oral and IV contrast
- Operative exploration and repair

Discussion

The prognosis for esophageal perforation depends on the location and timeliness of diagnosis and management. A long-standing perforation can result in mediastinitis, with a very high mortality rate. The patient is resuscitated in the emergency department and started on IV, broad-spectrum antibiotics. The patient is then quickly brought to the operating room and intubated with a double-lumen endotracheal tube. With the use of a left thoracotomy, the area of perforation is identified. Because this case has a relatively fresh perforation (only 3 hrs prior), treatment should be debridement of the area, closure of the esophageal perforation, and buttressing the closure with a pleural flap. Wide drainage of the mediastinum and thorax region is next accomplished with chest tubes.

- Had this been a perforation of longer duration (i.e., >24 hours), the prognosis would have been poorer regardless of treatment. Wide drainage, in addition to esophageal exclusion (e.g., an esophagostomy at the level of the neck and stapling off of the gastroesophageal junction), and a gastrostomy tube for feeding would have been indicated. These drastic measures are taken for the occasional patient with sepsis due to major esophageal leak and massive mediastinal contamination.

- Had this been a cervical esophageal perforation, the patient would be observed and kept NPO. Antibiotics would be administered. Neck exploration is reserved for the larger cervical perforations. Because this perforation is located in the thoracic esophagus, surgical exploration is mandatory.

An abdominal exam is important because pneumoperitoneum can "travel" up and create pneumomediastinum, so be sure the perforation is in the thorax and not abdomen before proceeding to operation.

There are 2 classic types of esophageal emergency that can occur after episodes of repeated, forceful vomiting following alcohol consumption or eating a rich meal:

- **Spontaneous rupture of the esophagus** (has no hematemesis)
- **Profuse upper GI bleeding** (Mallory-Weiss syndrome) from mucosal laceration at the gastroesophageal junction (has no pain and typically resolves without intervention)

The most common part of the esophagus that ruptures is the distal third, with the esophageal contents spilling into the mediastinum and/or left pleural space. Classic symptoms include dysphagia, odynophagia, fever, leukocytosis, tachycardia, tachypnea, and shock. Pain is retrosternal or epigastric and is usually very intense. "Crepitus" at the root of the neck or pneumomediastinum on chest x-ray with left pleural effusion can be seen. The gold standard of diagnosis is a water-soluble study (Gastrografin) or a barium swallow with extravasation of contrast in the mediastinum or pleural space. If diagnosis is still in doubt, an endoscopy can be used to see mucosal discoloration. CT scan can also be performed and would show an air–fluid level in the mediastinum.

An early intervention (<24 hrs from onset of symptoms) has a better outcome than a late one (>24 hrs). Treatment should proceed as follows:

1. Resuscitate with IV fluids and antibiotics

2. Diagnose with contrast study

3. Drain the pleural space with a chest tube

4. Explore: divert or repair

Final Diagnosis

Esophageal perforation

Esophageal Perforation

Sudden onset of severe chest pain after repeated, forceful vomiting following rich meal or an alcoholic binge

Suspect barotrauma to esophagus

Clinical signs are ↑ heart rate, ↑ respiratory rate, ↑ WBCs and fever, and crepitus in the neck

Chest x-ray left or right pleural effusion; pneumomediastinum

Gastrografin or barium swallow (gold standard of diagnosis) (extravasation of contrast to mediastinum or pleural space)

Endoscopy if contrast radiology is negative; CT scan of chest to see air-fluid level in mediastinum

Resuscitate with IV fluids and antibiotics

Drain pleural space and early operation for diversion or repair

CCS NOTE

Select gastrografin, a water-soluble contrast, and not barium. Barium can cause severe peritonitis and pleural inflammation if it extravasates through a perforation.

CASE 12

Chief Complaint

"I've been stabbed!"

History and Physical Examination

An 18-year-old man is brought to the emergency department by paramedics after being stabbed with an ice pick on the right side of the back, just left of the scapula. He complains of right-sided chest pain with inspiration and shortness of breath. No other injuries occurred. The patient is otherwise healthy. His tetanus immunization is up to date.

He is a healthy-appearing male in moderate distress. Vital signs are BP 120/70 mm Hg, pulse 110/min, and respirations 25/min. His head and neck are without evidence of injury; there is no jugular venous distension or crepitus. His heart is normal without any murmurs or muffling of heart sounds. Auscultation of the chest shows diminished breath sounds on the right side, but the left sounds normal. His abdomen is soft and nontender. On his back there is a 1-cm laceration just medial to the right scapula. There is no active bleeding or hematoma. There is no crepitus.

Differential Diagnosis

1. Pneumothorax

2. Mediastinal injury

Initial Management

Setting: emergency department

Diagnostic/Therapeutic Plan

- Continuous vital sign monitoring in the trauma evaluation area, including pulse oximetry

- Blood work: CBC, serum electrolytes, type and cross match

- Chest x-ray

Test Results

- Oxygen saturation 93% on 2 L nasal cannula

- Blood work: normal

- X-ray: 40% pneumothorax on the right side with a small pleural effusion; normal cardiac silhouette; normal mediastinum that is not wide and without pneumomediastinum

Assessment

Although the diagnosis of pneumothorax appears obvious from the history, stab wounds in this location of the back can potentially cause life-threatening mediastinal structure injuries. The lack of jugular venous distension on examination and the normal tracheal position on x-ray are inconsistent with a tension pneumothorax. Thus, this patient has a "simple" pneumothorax. The lack of crepitus and mediastinal air on x-ray help exclude esophageal perforation. The normal cardiac silhouette and normal-sized mediastinal shadow, along with normal (not muffled) heart sounds, make it unlikely that there is blood in the mediastinum or pericardium due to aortic or pericardial laceration.

Further Management Plan

- Oxygen administration: maintains adequate arterial oxygen levels, but also increases the oxygen content in the pleural space, which increases resorption

- Chest tube placement: with follow-up repeat chest x-ray to confirm lung re-expansion; if a significant amount of blood is evacuated, a traumatic hemothorax or iatrogenic injury must be considered.

- Analgesia

- Inpatient admission until air leak resolves and tube can be safely removed

CLINICAL PEARL

A flail chest is secondary to blunt trauma with multiple rib fractures.

Traumatic Pneumothorax

↓

Penetrating or blunt chest trauma
Decreased air entry to affected hemithorax
Tympanitic to percussion
Rib fracture that leads to tenderness, ecchymosis, or crepitus on palpation

Chest x-ray shows pneumothorax

Drain by chest tube if >20%
Observe if <20% (unless patient requires intubation or is symptomatic)

↓

Think of other injuries such as lung contusion, flail chest, or hemothorax

Discussion

Penetrating trauma to "the box" must be evaluated for a mediastinal vascular injury. This is preliminarily done as part of the Focused Abdominal Sonography for Trauma (FAST) in the evaluation for pericardial fluid. CT angiogram is the most sensitive test to rule out a major mediastinal vascular injury. The lack of air in the mediastinum would usually rule out esophageal injury, but an upper GI swallow is indicated if there is any clinical suspicion. If the stab occurs below the sixth to seventh intercostal space posteriorly, or below the fourth to fifth intercostal space laterally or anteriorly, then intraabdominal trauma must be ruled out, and laparotomy is indicated.

Follow-up Management and Prevention

Once the air leak resolves, the chest tube can be removed. A follow-up x-ray 4 hours later confirms no residual pneumothorax and the patient can be discharged home. No long term follow-up is necessary.

Final Diagnosis

Traumatic pneumothorax

For lung contusion and flail chest, admit the patient to a monitored bed and observe for desaturation and respiratory failure, with a low threshold for intubation and mechanical ventilation. Most contusions are self-limiting, so maintain a state of relative dryness (therefore, use caution when administering IV fluids).

Hemothorax requires immediate drainage to avoid post-traumatic fibrothorax. If initial chest tube drainage is >1500 mL of blood or 250 mL/hr for 4 consecutive hrs, operative exploration via thoracotomy is indicated.

"The box" is the anatomical region defined as the anterior chest between the nipples from the clavicles to the level of the costal margins, and the posterior chest between the scapular borders and the same cranial/caudal levels. Penetrating trauma to this region must be evaluated for a major mediastinal vascular injury.

Simple rib fractures are treated with analgesia utilizing local anesthesia, intercostal nerve blocks, or an epidural catheter if multiple ribs are involved. Aggressive pulmonary toilet is mandatory to resolve the inevitable atelectasis, which could lead to pneumonia, particularly in elderly patients.

Be aware of tension pneumothorax. Although most simple pneumothoraces are self-limiting, if the air leak persists for >72 hrs, a bronchopleural fistula may be present, possibly necessitating surgical repair.

CASE 13

Chief Complaint

Abdominal wall defect at birth

History and Physical Examination

At birth, a newborn presents with the bowel contents outside of the abdomen due to a defect of the abdominal wall.

Differential Diagnosis

1. Omphalocele

2. Gastroschisis

3. Umbilical hernia

Initial Management

Setting: emergency department

Diagnostic/Therapeutic Plan

- CBC and serum electrolytes

- IV hydration

Test Results

- CBC and serum electrolytes: normal

Assessment

This patient has a congenital abdominal wall defect and requires emergent surgical intervention, as the infant is at risk for sepsis from peritonitis and severe dehydration.

Further Management Plan

Move to the operating room for surgical closure: reduction of bowel contents and closure of the fascia and skin.

- If the fascia cannot be closed, close the skin and repair the resultant hernia at a later date.

- If neither the fascia nor the skin can be closed, perform a silo procedure (temporary prosthetic covering of the intestines) until the abdominal wall expands to a point where the fascia and/or skin can be closed; until that time, keep the child in ICU on antibiotics due to the risk of infection.

Discussion

- Omphalocele occurs centrally and the bowel contents have a peritoneal covering.

- Gastroschisis occurs laterally and the bowel contents have no covering, which causes significant edema of the intestines.

- Umbilical hernia is rarely seen at birth and has intact skin over the hernia. This is treated at a much later age.

Omphalocele is a "central or midline" anatomic defect in the abdominal wall where the midgut loop that forms much of the small intestines protrudes through the umbilical ring. An omphalocele has a peritoneal "covering," thus protecting the intestines from the amniotic fluid.

Gastroschisis is a "lateral" anatomic defect in the abdominal wall caused by a defect in lateral body folding to the right of the umbilical ring. It has no peritoneal covering, thus the intestines float in the amniotic fluid. It is commonly thought that amniotic fluid would be non-irritating to the intestines but that is not the case. It causes an intense inflammatory response and increases capillary permeability.

The intestines in omphalocele are protected from the amniotic fluid and look like fine spaghetti. The intestines in gastroschisis look like sausages and are very inflamed.

The surgical intervention for gastroschisis is usually more difficult because there is significant bowel edema, secondary to exposure of the intestines to the amniotic fluid, which causes inflammation. Gastroschisis is also associated with intestinal atresia.

Follow-up Management and Prevention

If only the skin can be closed over the defect, by definition a hernia will persist. This can be re-addressed at a later date when the infection and dehydration risks are lower.

True primary umbilical hernias are rarely present at birth, often close by age 5, and rarely incarcerate. Therefore, repair is often delayed until age 5.

Final Diagnosis

Abdominal wall defect, omphalocele versus gastroschisis

CASE 14

Chief Complaint

"The wound on my foot is getting worse."

History and Physical Examination

A 73-year-old woman who is in the hospital for management of her diabetes has a worsening foot ulcer. She has had hypertension and adult-onset diabetes for 20 years. Over the last few weeks an ulcerated lesion has developed on the first metatarsal-phalangeal joint of her right foot, which has grown to the size of a nickel. There is a small amount of cloudy drainage that she says hadn't changed much since she noticed it. She denies any pain in her calves and feet on either side. She wears regular shoes most of the time. She denies any trauma to the area. Her regular medications are insulin and a beta-blocker.

She is a well-appearing female in no apparent distress. She is afebrile with normal vital signs. Heart and lung examinations are normal. The abdomen is soft and nontender with no palpable masses. Examination of the lower extremities shows that the arterial pulses are intact and strong bilaterally at the femoral, popliteal, and both the posterior tibial and dorsalis pedis (the pedal pulses). On the ventral surface of her right foot, there is a 1×2 cm ulcer at the first metatarsal-phalangeal joint. There is a small amount of drainage. Probing the ulcer with a cotton-tipped swab demonstrates extension of the ulcer with a tract into the first metatarsophalangeal joint space. There is also a significant callous around the ulcer. There is minimal edema of the foot, and she has decreased sensation to pinprick bilaterally.

Differential Diagnosis

1. Diabetic foot ulcer

   • Most likely diagnosis based on history and physical exam

2. Possible foreign body

   • Can cause soft tissue infection with a similar presentation, and diabetic patients with decreased sensation (neuropathy) are at higher risk

3. Joint space infection (synovitis/osteomyelitis)

   • Possibly present given tracking of the ulcer into the metatarsal-phalangeal space and presence of drainage; it is unclear here if this is present, and if so, whether it is the primary or secondary problem

Initial Management

Setting: inpatient

Diagnostic/Therapeutic Plan

• Blood work: CBC, comprehensive metabolic panel, C-reactive protein, ESR, foot x-ray

• Broad spectrum antibiotics

• Insulin for blood glucose control

• Admission to inpatient setting

CLINICAL PEARL

C-reactive protein and ESR are general systemic markers of inflammation. Although not diagnostic, they would be expected to be elevated higher in osteomyelitis than in a simple soft tissue infection. More important, their trends can be used as an adjunct to evaluate response to treatment.

Test Results

- WBC: elevated at 15,000/μL

- Blood sugar: elevated at 350 mg/dL

- X-ray: soft tissue edema but no air; no foreign body present; periosteal changes concerning for osteomyelitis

Assessment

This patient most likely has a diabetic foot ulcer secondary to the peripheral neuropathy of diabetes. Despite strong pulses, the microvascular angiopathy adds an additional risk of infection seen in diabetics. The lack of sensation may add to the risk of an unknown foreign body that the patient stepped on but could not feel; however, this is visualized on x-ray. The mild periosteal changes consistent with osteomyelitis and the extension of the ulcer tract into the joint make this a serious infection requiring immediate attention.

Further Management Plan/Results

- MRI scan is optimal to evaluate for osteomyelitis. Bone scan is less sensitive and is not the first choice to evaluate for osteomyelitis.

- Surgical debridement with possible amputation of the great toe and metatarsal head or more proximally; send tissue for culture and antibiotic sensitivity.

Discussion

The most common causes of ulcers in the lower extremities are **arterial insufficiency**, **venous insufficiency**, and **DM**.

- **Ulcers from arterial insufficiency** are characterized by chronic ischemia, a history of claudication/rest pain, and diminished or absent pulses. These ulcers are usually located on the tips of digits.

- **Ulcers of venous insufficiency** are characterized by hyperpigmentation of the skin, location in the gaiter area (the lower half of the leg above and around the ankle), chronic edema, and varicose veins, most commonly anterior to the medial malleolus (great saphenous vein).

- **Ulcers which result from DM** usually have associated neuropathy and vasculopathy. The most common site is the first metatarsal-phalangeal joint followed by the calcaneus.

Basic Science Correlate

Nerves have the GLUT-1 transporter, which is not insulin-dependent. High plasma glucose results in high levels of glucose in the neurons, which in turn disrupts the normal metabolism. Ultimately, neuropathy will result.

Note that hyperglycemia results in protein glycation, impairing host proteins involved in the following:

- Complement activation

- Bacterial uptake

- Phagocytic killing

Hyperglycemia changes the binding of host surface receptors for pathogens. The resulting macrophage dysfunction further enhances the virulence of pathogens, causing serious and progressive soft tissue infections.

Peripheral neuropathy is the most important cause of diabetic foot ulcers. Patients are not aware of the injury because they feel no pain. Stepping on a nail or wearing ill-fitting shoes commonly causes the initial infection, and the secondary infection allows the injury to progress. Motor neuropathy can cause abnormal weight bearing results, as seen in Charcot joints, and deformities, like hammertoes or hallux valgus, which shift weight bearing proximal to metatarsal heads. Ulcers develop on the dorsal aspect of hammertoes.

With ischemia, distal pulses may or may not be diminished in diabetes, but the microangiopathy results in poor microcirculation of the distal tissue of toes and feet, enhancing the life of ulcers. Most commonly, ulcers erode to the joint spaces, exposing cartilage and causing osteomyelitis. MRI or bone scan (less optimal) can confirm the diagnosis of osteomyelitis. In such cases, if antibiotic treatment is unsuccessful, the only salvage is amputation of the affected toe, debridement of cartilage and bone, and healing by the secondary intention.

Diabetics should be evaluated for good perfusion of distal extremities by noninvasive vascular studies (toe pressure and tissue-oxygen content) to predict amputation site before surgery. If arterial pressures are poor, revascularization by bypass surgery or an endovascular intervention is indicated prior to amputation. If the wound is grossly infected and an abscess is present, or if there is crepitus in soft tissues with cellulitis, an emergent debridement of infection should be performed to prevent necrotizing fasciitis (guillotine-open amputation). Absolute non-weight bearing is the key to healing diabetic ulcers.

Infected foot ulcers in diabetics are dangerous and can be underdiagnosed due to neuropathy.

- The most common location is the base of the first toe at the first metatarsophalangeal joint, due to the repetitive pressure and weight during ambulation.

- Extension of the infection into deep tissues requires immediate extensive debridement and drainage with probable amputation of the affected toe or proximally.

In this patient, the clinical finding of extension of the wound into the joint space mandates amputation of the toe, the joint, and the metatarsal head. Failure to do so could result in extension of the infection along fascial planes, leading to a foot or more proximal amputation. Broad-spectrum antibiotics should be used because most diabetic foot infections are of mixed flora. Operating room cultures should be taken and the information used to tailor the antibiotic regimen based on sensitivities.

Blood sugar control is crucial, as all patients–even those without diabetes–will have elevated glucose in the face of infection, and insulin requirements may increase temporarily. Ischemia of an extremity due to associated vascular disease should be assessed, as that affects healing and the delivery of IV antibiotics to the site of infection. If distal pulses are intact and strong, likelihood is good for healing. If they are poor, noninvasive and invasive vascular evaluation should be initiated with possible intervention.

CLINICAL PEARL

If osteomyelitis is present and proves to be refractory to antibiotics and surgical debridement, amputation may be necessary. It is crucial to evaluate the patient's large vessel anatomy before amputation to ensure sufficient blood flow to heal a major amputation.

Follow-up Management and Prevention

Follow-up management of diabetic foot ulcers involves a combination of wound care and antibiotics. Wound care is determined by depth of wound, presence of infection, vascular supply allowing healing, and extent of surgical debridement. If infected tissue is still present, e.g., clinical osteomyelitis when infected bone is exposed, long term IV antibiotics may be necessary.

The key to chronic management of diabetic foot ulcers is prevention. Rigorous diet and medical maintenance of glucose are essential in preventing progression of disease and the neuropathy which leads to foot ulcers and chronic wounds. Regular podiatry evaluation is crucial to evaluate for wounds before they progress and provide appropriate off-loading footwear to prevent skin and soft tissue breakdown from otherwise normal pressure points.

Final Diagnosis

Infected diabetic foot ulcer

CASE 15

Chief Complaint

"I feel something pulsating in my belly."

History and Physical Examination

A 68-year-old man with hypertension comes to the clinic because he "feels a pulsating mass in my abdomen." He denies any abdominal/back pain, pain in the legs while walking, shortness of breath, and chest pain. His current medications include a calcium-channel blocker and beta-blocker. He had a myocardial infarction 20 years ago. He appears well and in no apparent distress. His blood pressure is 185/125 mm Hg, equal in both arms, and pulse is 68/min.

Heart and lung examinations are within normal limits. The abdomen is soft and not tender. There is a 6-cm pulsatile mass palpable in the mid-abdomen. Rectal exam shows guaiac-negative stool and is negative for masses. The prostate is large and rubbery with no palpable masses. Examination of the extremities shows no evidence of ischemic changes; femoral, popliteal, and pedal pulses are strong and equal.

Differential Diagnosis

1. Abdominal aortic aneurysm (AAA)

2. Intra-abdominal or retroperitoneal tumor

Initial Management

Setting: outpatient

Diagnostic/Therapeutic Plan

- Blood work: CBC, serum electrolytes

- EKG

- Chest x-ray

- CT scan (abdomen and pelvis) with IV contrast

Test Results

- Blood work: normal

- EKG: evidence of an old myocardial infarction but no acute changes

- Chest x-ray: normal

- CT scan (abdomen and pelvis): >6 cm pulsatile mass appearing to arise from the infrarenal aorta

Assessment

The history of vascular disease, as evidenced by a prior myocardial infarction, suggests other locations of vascular pathology. The pulsatile mass found on examination is either an abdominal aortic or iliac artery aneurysm, and the diagnosis is made with CT scan. Although some colon tumors may feel pulsatile on exam, the negative stool guaiac and normal CBC help exclude this.

CLINICAL PEARL

Although AAA's are usually appreciable on physical exam, they may not be in obese patients. It should be considered in the differential diagnosis for abdominal or back pain, especially in patients with a cardiac or vascular history.

Basic Science Correlate

The presence of vascular pathology in one location is a marker for disease in others. The combination of genetics, smoking, and elevated LDL results in systemic atheromatous disease due to LDL oxidation and macrophage-proteoglycan mediated plaque formation. In the coronary and peripheral arteries this leads to ischemia and possible aortic ulceration and media weakening.

Discussion

An abnormal aortic aneurysm is predominantly a male disease (M:F = 3–8:1). Familial clustering is observed. Ninety percent are secondary to atherosclerosis and 5% are inflammatory; 95% are infra renal; and 75% are asymptomatic and discovered incidentally. The rest are symptomatic or result in a rupture. Symptoms include body aches and flank or abdominal pain. An abnormal aortic aneurysm can be confused with renal colic, perforated sigmoid diverticulitis, sciatica, osteoarthritis of the spine, pancreatitis, thromboembolic phenomena, or compression of the duodenum.

Although U/S can identify large AAAs, it is limited by user subjectivity, patient body habitus, and intraluminal thrombus. The gold standard of diagnosis is CT scan with IV contrast.

Indications for surgery include the following:

- Size >5 cm
- Growth >0.5 cm per year
- Symptomatic presentation
- Rupture

The most common cause of preoperative mortality is myocardial infarction. Other complications include renal insufficiency, lower extremity ischemia, ischemic colitis, aortoenteric fistula, sexual dysfunction, and paraplegia secondary to spinal cord ischemia. U/S is now commonly used for screening AAA. If you suspect AAA, the first diagnostic test should be CT scan.

Follow-up Management and Prevention

Pre-operative cardiopulmonary assessment is required, followed by elective AAA repair (either open or endovascular, depending on vascular anatomy and comorbidities). Goldman classification is used to assess cardiac risk.

- Class I and II patients, with careful perioperative monitoring, have a low risk
- Higher-risk patients need a coronary artery workup and management.
- Perioperative risks include bleeding, infection, myocardial infarction, renal, hepatic, and respiratory failure, lower extremity or intestinal ischemia, paralysis, and death.

Although this list is extensive, the overall risk of morbidity for elective AAA surgery is 10–20% and mortality around 2%, whereas with unrepaired rupture the risk of mortality nears 100%. The risk of rupture increases with size, with aneurysms >6 cm carrying a 10–20% risk of rupture per year.

For this reason, even small aneurysms (<4 cm) must be evaluated regularly, with annual U/S and/or CT scan.

Final Diagnosis

Abdominal aortic aneurysm

CASE 16

Chief Complaint

"I have blood coming out of my nipple."

History and Physical Examination

A 36-year-old woman comes to the clinic complaining of intermittent bloody discharge from her right nipple over the last 2 months. It is spontaneous in nature without any relation to her menses. She is not currently sexually active. She does not take any medications or use birth control pills. She denies any associated breast mass with the discharge. She denies trauma. In general, she is a well appearing female in no apparent distress with stable vital signs.

Physical examination shows that both breasts are symmetrical with no evidence of nipple retraction. There is no axillary adenopathy. Both nipples appear normal with no evidence of any lesions. At the 2 o'clock position of the right nipple, a small, pea-sized nodule is palpable, and a small amount of serosanguineous discharge can be expressed when palpating this region. The left nipple has no palpable masses. The remaining breast tissue is without discrete masses bilaterally. The remainder of the examination is normal.

Differential Diagnosis

1. Intraductal papilloma

   • Most common cause of bloody nipple discharge, but you must always rule out cancer

2. Breast carcinoma

   • Must always be considered with any breast pathology including mass and discharge

3. Trauma

   • Patient denies history but could be unaware; can lead to hematoma presenting as a mass

4. Breast abscess

   • Palpable nodule can be an abscess, less likely due to absence of fever, erythema, or fluctuance

Initial Management

Setting: outpatient

Diagnostic/Therapeutic Plan

• Mammography

• U/S

Test Results

• Mammography: negative for any suspicious lesions

• U/S: small solid mass in palpable area

CLINICAL PEARL

The #1 risk factor for breast cancer is a personal history of cancer in the contralateral breast. The second most common risk factor is a positive family history.

CLINICAL PEARL

MRI is more sensitive than mammography especially in women age <40 where the breasts are usually dense. In this case, however, there is a strong clinical suspicion of intraductal papilloma with a palpable mass, so regardless of MRI findings one must biopsy the mass. If a mass was not palpable, MRI or ductogram would be indicated.

Assessment

Palpable masses and nipple discharge may be associated with intraductal papilloma or a true breast malignancy. Although mammogram is somewhat helpful, 15% may be negative despite the presence of a significant lesion. This is especially true in premenopausal women who have denser breast tissue, making the mammogram more difficult to read.

The final diagnosis cannot be made without histologic analysis of the mass.

Further Management Plan

Excisional biopsy of mass: benign intraductal papilloma

Discussion

In premenopausal women, bloody discharge is most often associated with intraductal papilloma, unless there is a significant family history of early breast cancer. Intraductal papilloma is a benign lesion, and no further treatment is necessary once the tissue diagnosis has been made. The patient should continue with self-breast exams and yearly clinical exams thereafter.

For most women, mammography is recommended as a baseline study beginning age 40. It is done earlier if there is a strong history of breast or ovarian cancer in first-degree relatives, or if the patient presents with suspicious symptoms of a persistent lump, discharge, or skin changes.

Breast carcinoma can be either in situ or infiltrating. In situ carcinomas can also be lobular or ductal. Infiltrating carcinoma can be lobular or ductal, inflammatory, mucoid, or colloid.

Ductal carcinoma in situ (DCIS) is treated as a malignancy.

- Malignant cells usually have not infiltrated the basement membrane. They appear as clustered, pleomorphic calcifications on the mammogram.
- Because most lesions are not palpable, a needle localization or stereotactic biopsy is required to obtain pathologic samples.
- Treatment is simple mastectomy or breast conserving therapy with radiotherapy.
- No chemotherapy is needed.

Lobular carcinoma in situ (LCIS) is an incidental pathologic finding in a breast biopsy sample that has been done for some other reason.

- Not a cancer in itself but rather a marker for increased cancer risk at 1% per year.
- The cancer can be either ductal- or lobular-infiltrating, and can occur in either breast.
- Treatment is close surveillance or bilateral mastectomy in cases with strong family history of breast cancer (BRCA1 positive).

Invasive breast cancer is considered a **systemic disease**. It is the lack of this understanding that led to a century of failed treatments and death related to recurrence years after the surgery, as most thought surgery alone was the only treatment. Chemotherapy was reserved for select advance cases that were node-positive. Obviously, that was ineffective in curing cancer.

Today breast cancer is considered a systemic illness, having 2 components from the start:

- Loco regional
- Systemic

Loco regional disease is treated by surgery (modified radical mastectomy) or breast conservation treatment (lumpectomy with radiotherapy to breast). Outcome is the same for both approaches; thus, the majority of women (90%) opt for breast conservation.

Systemic cancer is present even if not visualized by scans or proved by nodal histology, due to the biology of the tumor and consistent historical failure to cure breast cancer over the decades past. Hence, systemic load of cancer is assumed in all cases of invasive cancer. Treatment is chemotherapy and hormonal therapy as well if receptor-positive.

The only women who should not receive chemotherapy for invasive breast cancer are those who fulfill **all the following** 4 criteria.

- Post-menopausal
- Sentinel node negative for metastasis
- Estrogen-receptor positive/progesterone-receptor positive
- Tumor size <2 cm

In these cases the systemic component of the disease is assumed to be very limited, and hormonal therapy alone is considered adequate treatment.

Locally advanced breast cancer should initially be staged by bone scan and CT of the chest and abdomen. If >4 nodes are positive, consider high-dose chemotherapy or autologous bone marrow transplant.

Management of recurrent breast cancer depends on the site of recurrence and initial management. After breast-conserving therapy, salvage is through mastectomy.

- Recurrence in the axilla is managed with radiotherapy.
- Recurrence in the chest wall after mastectomy is treated with surgical excision with radiotherapy.

Follow-up Management and Prevention

- No further treatment
- Continued observation with monthly self breast examinations and yearly mammography

Final Diagnosis

Intraductal papilloma

CASE 17

Chief Complaint

"I have a lump in my neck."

History and Physical Examination

A 42-year-old woman comes to the office with a lump in her anterior neck. She states that she has been in her usual health when she noticed a small lump at the base of her neck on the right side. Over the course of 1 month, it has not changed. She denies any associated symptoms such as palpitations, hot flashes, and jitteriness. She denies any history of cancer in the head/neck and any history of radiation to her neck. She denies any change in voice and hoarseness. She does not smoke.

In general, she appears healthy and is in no apparent distress. Examination shows a 2-cm, soft, fixed nodule in the right lobe of the thyroid. There is no evidence of any other adenopathy in the neck. The remainder of the physical examination is unremarkable.

Differential Diagnosis

1. Nodular goiter

2. Thyroid cancer

3. Thyroid adenoma

Initial Management

Setting: outpatient

Diagnostic/Therapeutic Plan

- Thyroid function tests (TFTs)

- Fine needle aspiration (FNA); ultrasound-guided if necessary

Test Results

- TFTs: normal

- FNA: highly suspicious papillary cells

Assessment

A 42-year-old woman with no significant past medical history presents with a neck mass. Physical exam suggests a thyroid origin, and further workup with TFTs and FNA are consistent with papillary thyroid cancer.

Further Management Plan/Results

- Chest x-ray: no evidence of metastatic disease

- Total thyroidectomy, with possible limited lymph node dissection

Discussion

A thyroid mass can be an adenoma, nodular goiter, or malignancy. A single mass is more suggestive of malignancy.

- If TFTs are normal, a radioactive iodine nuclear scan is rarely helpful and so workup should proceed to FNA.

- If TFTs are abnormal, a scan may be helpful in assessing risk.
  - A "hot" nodule (increased radioactive iodine uptake) is typically associated with benign lesions.
  - A "cold" nodule (no uptake) is more likely to be malignant.

CLINICAL PEARL

"Hot" or benign thyroid nodules can be suppressed with iodine treatment.

FNA with evaluation of cytology is the first step in the evaluation of a thyroid mass. It is minimally invasive with low morbidity and is 96–100% accurate for papillary cancer.

However, it is not as reliable for other types of thyroid tumors, e.g., follicular cancer versus benign follicular adenoma, as cytology alone cannot differentiate benign from malignant follicular cells.

If a diagnosis of thyroid cancer has been made, evaluation for metastatic disease should be performed using chest x-ray. If cervical lymph nodes are palpated on physical exam or there is concern for airway or recurrent laryngeal nerve involvement, neck CT is indicated.

Basic Science Correlate

The worst prognostic factor is capsular invasion, not lymph node metastasis.

Thyroid carcinoma can be papillary, follicular, medullary, or anaplastic. Risk factors for thyroid carcinoma include:

- Elderly age

- History of ionizing radiation

- Family history of thyroid cancer

- Rapid nodular growth

- Compressive symptoms

- Hoarseness of voice

- Presence of a firm, irregular, fixed nodule or cold nodule on thyroid scan

Papillary thyroid cancer is the most common type (60–70%) and is associated with radiation exposure. Women are affected by papillary carcinoma 2–3× more than men.

- There is a bimodal frequency, and peaks occur in the second and third decades and again later in life.

- This tumor grows slowly and spreads via lymphatics after many years.

- Treatment is surgical resection.

  - Lobectomy alone may be sufficient for small (<1 cm), low-risk, unifocal, intrathyroidal papillary carcinomas with no evidence of cervical nodal involvement. This procedure is well tolerated with a low risk of morbidity, but 5–10% of patients will have a recurrence in the thyroid. Accordingly, **total thyroidectomy** is recommended due to the high incidence of multicentric involvement and possibility of dedifferentiation of any residual tumor to the anaplastic cell type.

Patient Safety Note

The most significant complication of thyroid surgery is injury to the recurrent laryngeal nerve. Great care must be taken during the dissection to visualize and preserve the nerve. Some guidelines advocate the use of intra-operative nerve monitoring, although its ability to prevent injury has not been proven. The most likely place where nerve injury occurs is not during ligation of the inferior thyroid arteries, but more often during division of the suspensory ligament of Berry. Injury to the recurrent laryngeal nerve leads to vocal cord paralysis and if bilateral, it may lead to airway occlusion secondary to the vocal cords being paralyzed in adduction. This will require a permanent tracheostomy.

Another important complication after surgery is post-op stridor and hypoxia in the recovery room due to a hematoma under the deep cervical fascia. If found, patients need evacuation of the hematoma by opening the wound at bedside in the recovery room to prevent hypoxic insult to the brain.

Follicular carcinoma (15% of all thyroid cancers) occurs mostly in elderly patients. Women are affected more than men. This tumor is more aggressive than papillary carcinoma. Follicular carcinoma spreads hematogenously with distant metastasis to the lung and bone. Treatment requires total thyroidectomy with postoperative radioiodine ablation. Again, FNA cytology alone cannot differentiate between benign and malignant tumors.

Anaplastic carcinoma (10% of all thyroid cancer) occurs mostly in elderly patients. Women are affected more than men. This is highly malignant with rapid and painful enlargement. Eighty percent of patients die within 1 year of diagnosis. Treatment is not surgical, except for palliation (e.g., tracheostomy).

Medullary carcinoma (5% of all thyroid cancer) occurs as a sporadic or familial form. Its tumor arises from parafollicular cells of the thyroid and is more malignant than follicular carcinoma. The tumor often produces calcitonin as a tumor marker.

Medullary carcinoma is the component of 2 types of MEN (multiple endocrine neoplasia):

- MEN Type 2A (Sipple syndrome): pheochromocytoma, medullary thyroid carcinoma, and (in 50% of cases) parathyroid hyperplasia
- MEN Type 2B: pheochromocytoma, medullary carcinoma, and neuromas

Medullary carcinoma may also occur in families without other associated endocrine dysfunctions. The only effective therapy is thyroidectomy, which should be performed after pheochromocytoma resection if an MEN syndrome is present.

Follow-up Management and Prevention

Thyroid cancer staging is typically done after total thyroidectomy. As this is the only tissue in the body which uptakes and concentrates iodine, total body radioiodine scan offers a unique opportunity to stage the disease for distant metastasis. The premise is that if the entire thyroid gland is removed, radioiodine injected will not be taken up by any part of the body unless there is a metastatic focus of thyroid tissue.

If the scan is indeed positive with metastatic foci, therapeutic dose of radioiodine is injected that will selectively be absorbed by metastasis and in the process the cancer foci in the body will be ablated. This is a very good example of highly selective anti-cancer therapy that will only destroy cancer without affecting normal tissue.

Follow up for future cancer recurrence will be based on serial estimation of thyroglobulin protein, which is only produced by thyroid follicles. After thyroidectomy, its levels are undetectable. Recurrence is suspected when the thyroglobulin begins to rise in the serum.

Final Diagnosis

Papillary thyroid cancer

CASE 18

Chief Complaint

"I have a hard time swallowing food."

History and Physical Examination

A 65-year-old man comes to the office complaining of difficulty swallowing. The patient was in his usual state of health until approximately 1 month ago, when he noted difficulty swallowing, especially solid foods. He does not seem to have a problem swallowing liquids. He also notes a 10-lb weight loss in the last few weeks. His temperature is 37.0 C (98.6 F), and blood pressure is 125/80 mm Hg.

The patient has a 50-pack-year smoking history and drinks 3–4 ounces of vodka a night. He had an episode of pneumonia about 8 months ago. He is a thin man in no apparent distress. Upon physical examination there is some evidence of bitemporal wasting. There is no head and neck adenopathy. The lungs are clear to auscultation, and cardiac exam is normal. The abdomen is soft with no palpable masses. Rectal examination reveals guaiac-positive stool and no palpable masses.

Basic Science Correlate

Cachexia related to cancer is due to the high metabolic activity of tumors and the release of tumor necrosis factor alpha (TNFα).

CLINICAL PEARL

Temporal wasting is a sign of significant weight loss and is a suggestion for cancer.

Differential Diagnosis

1. Esophageal cancer
   - Explains presenting symptoms and patient's history puts him at high risk
2. Gastric cancer
   - Explains presenting symptoms and patient's history puts him at high risk
3. Gastroesophageal reflux disease (GERD) with stricture
   - Weight loss may be from reduced oral intake
4. Esophageal diverticulum
   - Weight loss may be from reduced oral intake

Initial Management

Setting: outpatient

Diagnostic/Therapeutic Plan

- Blood work: CBC, comprehensive metabolic panel
- Chest x-ray
- Upper GI swallow

Test Results

- Hemoglobin 10 g/dL (normal 13–15 g/dL), electrolytes and liver function panel normal

- X-ray: no masses identified, normal cardiac silhouette

- Upper GI swallow: ~3 cm-long mass in distal esophagus just proximal to the esophagogastric junction

Assessment

Based on the anemia, weight loss, and results of the upper GI swallow, this is likely carcinoma of the distal esophagus. The appearance of a mass on the upper GI swallow effectively excludes a benign condition such as a stricture or diverticulum, and localizes the lesion to the esophagus rather than the stomach.

Biopsy is essential to confirm the diagnosis and histology.

Further Management Plan/Results

- Upper endoscopy with biopsy: squamous cell carcinoma

- CT scan of the chest and abdomen: negative for adenopathy or distant lesions

- Endoscopic U/S: T3N0 lesion confined to the distal esophagus

- PET scan

- Cardiopulmonary assessment: WNL

- Surgical resection: esophagectomy

Discussion

Years ago most malignant esophageal malignancies were squamous cell carcinomas and often associated with cigarette smoking and prolonged alcohol abuse. Today, adenocarcinomas are more common and associated with GERD (the fast food culture of pizza and soda drinks, burgers and fries is rampant and responsible for GERD, epidemic in the United States). The treatment of choice for a patient with a localized distal esophageal cancer is surgical resection. Depending on the location of the tumor and presence/absence of lymph node involvement, neoadjuvant chemotherapy and radiation may be indicated.

There are several approaches to the surgical procedure: transhiatal with neck incision; laparotomy and right thoracotomy ("Ivor-Lewis"); laparotomy, right thoracotomy, and neck incision ("McKeown"); and left thoracoabdominal. In the workup of esophageal cancer, one must also consider bronchoscopy for lesions in the mid or proximal esophagus because of the potential of invasion of the tracheobronchial tree.

For unresectable esophageal cancer, dysphagia can be palliated by dilation, laser therapy, or stenting. Radiation therapy and chemotherapy are used but increased overall survival has yet to be proven.

CLINICAL PEARL

The best test to assess local invasion of a tumor of the GI tract is endoscopic U/S, a minimally invasive procedure. It can assess the presence and depth of adenopathy, and thus essential in the workup of esophageal and rectal carcinoma.

Follow-up Management and Prevention

Esophageal carcinoma is restaged pathologically after surgical resection. The presence/absence of residual tumor and lymph node involvement dictates adjuvant therapy, typically with platinum-based chemotherapy after appropriate recovery. Nutrition is of utmost importance in the post-operative patient, with the majority of surgeons placing an enteral feeding distal to the pylorus at the time of resection, most commonly with a feeding jejunostomy.

Modifiable risk factors for esophageal carcinoma include smoking and alcohol consumption, both of which are modifiable and should be addressed with every patient at risk. Barrett's esophagus is the presence of metaplasia of the esophagus from the normal stratified squamous epithelium to a columnar epithelium with goblet cells due to chronic gastric acid reflux. Patients with Barrett's are screened regularly with upper endoscopy with random biopsies. The presence of high-grade dysplasia is an indication for surgical resection as this histology is highly predictive of progression to carcinoma.

Final Diagnosis

Esophageal cancer, squamous cell

CASE 19

Chief Complaint

Right upper quadrant pain

History and Physical Examination

A 64-year-old man comes to the office complaining of epigastric and right upper quadrant (RUQ) pain. He was in his usual state of health until approximately 2 months ago, when he started noticing epigastric pain that radiated to the RUQ and to the back. He has also had a 6-lb weight loss and has noticed a darkening of his urine. His past medical history is significant for stable angina. His temperature is 37.0 C (98.6 F) and BP 150/80 mm Hg. His sclera is mildly icteric. His lungs are clear and heart has a regular rate and rhythm. His abdomen is soft, non-tender, and non-distended. There is fullness appreciated upon palpation of the RUQ. Rectal examination shows guaiac-negative stool and no palpable masses.

Differential Diagnosis

1. Intrinsic obstruction of common bile duct: choledocholithiasis, cholangiocarcinoma, or biliary stenosis

2. Extrinsic compression of common bile duct: pancreatic mass, duodenal mass or inflammation, or lymph nodes

Initial Management

Setting: outpatient

Diagnostic/Therapeutic Plan

- Blood work: serum electrolytes, LFTs, CBC, coagulation profile
- RUQ U/S

Test Results

- LFTs: significant for a direct bilirubin of 5 mg/dL, alkaline phosphatase 420 U/L; electrolytes, CBC, albumin and coagulation profile all normal
- U/S: dilated gallbladder and common bile duct; fullness in region of the head of the pancreas, no stones

Basic Science Correlate

Bile is necessary to absorb fat-soluble vitamins A, D, E, and K. Vitamin K is necessary for hepatic synthesis of clotting factors, so patients with obstructive jaundice can present with coagulopathy. This is especially important to assess in considering an operative intervention of any sort (including an ERCP for sphincterotomy).

CLINICAL PEARL

Endoscopic U/S is useful for assessing the extent of a mass. It can guide biopsy as well, although when surgical resection is being considered, plan carefully, as seeding of the area with tumor can possibly worsen prognosis. Similarly, routine biliary stenting by ERCP should not be performed as it is associated with increased post-operative infection and overall morbidity, and offers little benefit outside of an acute obstructive process or cholangitis.

Assessment

The elevated bilirubin and sonographic findings suggest obstructive jaundice secondary to a pancreatic mass. The possibility of obstructive jaundice secondary to a benign process, such as common bile duct stones, is less likely with a sonogram suggesting "fullness" at the head of the pancreas. The pain radiating to his back is also common in a pancreatic process. The finding of a painless palpable gallbladder (i.e., Courvoisier's sign) is associated with a proximal pancreatic mass.

Further Management Plan/Results

- CT scan of abdomen with IV contrast: mass in the head of the pancreas; dilated common bile duct, pancreatic duct and gallbladder; no evidence of any other masses in the liver
- ERCP: no intraductal mass identified
- Serum CA 19–9: 100 U/mL (normal <40 U/mL)
- Pancreaticoduodenectomy (Whipple procedure)

Discussion

This patient has a malignant mass localized to the head of the pancreas, and ERCP shows no involvement of the ducts. Surgical exploration, i.e., the Whipple procedure, in an attempt to entirely resect the cancer is the treatment of choice. If at the time of exploration distant metastases are identified, then a palliative surgical bypass of the common bile duct should be considered. Similarly, if impending obstruction of the gastric outlet is identified, bypass with a gastrojejunostomy should also be considered. Palliation can also be accomplished with percutaneous transhepatic drainage. Percutaneous endoscopic gastrostomy can also be used for GI decompression for palliation. A celiac axis block at the time of operative exploration can also be performed for palliation.

Pancreatic cancer is the fifth most common cause of cancer-related death. It is associated with smoking, benzidine, alcohol, diabetes, and chronic pancreatitis. Eighty percent are ductal cell adenocarcinoma, and 80% involve the pancreatic head. Pancreatic cancer is characterized by painless jaundice, anemia, and weight loss. Pain is more commonly seen with body/tail tumors, often with celiac plexus involvement.

Courvoisier's sign is seen in about 50% of pancreatic tumors at the head of the pancreas. Other possible findings are cholangitis and migratory thrombophlebitis. Laboratory tests show elevated LFTs with predominant direct hyperbilirubinemia and increased alkaline phosphatase. The tumor marker is CA 19–9. The gold standard for diagnosis is a CT scan, but ERCP and MRCP are also useful. Duplex U/S can add additional helpful information in assessing vessel encasement and therefore operability.

A mass is considered unresectable if:

- Encasing of a vessel or lymph node is positive in the hilum of the liver
- There are liver metastases or multiple peritoneal metastases.

In these cases, palliate by drainage of the biliary tree via stent or open surgery, and percutaneous endoscopic gastrostomy.

If resectable (confirmed to pancreas and not encasing portal vein), the procedure of choice is the Whipple procedure. Consider postoperative chemotherapy for cases involving systemic disease. There is an approximate 5–20% chance of a 5-year survival. If the tumor size is <2 cm and confined to the pancreas, then the 5-year survival rate is 40%.

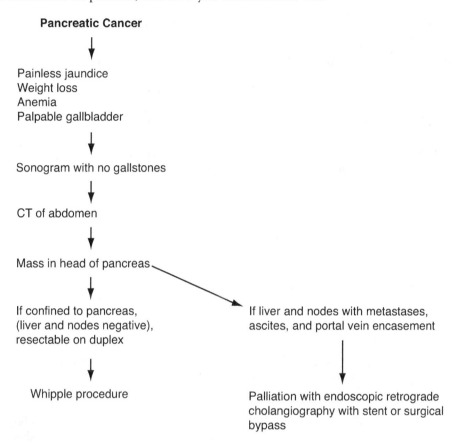

Pancreatic Cancer

Painless jaundice
Weight loss
Anemia
Palpable gallbladder

Sonogram with no gallstones

CT of abdomen

Mass in head of pancreas

If confined to pancreas, (liver and nodes negative), resectable on duplex

If liver and nodes with metastases, ascites, and portal vein encasement

Whipple procedure

Palliation with endoscopic retrograde cholangiography with stent or surgical bypass

Follow-up Management and Prevention

Systemic chemotherapy is not very effective with pancreatic cancer, but is the only option in late stage disease. It should be considered in the adjuvant setting based on lymph node staging. Unfortunately there is no effective screening tool for pancreatic cancer.

Final Diagnosis

Pancreatic cancer

CASE 20

Chief Complaint

Left lower quadrant abdominal pain and fever

History and Physical Examination

A 60-year-old man, otherwise healthy, is brought to the emergency department because of a sudden onset of severe left lower quadrant (LLQ) abdominal pain. He has no nausea, vomiting, or recent changes in bowel habits. On physical examination his vital signs are: temperature 38.3 C (101 F), pulse 100/min, BP 120/80 mm Hg, and respirations 22/min. On abdominal exam, the patient has a moderately distended abdomen, with tenderness to palpation and guarding in the LLQ. There are no hernias. The rectal exam is negative. Stool is negative for occult blood.

Differential Diagnosis

1. Acute diverticulitis

   - Most consistent with the patient's history and physical; no information is given regarding the patient's history of previous episodes, family history, or colonoscopy, but this is still the leading diagnosis.

2. Perforated colon carcinoma

   - Given the patient's age, this is a significant concern and if perforated, can present similar to an acute episode of diverticulitis.

3. Inflammatory bowel disease (IBD)

   - An acute exacerbation with possible bowel perforation could explain the findings, and ulcerative colitis does have a second peak in 6th decade of life, making this a possible diagnosis.

Initial Management

Setting: emergency department

Diagnostic/Therapeutic Plan

- Blood work: CBC with differential, serum electrolytes
- Chest x-ray
- CT scan of abdomen and pelvis with IV contrast

Test Results

- WBC 12,000/mL; electrolytes normal
- Chest x-ray: no pneumoperitoneum
- CT scan: significant LLQ phlegmon

Assessment

Any of the diagnoses in the differential could cause this abdominal pain and explain the CT scan findings. Without any prior GI symptoms, diverticulitis would be most likely.

If the patient had prior GI symptoms such as altered bowel habits, bleeding per rectum, and weight loss, the more likely diagnosis will be colon cancer or IBD. A family history would be helpful as well.

Further Management Plan

1. NPO
2. IV hydration
3. IV antibiotics

Discussion

If the patient responds to the above treatment and this is the first episode, no further treatment is necessary except for dietary fiber intake. He will absolutely need a colonoscopy in approximately 6 wks to evaluate for a malignancy. Colonoscopy is not performed in the acute setting for potential perforation risk.

If the patient responds to the above treatment but this has been one of multiple episodes, consideration should be toward elective resection of the involved colon. If the patient does not respond or worsens, intervention is necessary. If CT scan demonstrates a pericolic abscess, percutaneous drainage should be performed to potentially avoid a surgical intervention. Surgical intervention usually involves resection with end colostomy (Hartmann's procedure).

Management of Acute Diverticulitis

IV antibiotics, IV fluids, bowel rest

Pain improves → Colonoscopy 4 weeks later

If colonoscopy is positive for cancer (not commonly coexistent with acute diverticulitis) → Sigmoid resection (6 weeks) → Chemotherapy

If diverticulitis without mucosal lesion (cancer) → Sigmoid resection electively

Pain worsens, peritonitis progresses → Emergent laparotomy, Hartman procedure → (6 weeks) Reversal of Hartman procedure

Follow-up Management and Prevention

If the patient recovers from this episode without surgery, colonoscopy is performed no sooner than 6 weeks later to evaluate for malignancy, either at the site of perforation or a synchronous lesion elsewhere in the large intestine. If the patient undergoes surgery, pathological assessment of the specimen will dictate further management. If malignancy is present, degree of local invasion and further evaluation for metastatic disease will determine whether systemic chemotherapy is warranted. Colostomy reversal should be considered at a later time after adequate recovery from the acute process and/or systemic antineoplastic therapy, if indicated.

Final Diagnosis

Acute diverticulitis of the sigmoid colon

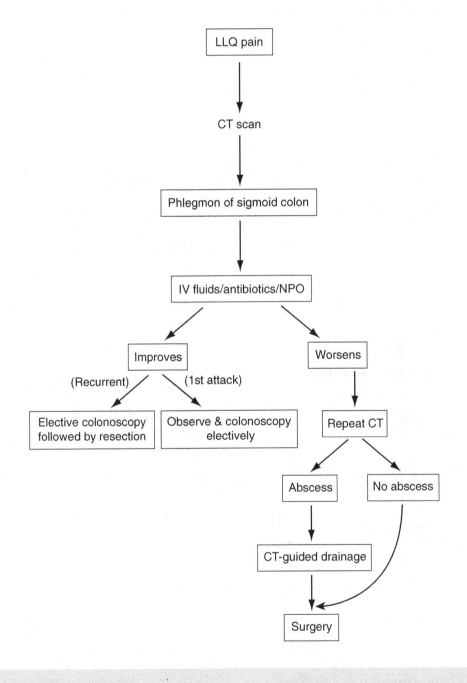

CASE 21

Chief Complaint

Bulge with tenderness in the abdominal wall

History and Physical Examination

A 40-year-old man with previous history of emergent laparotomy for perforated peptic ulcer now presents with a 6-month history of an enlarging tender bulge of his abdominal wall. It is made worse by coughing, sneezing, or straining. There are no other GI complaints. On physical exam, the patient is afebrile and has normal vital signs. Examination is normal except for his abdomen, which has a midline scar and a reducible, slightly tender hernia. The overlying skin is normal.

Differential Diagnosis

1. Ventral incisional hernia

   • Most common cause of ventral hernia

2. Epigastric hernia

3. Diastasis recti

   • Not a true hernia

Initial Management

Setting: outpatient

Diagnostic/Therapeutic Plan

• Blood work: CBC and electrolytes

Test Results

• Blood work WNL

Assessment

An uncomplicated, symptomatic ventral incisional hernia should be repaired surgically. The approach is at the discretion of the surgeon and can be open or laparoscopic and commonly includes the use of mesh or a primary suture repair. No one approach has been demonstrated to be more superior.

Should the patient have associated GI complaints, a CT scan should be obtained to rule out underlying intra-abdominal pathology. If the patient has evidence of incarceration (inability to reduce the hernia) or strangulation (compromised blood flow with overlying skin changes), emergent surgical intervention is required.

Further Management Plan

• CT scan: fascial defect without any other abnormalities

• Surgical repair

Discussion

Ventral hernias are most commonly secondary to prior abdominal operations. The decision whether to do a laparoscopic or open approach, with or without mesh, is at the discretion of the surgeon. If the hernia is secondary to an intra-abdominal pathology (carcinoma), this should be addressed first.

Epigastric hernias are spontaneous hernias not due to prior surgical intervention. Diastasis recti is not a true hernia (no fascial defect), but rather, a separation of the rectus abdominis at the linea alba. It needs no surgical intervention.

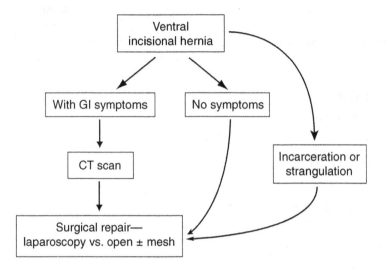

Final Diagnosis

Ventral incisional hernia

CASE 22

Chief Complaint

Pain and tingling in fingers

History and Physical Examination

A 30-year-old female computer programmer has had progressive symptoms of pain and tingling in the thumb, index finger, long finger, and ring finger of her right hand for one year. This is made worse when she spends long hours typing and at night. She is otherwise healthy.

On physical examination the patient is afebrile and vital signs are normal. Examination is normal except for right hand and wrist, which reveal decreased sensation over the median nerve distribution. Motor function is intact. Pulses are normal. There is no muscle atrophy or skin changes. Tinel's and Phalen's signs are both positive.

Differential Diagnosis

1. Carpal tunnel syndrome
2. Cervical radiculopathy
3. Osteoarthritis
4. Tendonitis

Initial Management

Setting: outpatient

Diagnostic/Therapeutic Plan

- Blood work: CBC and electrolytes
- Wrist x-rays, AP and lateral views
- Cervical x-rays if indicated

Test Results

- Blood work: normal
- X-rays: normal

Assessment

Carpal tunnel syndrome due to median nerve compression

CLINICAL PEARL

Tinel's sign is replication of symptoms by tapping the median nerve at the wrist.

Phalen's sign is replication of symptoms caused by flexion of the wrist joints for 2 min.

Further Management Plan

1. Rest to the wrist joint

2. Orthotic splints

3. NSAIDS

4. Steroidal injections

Discussion

Usually non-operative treatment of carpal tunnel syndrome is successful. Should it fail, surgical intervention with decompression of the carpal tunnel is indicated. Nerve conduction velocities (NCV) and electromyography (EMG) are mandatory prior to surgery to confirm the diagnosis.

Final Diagnosis

Carpal tunnel syndrome

CASE 23

Chief Complaint

Pain in the wrist after fall

History and Physical Examination

A 30-year-old woman slipped and fell and landed on her outstretched hand, resulting in immediate pain in the wrist. She is otherwise healthy with no complaints. On physical examination the patient is afebrile with normal vital signs. She has exquisite tenderness in the wrist at the anatomical snuffbox. Neurovascular exam is normal. There is no obvious deformity of the wrist joint and there is a full range of motion.

Differential Diagnosis

1. Scaphoid fracture

2. Colles' fracture: fracture of the distal radius and ulnar styloid

3. Supracondylar fracture of the humerus

Initial Management

Setting: outpatient

Diagnostic/Therapeutic Plan

- Blood work: CBC and electrolytes

- Anteroposterior and lateral x-ray of the wrist

Test Results

- Blood work: CBC and electrolytes: normal

- X-ray: scaphoid fracture

Assessment

Scaphoid fracture

Further Management Plan

Immobilization (splint and/or cast)

Discussion

Not all scaphoid fractures are immediately visualized on initial x-ray evaluation. Failure to make this diagnosis can result in avascular necrosis of the scaphoid, which can result in severe disability. Therefore, if the x-rays are negative and the clinical suspicion is high, treatment is performed as if this is a scaphoid fracture.

Subsequent follow-up should include one of the following:

- Repeat x-ray in 1–2 wks

- Bone scan

- MRI (most sensitive of these tests) to confirm or rule out the diagnosis

Follow-up Management and Prevention

Repeat x-rays in 1–2 weeks to assess healing of the fracture. If x-ray is indeterminate, MRI is indicated.

Final Diagnosis

Scaphoid fracture

CASE 24

Chief Complaint

Abdominal pain and fullness

History and Physical Examination

A 55-year-old man has noticed for the past 2 months progressive discomfort and fullness in his abdomen. He also complains of early satiety. Three months ago he was involved in a severe motor vehicle accident, where he had a steering wheel injury to his chest and abdomen. He has no other GI symptoms. He does not drink alcohol and has no history of biliary tract disease.

On physical examination the patient is afebrile with normal vital signs. He is anicteric. Examination is normal except for the abdomen, which reveals epigastric fullness with moderate tenderness. Bowel sounds are normal and there are no hernias. There are no discrete masses or organomegaly. Rectal examination is negative.

Differential Diagnosis

1. Pancreatic pseudocyst
2. Intra-abdominal malignancy
3. Bowel obstruction
4. Biliary tract disease

Initial Management

Setting: inpatient

Diagnostic/Therapeutic Plan

- Blood work: CBC, serum electrolytes, LFTs, lipase, amylase
- Chest and abdominal x-ray
- Abdominal U/S
- CT scan of the abdomen with oral and IV contrast

Test Results

- Blood work: normal except for slight lipase elevation
- X-ray: no pneumoperitoneum, no dilated loops of bowel
- U/S: no gallstones; ill-defined cystic mass in the area of the mid-pancreas
- CT scan: 8 cm cystic mass in mid-portion of the pancreas

Assessment

Most likely this represents a pancreatic pseudocyst secondary to blunt abdominal trauma. This could represent a cystic pancreatic neoplasm, but this is less likely, given the history of trauma.

Further Management

Internal surgical drainage (cystogastrostomy, cystoduodenostomy, cystojejunostomy).

Discussion

Pancreatic pseudocyst can occur from pancreatitis due to any cause. In this case, the history of trauma is suspect. However, cystic neoplasms of the pancreas must always be considered, as the traumatic incident may not be related. Complications from pancreatic pseudocyst include extrinsic obstruction, infection, and hemorrhage.

Pancreatic pseudocysts that are asymptomatic and small can be observed and followed by imaging studies. Maturation of the pseudocyst (satisfactory thickness of the pseudocyst wall to hold sutures) must be present (determined by CT scan and may take as long as 6–8 weeks) before surgical intervention. In general terms, the management of pancreatic pseudocysts is 6 cm diameter, 6 mm thick wall, and 6 weeks old before surgery is considered.

As noted, internal drainage is the best treatment, but if the cyst is infected, percutaneous drainage is the right thing to do.

Final Diagnosis

Pancreatic pseudocyst

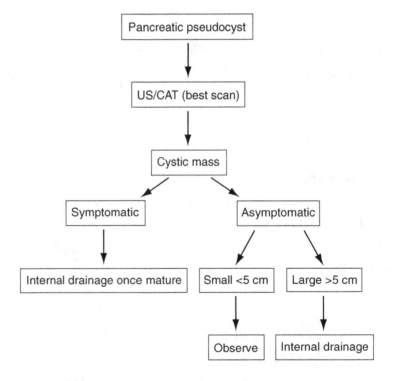

CASE 25

Chief Complaint

Newborn in severe respiratory distress

History and Physical Examination

A newborn presents with severe respiratory distress following a normal pregnancy and delivery. On physical exam, the infant is afebrile with marked tachypnea and using all accessory muscles of respiration. There is no evidence of cyanosis. HEENT is normal with trachea in the midline. There are decreased breath sounds in left chest but normal breath sounds in right chest. Heart has no murmurs or gallops. Abdomen is scaphoid, soft, no masses, or organomegaly. There are normal bowel sounds.

Differential Diagnosis

1. Congenital diaphragmatic hernia (CDH)
2. Spontaneous pneumothorax
3. Chylothorax

Initial Management

Setting: emergency department

Diagnostic/Therapeutic Plan

- Blood work: CBC and electrolytes
- Continuous pulse oximetry
- Serial arterial blood gases
- Chest x-ray

Test Results

- Blood work: normal
- Oximetry: O_2 saturation in mid 80%s
- Blood gases: severe hypoxia and acidosis
- X-ray: air fluid levels in left chest; absence of significant lung markings

Assessment

Acute respiratory distress secondary to CDH

Further Management

1. ABCs of resuscitation, including emergent endotracheal or nasogastric intubation

2. NG tube decompression

3. Operative repair of diaphragmatic hernia

Discussion

As there was clear evidence of bowel in the chest and no evidence of pneumothorax or chylothorax, the diagnosis is CDH. This infant needs emergent surgical intervention. The repair of the diaphragm is done through the abdomen and is in fact not difficult to do.

The complications of this disease do not relate to the surgery but to the hypoplasia of bilateral lungs. The subsequent inability to ventilate this infant because of the lung hypoplasia is the major contributor of this infant's morbidity and mortality. Extracorporeal membrane oxygenation may be helpful to oxygenate the infant until the lungs develop further and recover. Prior to delivery, CDH can only be diagnosed in utero by U/S.

Final Diagnosis

CDH

PART IV

EPIDEMIOLOGY AND BIOSTATISTICS

KEY DEFINITIONS

Epidemiology. Study of the distribution and determinants of health-related states within a population. It refers to the patterns of disease and the factors that influence those patterns.

Clinical epidemiology. Study and application of population-based data with patient decision-making.

Endemic. The usual, expected rate of disease over time. The disease is maintained without much variation within a region.

Epidemic. Occurrence of disease in *excess* of the expected rate. Epidemiology is the "study of epidemics." Usually presents in a larger geographic span than endemics.

Pandemic. A worldwide epidemic.

Epidemic curve. A visual description of an epidemic curve is disease cases plotted against time. The classic signature of an epidemic is *a "spike" in time.*

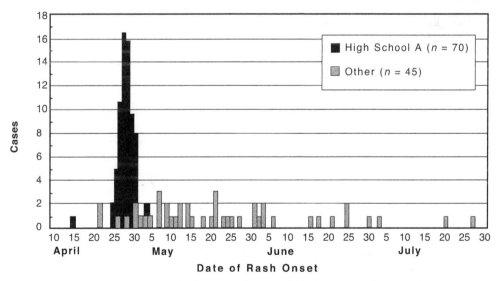

Reported measles cases by date of rash onset, Elgin, Illinois, April 15 to July 28, 1985

Measles Outbreak

An explosive point-source outbreak of measles in an Elgin, Illinois school caused by a single index case whose hacking cough produced an aerosol of measles virus.

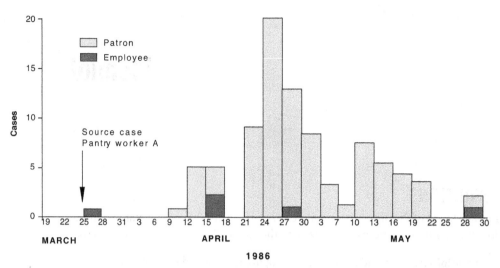

Onsets of illness in patrons and employees: hepatitis A outbreak on a floating restaurant, Florida.

Food-Borne Outbreak

A food-borne outbreak of hepatitis A among patrons of a Fort Lauderdale, Florida restaurant.

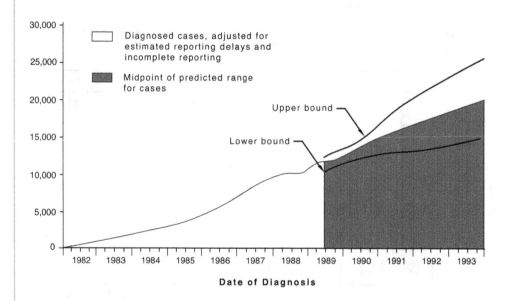

Multiple-Year Increase in AIDS Cases in the United States

Continuous increase in U.S. AIDS cases from the original report of 5 cases in 1981 through the 500,000th case reported in 1995, and beyond.

TYPES OF PREVENTION

Prevention goals in medicine promote health, preserve health, restore health when it is impaired, and minimize suffering and distress. These goals aim to minimize both morbidity and mortality.

Primary prevention is the promotion of health at both individual and community levels by facilitating health-enhancing behaviors, preventing the onset of risk behaviors, and diminishing exposure to environmental hazards. *Primary prevention efforts decrease disease incidence.*

Secondary prevention is the screening for risk factors and early detection of asymptomatic or mild disease, permitting timely and effective intervention and curative treatment. *Secondary prevention efforts decrease disease prevalence.*

Tertiary prevention is the reduction of long-term impairments and disabilities and prevention of repeated episodes of clinical illness. The goals of tertiary prevention are to prevent recurrence and to slow progression.

Examples of Prevention for Coronary Heart Disease

Primary prevention	Health education programs to promote healthy lifestyles and prevent onset of heart disease risk factors. An example would be the "Hearty Heart" nutrition program for elementary school children.
Secondary prevention	Community blood pressure screening. Physician support to quit smoking cigarettes.
Tertiary prevention	Graded aerobic physical activity program prescribed to patients during recovery from first myocardial infarction.

REVIEW QUESTIONS

Prevention and Key Definitions

Response options for **Questions 1–4**:

    A. Health promotion

    B. Primary prevention

    C. Secondary prevention

    D. Tertiary prevention

    E. Palliative care

1. Breast self-examination.

2. Physical therapy/rehabilitation and ergonomic training program for blue-collar workers recovering from severe back strain injury sustained on the job.

3. School-based sexual health education program for middle school students.

4. Confidential PPD testing to detect latent tuberculosis infection conducted at community clinics by county health department personnel.

Response options for **Questions 5–7**:

    A. Hypoendemic

    B. Endemic

    C. Epidemic

    D. Hyperendemic

    E. Pandemic

    F. Holoendemic

5. A multinational outbreak of influenza

6. The rapid rise in AIDS cases among drug injectors in Bangkok in the late 1980s

7. The long-term, relatively constant rate of occurrence of colorectal cancer in U.S. women

---

1. **Answer: C.** Self-screening for early detection leading to early diagnosis and effective, life-saving treatment.

2. **Answer: D.** Rehabilitation following an episode of injury with a concurrent focus on preventing subsequent injury.

3. **Answer: B.** Prevention of onset of risky sexual behaviors.

4. **Answer: C.** Screening to detect tuberculosis (TB) infection, to be followed by therapy to prevent progression to active TB.

5. **Answer: E.** A pandemic is an epidemic that crosses national borders.

6. **Answer: C.** AIDS appeared suddenly, and the epidemic increased exponentially.

7. **Answer: B.** When disease cases are plotted over time, a flat horizontal line depicts an endemic pattern.

MEASURES OF MORBIDITY AND MORTALITY

Rates

Rate is the frequency of occurrence of epidemiologic events in a population. It is used to compare epidemiologic events among populations.

Rate allows direct comparison of "events per identical number of people" in different populations, or of epidemiologic events in a single population assessed at different points in time.

Rate Equation

$$\text{Rate} = \frac{\text{Numerator}}{\text{Denominator}} \times \text{Multiplier}$$

where the *numerator* is the number of epidemiologic events, the *denominator* is the number of people in the population of interest, and the *multiplier* is selected so that the result of the rate computation generally yields a number in the range from 1 to 100.

Multipliers

For major vital statistics, such as birth rate, death rate, and infant mortality rate, the preferred multiplier is 1,000. The result is expressed as a "rate per 1,000."

For individual diseases, the most common multiplier is 100,000. The result is expressed as a "rate per 100,000."

Matching Numerator and Denominator

- Essential rule: Match the numerator with the denominator.
- Match on person, place, and time characteristics.

$$\text{Rate} = \frac{\text{Epidemiologic events occurring in a population of persons at a given place at a given time}}{\text{Defined population of persons at a given place at a given time}} \times \text{Multiplier}$$

SPECIFIC AND ADJUSTED RATES

Specific Rates

Specific rates "specify" a subset of the total population that is singled out for special examination or comparison with other subsets of the population. Use the following formula:

$$\text{Specific rate} = \frac{\text{All events in specified subpopulation}}{\text{Specified subpopulation}} \times \text{Multiplier}$$

Common demographic variables used for specific rates:

- Age group
- Gender
- Race/ethnicity
- Highest level of education attained
- Marital status
- Socioeconomic status

NOTE

Populations can be stratified on 2 or more demographic variables at a time.

Matching numerator and denominator is the most important concept for computing specific rates. Example:

"Event" of interest:	Cancer deaths
Place:	State of Nevada
Time:	Calendar year, 1996
Rate of interest:	Age-specific rate* for ages 45–64
Formula:	$\dfrac{\text{Deaths from cancer among persons ages } 45-64 \text{ in Nevada during 1996}}{\text{Population of Nevada residents ages } 45-64, \text{ midyear 1996}} \times 100,000$

*Age-specific rate: a rate for a specified age group

Adjusted Rates (or Standardized)

Definition: Rates calculated after using statistical procedures to minimize demographic differences between populations being compared. Comparisons of rates between two groups may be misleading if the composition of the groups differs on important demographic characteristics. Adjustment improves the validity of the comparison.

The following two cases are examples of comparisons between groups where rate adjustment is clearly essential.

The rate of alcoholism and alcohol abuse is found to be higher among workers in an automobile assembly plant compared with same-age workers at a textile mill in the same city.

Adjustment for gender differences is warranted. *First, the two populations differ on a demographic characteristic:* Automotive workers tend to be men; textile workers tend to be women. *Second, the disease/disorder is related to the same demographic:* Alcohol problems are more prevalent in men. The higher observed rate in automotive workers may be due to the marked differences in gender in the two employee populations.

> The rate of lung cancer is found to be higher among male factory workers ages 50–64, than among male computer programmers ages 50–64, in the same company.

Adjustment for level of education is warranted. *First, the two populations differ on a demographic characteristic:* Factory workers tend to have a low level of education; computer programmers are likely to be college graduates. *Second, the disease/disorder is related to the same demographic:* The major cause of lung cancer is cigarette smoking. People with lower levels of education have higher smoking rates; college graduates have the lowest smoking rates. The differences in lung cancer rates may reflect expected differences in smoking prevalence rates for workers with different levels of education.

Properties of a board-style adjusted rate problem:

- A significant difference in the rate of disease is declared to exist between two groups. The compared rates are unadjusted.

- The two groups differ on a key demographic variable.

- The disease is known to be related to the same demographic variable.

- *Adjustment will tend to make the observed difference between unadjusted rates disappear.*

Disease Rates Positively Correlated with Age

		Population A		Population B		Population C	
		Cases	**Population**	**Cases**	**Population**	**Cases**	**Population**
Younger	1/1,000	1	1,000	2	2,000	3	3,000
Intermediate	2/1,000	4	2,000	4	2,000	4	2,000
Older	3/1,000	9	3,000	6	2,000	3	1,000
		14	6,000	12	6,000	10	6,000
Crude Rates	Per/1,000	2.3		2.0		1.6	

REVIEW QUESTIONS

Adjusted Rates

8. In the United States, the suicide rate for physicians is significantly higher than the corresponding rate for the general population. What is the most appropriate interpretation of this finding?

   A. Higher suicide rates in physicians are likely to be related to job stress, including life-and-death decision making for patients in the care of the physician.

   B. Higher rates of suicide in physicians are likely to be related to constant exposure to human suffering, trauma, and death.

   C. Physicians have higher rates of suicide than the general population; no further interpretation is possible from the information presented.

   D. While the unadjusted rate of suicide is higher for physicians, failure to adjust for differences between physicians and the general population on socioeconomic status precludes meaningful interpretation of this finding.

   E. The finding of statistical significance proves that physicians are at higher risk for suicide than nonphysicians.

8. **Answer: D.** When a significant relationship is stated but the comparison groups have some obvious demographic difference, look for the answer that suggests conclusions may be invalid unless rates are "adjusted" or "standardized" to compensate for the demographic disparities.

   In this instance, physicians are generally a higher socioeconomic status (SES) group relative to the general population. Suicide rates are elevated for high-SES people. Once adjusted for SES differences, the finding of higher suicide rates in physicians no longer stands.

   Note: Strongly suspect any response that claims that "proof" has been demonstrated. No single study can achieve proof. Furthermore, no investigator would be so self-aggrandizing as to claim to have conducted the definitive study. Such a response option ("distractor") is almost always wrong.

MEASURES OF MORBIDITY

Incidence and Prevalence

Prevalence Rate: All Cases

Prevalence rate is the proportion of individuals with existing disease at a point in time (point prevalence). It is the proportion of individuals with existing disease during a period of time (period prevalence).

- The focus is on chronic conditions.
- The numerator refers to ALL individuals who have the illness at the time(s) in question.

$$\text{Prevalence rate} = \frac{\substack{\text{Persons with existing disease} \\ \text{at a given place at a given time}}}{\substack{\text{Population of persons at risk for} \\ \text{disease at a given place at a given time}}} \times \text{Multiplier}$$

Incidence Rate: New Cases Only

- The incidence rate is the proportion of individuals developing new disease during a period of time.

- It is the rate of new disease events in a population during a period of time.

- Incidence rates can be calculated only over a period of time, not at a single point.

- The focus is on acute conditions.

$$\text{Incidence rate} = \frac{\text{Persons with disease onset at a given place at a given time}}{\text{Population of persons at risk to catch disease at a given place at a given time}} \times \text{Multiplier}$$

Attack rate is a type of incidence rate that focuses on a known exposure or risk. For example, if 10 of 100 children who attend daycare A, and 40 of 100 children who attend daycare B develop diarrhea, the attack rate would be 10% for attendance at daycare A and 40% for attendance at daycare B.

"Prevalence Pot"

A "prevalence pot" is a common portrayal of the concept of prevalence and its relationship to incidence. At the first moment of observation, the count of cases "in the pot" provides an estimate of point prevalence. Incident cases are observed over time. These new cases are added to the pre-existing cases. As long as clinical illness persists, cases remain in the pot. Cases leave the prevalence pot in one of two ways, through recovery or death. *Changes in prevalence over time can be determined by monitoring trends in incidence, recovery, and death.*

Incident cases

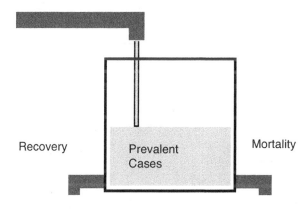
Recovery   Prevalent Cases   Mortality

Prevalence Pot Diagram

Number needed to treat (NNT): number of people in the general population who need to be treated in order to prevent one case

- The *inverse* of the incidence rate

- If incidence = 16 per 1,000 = 16/1,000

- Inverse = 1,000/16 = 625 = NNT

CCS NOTE

Relationship between Incidence and Prevalence:

- Prevalence = Incidence × Duration (conceptual formula, not computational)

- Duration $= \dfrac{\text{Prevalence}}{\text{Incidence}}$

- Changes in incidence, duration, or both will ultimately affect prevalence.

Equations for Common Epidemiological Measures

Measure	Equation	Notes
Incidence rate	$$\dfrac{\text{New cases}}{\text{Total population at risk to catch disease during period of time}}$$	• Acute cases • New cases only
Prevalence rate	$$\dfrac{\text{Total cases}}{\text{Total population at risk during period of time*}}$$	• Chronic cases • Do not include in numerator any deaths or cases that recovered from disease, as they are no longer existing cases of illness
Prevalence	Incidence × duration	• Assuming incidence and duration are stable
Duration	$$\dfrac{\text{Prevalence}}{\text{Incidence}}$$	
Number needed to treat	$$\dfrac{1}{\text{Absolute risk reduction}}$$	• Inverse of incidence rate

*Point prevalence will have denominator at a specific point in time, whereas period prevalence will include a specific period of time.

REVIEW QUESTIONS

Incidence and Prevalence

9. A pharmaceutical corporation completes trials on a vaccine for a severe strain of influenza virus demonstrating high vaccine efficacy. The Food and Drug Administration approves the vaccine for use in the U.S. As the influenza pandemic approaches U.S. borders, the Centers for Disease Control and Prevention launches a nationwide campaign to vaccinate the population using local public health department personnel throughout the country to ensure that the vaccine is available, free of charge, to all people. Assuming that a high degree of vaccine coverage is achieved, what is the expected impact of this major public health initiative?

   A. Decreased duration of influenza illness leading to decreased prevalence

   B. Decreased incidence of influenza illness leading to decreased prevalence

   C. Decreased incidence offset by increased duration: no change in prevalence

   D. No change in observed incidence or duration: no change in prevalence

   E. Effects on prevalence cannot be determined from the information provided

10. A new, effective treatment for a common disease, leading to complete cure, is developed. Which of the following impacts on disease occurrence is expected?

   A. Decreased duration of illness, leading to decreased prevalence

   B. Decreased incidence of illness, leading to decreased prevalence

   C. Decreased incidence and duration of illness, leading to decreased prevalence

   D. No change in observed incidence or duration: no change in prevalence

   E. Effects on prevalence cannot be determined from the information provided

Questions 11–14

Among 245 college students who dedicated one month of summer break to building homes for Habitat for Humanity, 12 developed back strains on the job. Based on the diagram of these 12 episodes of back strain, answer the following questions:

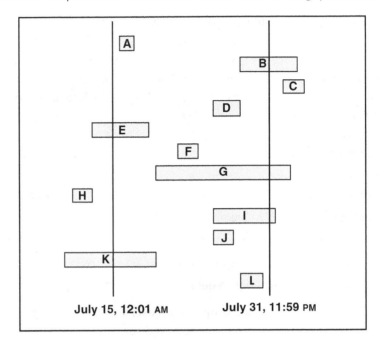

Response options for **Questions 11–14**:

A. 2/242

B. 2/244

C. 2/245

D. 3/242

E. 3/245

F. 8/242

G. 8/244

H. 8/245

I. 10/244

J. 10/245

K. 12/245

11. What is the point prevalence rate on July 15, 12:01 AM?

12. What is the point prevalence rate on July 31, 11:59 PM?

13. What is the incidence rate for the period July 15–July 31?

14. What is the period prevalence for July 15–July 31?

9. **Answer: B.** Vaccination decreases the likelihood of development of new infection and clinical disease. In turn, the prevalence during the peak of the influenza season will be decreased.

10. **Answer: A.** An effective treatment will move people more quickly toward recovery. Average duration of illness will decrease. Prevalence, the proportion of people ill with the disease at a point in time, will also decrease. This will apply to both acute and chronic diseases. When implementing a new treatment, incidence is not affected for a chronic disease. Also, the treatment per se will not affect incidence for an acute disease.

11. **Answer: C.** On July 15, two students had symptoms of back strain (E, K).

12. **Answer: E.** On July 31, three students had symptoms of back strain (B, G, I).

13. **Answer: H.** Eight new cases of back strain had onset between July 15 and July 31 (A, B, D, F, G, I, J, L).

14. **Answer: J.** A total of 10 students had symptoms of back strain at some time during the period July 15–July 31, including two with onset prior to July 15 (E, K) and eight with onset during the period July 15–31 (A, B, D, F, G, I, J, L).

VITAL STATISTICS AND RATES

Birth Rate

Definition: Rate of live births in a population during a time period (usually the calendar year).

$$\text{Simple formula: } \frac{\text{Live births}}{\text{Population}} \times 1{,}000$$

Interpretation: "Births per 1,000 population"

Fertility Rate

Definition: Rate of live births among women of childbearing age (ages 15–44) in a population during a time period (usually the calendar year).

$$\text{Simple formula: } \frac{\text{Live births}}{\text{Women of childbearing age}} \times 1{,}000$$

Interpretation: "Births per 1,000 women of child-bearing age"

Mortality Rate

Definition: Rate of deaths in a population during a time period (usually the calendar year).

$$\text{Simple formula: } \frac{\text{Deaths}}{\text{Population}} \times 1{,}000$$

Interpretation: "Deaths per 1,000 population."

Synonyms: death rate, crude death rate

Infant Mortality Rate

Definition: Yearly rate of deaths among children age <1 in relation to the number of live births during the same year. Within a population, the infant mortality rate is a key indication of the population's health status.

$$\text{Simple formula: } \frac{\text{Infant deaths}}{\text{Live births}} \times 1{,}000$$

Interpretation: "Infant deaths per 1,000 live births"

$$\text{Neonatal mortality rate: } \frac{\text{Infant deaths prior to day 28}}{\text{Live births}} \times 1{,}000$$

$$\text{Postneonatal mortality rate: } \frac{\text{Infant deaths from day 28 through day 365}}{\text{Live births}} \times 1{,}000$$

Infant mortality rate: neonatal mortality rate + postneonatal mortality rate

Perinatal mortality rate: Stillbirths and deaths in the first week of life/Live births × 1,000

Infant Mortality

The infant mortality rate of a country is the number of infant deaths for every 1,000 live births. It reflects the overall health of the society. In the United States, the rate in 2020 was 5.4 deaths per 1,000 live births, i.e., 20,000 infants died that year. The leading causes of infant death are:

- Birth defects
- Preterm birth and low birth weight
- Sudden infant death syndrome (SIDS)
- Injury (e.g., suffocation)
- Maternal pregnancy complications

Other facts

Mortality rates are higher than average among infants born to mothers who are Black, American Indian, Alaska Natives, and Pacific Islanders.

- SIDS rates reduced sharply by avoiding having infants sleep on their stomachs.

Sociologic risk factors for children

- Maternal immaturity: Risk of premature birth increases dramatically below age 19
- Poverty is a major risk factor for prematurity and other unfavorable outcomes.
- The single-parent family is also correlated with child abuse, childhood suicide, truancy, and delinquency.

Facts about adolescent pregnancy

Roughly, one million U.S. teenage girls (10% of total) become pregnant each year. Fifty percent have the child, 20% have spontaneous abortions, and 30% have an elective abortion.

- Over 50% of teens do not use contraceptives the first time they have intercourse.
- Teen mothers often drop out of school; may never work; and become welfare-dependent.
- Neonatal deaths and prematurity are common.

Adolescent sexual behavior

- Eighty percent of boys and 70% of girls are sexually active by the age of 18.
- More than 20% of all sexually active girls become pregnant at least once before the age of 20 years.
- *Pregnancy is the leading cause of school dropout among girls.*
- Roughly 80% of sexually active adolescents do not use birth control.
- *One out of five teenagers will have a sexually transmitted disease.*

Maternal mortality rate

Definition: Yearly rate of deaths in women from causes associated with childbirth in relation to the number of live births during the same year.

$$\text{Simple formula: } \frac{\text{Maternal deaths}}{\text{Live births}} \times 10,000$$

Interpretation: "Maternal deaths per 100,000 live births"

Case fatality rate (CFR)

Definition: Percentage of cases of an illness or medical condition that results in death within a specified time period.

$$\text{Simple formula: } \frac{\text{Deaths}}{\text{Cases}} \times 100$$

Interpretation: Proportion of cases that end in death (fatality)

Example: In a population of 200 people, 25 become ill, and 5 die from the illness.

$$\text{CFR} = \frac{5\text{ Deaths}}{25\text{ Cases}} \times 100 = 20\%$$

Proportionate mortality rate (PMR)

Definition: Percentage of deaths from all causes that are due to a specified cause during a specified time period.

$$\text{Simple formula: } \frac{\text{Deaths from a specified cause}}{\text{Total deaths}} \times 100$$

Interpretation: Proportion of deaths from a specific cause.

The PMR is used for the most common causes of death in a population.

Types of Measured Rates

Crude mortality rate	Deaths per population
Cause-specific mortality rate	Deaths from a specific cause per population
Case-fatality rate	Deaths from a specific cause per number of persons with the disease
Proportionate mortality rate (PMR)	Deaths from a specific cause per all deaths

REVIEW QUESTIONS

Rates

Response options for **Questions 15–17:**

    A. Birth rate

    B. Fertility rate

    C. Infant mortality rate

    D. Maternal mortality rate

    E. Age-adjusted rate

    F. Case-fatality rate

    G. Sex-adjusted rate

    H. Proportionate mortality rate

    I. Age-specific rate

    J. Sex-specific rate

    K. Age- and sex-specific rate

    L. Age- and sex- and race/ethnicity-specific rate

15. Rate of live births among women of childbearing age.

16. The proportion of cases of a disease that die from that disease.

17. Prevalence rate of obesity in women, ages 45–64.

---

15. **Answer: B.** Restatement of definition of fertility rate.

16. **Answer: F.** Restatement of definition of case-fatality rate.

17. **Answer: K.** Age- and sex-specific rate; prevalence rate restricted to women in the age range 45–64.

Table for **Questions 18 and 19:**

Incidence and Mortality of Disease

Age	Disease A		Disease B		Total	
Groups	Cases	Deaths	Cases	Deaths	Deaths	Population
0–12	2	1	300	1	40	22,000
13–24	101	34	267	0	30	18,000
25–64	50	42	1,042	2	125	50,000
>64	0	0	986	95	303	30,000
Totals	153	77	2,595	98	498	120,000

18. The case-fatality rate for Disease A is

    A. $77/120,000 \times 1,000$

    B. $77/120,000 \times 100,000$

    C. $153/120,000 \times 100,000$

    D. $153/498 \times 100$

    E. $77/153 \times 100$

19. The proportionate mortality rate for Disease B is

    A. $98/120,000 \times 100,000$

    B. $2,595/120,000 \times 100,000$

    C. $98/2,595 \times 100$

    D. $98/498 \times 100$

    E. Cannot be determined

---

18. **Answer: E.**

19. **Answer: D.**

YEARS OF POTENTIAL LIFE LOST AND SURVIVAL ANALYSIS

Years of Potential Life Lost (YPLL) (indicator of premature death):

The YPLL for a particular cause of death is the sum, over all persons dying from the cause, of the years that these persons would have lived had they experienced normal life expectancy. Assume life expectancy is 75 years. A person who dies at age 65 would be dying 10 years prematurely ($75 - 65 = 10$ YPLL). For 100 such people, the YPLL calculation would be: $100 \times (75 - 65) = 1,000$ YPLL. In the United States, the leading cause of YPLL is **unintentional injury** before age 65.

Survival Analysis

Survival analysis is a class of statistical procedures for estimating the proportion of people who survive in relation to the length of survival time. The starting point is 100% survival. In 2000, the median survival time was 78 years.

A survival curve is a curve that starts with 100% of the study population and shows the percentage of the population still surviving at successive times for as long as information is available.

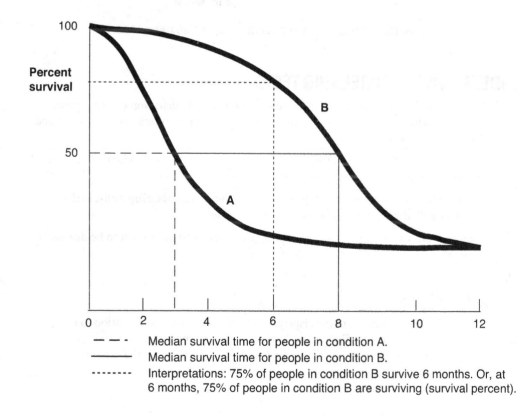

- – – - Median survival time for people in condition A.
——— Median survival time for people in condition B.
- - - - - - Interpretations: 75% of people in condition B survive 6 months. Or, at 6 months, 75% of people in condition B are surviving (survival percent).

Survival Curve

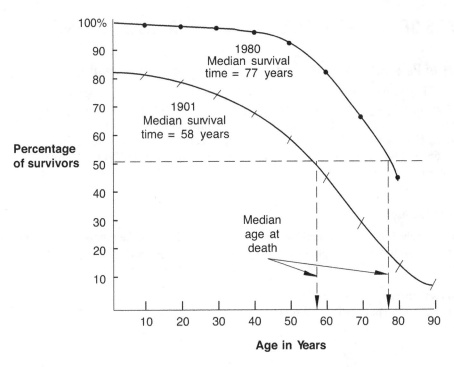

Percentage of Survivors at Specified Ages, 1901 and 1980

UNDERSTANDING SCREENING TESTS

Definition. Screening is the process of using tests to permit early detection of risk factors, asymptomatic infection, or early stages of clinical disease, thus permitting early diagnosis and early intervention or treatment.

- Screening is usually applied to populations of apparently well individuals. Illness, if present, is asymptomatic (subclinical, inapparent).

- Screening tests allow for earlier detection and earlier diagnosis. Hopefully, earlier treatment will affect a more favorable clinical course.

- Screening test results are classified as "positive" (presumed by the test to be diseased) or "negative" (presumed by the test to be well).

Classic 2 × 2 Table

The 2 × 2 table is the standard form for displaying screening test results in relation to disease status. Disease status categories (diseased and well) are diagrammed in the vertical columns. Screening test results (positive, negative) are diagrammed in the horizontal dimension.

Classic 2 × 2 Table

	Disease	No Disease	Totals
Positive	True Positive [TP]	False Positive [FP]	TP + FP
Negative	False Negative [FN]	True Negative [TN]	TN + FN
Totals	TP + FN	TN + FP	TP + TN + FP + FN

Cells in the 2 × 2 Table

- Positive (P) and Negative (N) refer to the actual screening test results.
- True (T) and False (F) refer to the agreement of screening test results with the "gold standard."
  - **TP** is a diseased person who is correctly classified as positive.
  - **TN** is a healthy person who is correctly classified as negative.
  - **FP** is a healthy person who is misclassified as positive.
  - **FN** is a diseased person who is misclassified as negative.

Screening Results in a 2 × 2 Table

		Disease				Totals
		Present		**Absent**		
Screening Test Results	Positive	TP	80	FP	40	TP + FP
	Negative	FN	20	TN	60	TN + FN
	Totals	TP + FN		TN + FP		TP + TN + FP + FN

Measures of Screening Test Performance

Sensitivity and Specificity

1. **Sensitivity:** The proportion of people with disease who are correctly classified by the screening test as positive.
   - Sensitivity = TP/All people with disease
   - *Sensitivity = TP/(TP + FN)*
   - Location on 2 × 2 table: left column
   - Highly sensitive tests identify most, if not all, possible cases
   - Considered when there is a consequence associated with missing the detection of disease

2. **Specificity:** The proportion of well people who are correctly classified by the screening test as negative.

   - Specificity = TN/All well people

   - *Specificity = TN/(TN + FP)*

   - Location on 2 × 2 table: right column

   - Highly specific tests identify most, if not all, well people (i.e., not diseased), will give few FP results

   - Considered when FP results can harm the patient

3. **Predictive Values:** A measure of the test which represents the percentage of test results that match the diagnosis of the patient. These values are predicted by the disease prevalence in the given population.

   a. **Positive Predictive Value (PPV):** The proportion of people with a positive screening test result who are diseased. (i.e., that a person with a positive test is a true positive)

      - Positive Predictive Value = TP/All people with a positive test result

      - Positive Predictive Value = TP/(TP + FP)

      - Location on 2 × 2 table: top row

      - ↑ specificity = ↑ PPV

   b. **Negative Predictive Value (NPV):** The proportion of people with a negative screening test result who are well. (i.e., that a person with a negative test is a true negative)

      - Negative Predictive Value = TN/All people with a negative test result

      - *Negative Predictive Value = TN/(TN + FN)*

      - Location on 2 × 2 table: bottom row

      - ↑ sensitivity = ↑ NPV

4. **Accuracy:** The proportion of all screened people who are correctly classified by the screening test.

   - Accuracy = (TP + TN)/All screened people

   - *Accuracy = (TP + TN)/(TP + TN + FP + FN)*

   - Location on 2 × 2 table: main diagonal

   - Can be used to summarize overall value of a test

5. **Prevalence:** The proportion of screened people who have disease.

   - Prevalence can be estimated only if the entire population or a representative sample of the population is screened.

   - *Prevalence = (TP + FN)/(TP + TN + FN + FP)*

   - ↑ prevalence of a disease usually equals ↑ PPV and ↓ NPV

   - ↓ prevalence of a disease usually equals ↓ PPV and ↑ NPV

6. **Likelihood ratio:** The expression of how many more (or less) likely a test result is to be found in nondiseased (or diseased) compared with diseased (or nondiseased).

- Positive likelihood ratio (LR+) is the proportion of diseased people to that of non-diseased people with a positive test result

$$LR+ = \frac{Sensitivity}{1-specificity} \quad OR \quad \frac{Sensitivity}{FP/(TN + FP)}$$

- Negative likelihood ratio (LR-) is the proportion of diseased people to that of non-diseased people with a negative test result

$$LR- = \frac{1-sensitivity}{Specificity} \quad OR \quad \frac{FN/(TP+FN)}{Specificity}$$

Screening Test Diagram

The screening test diagram displays the distributions of the screening test measure separately for people with disease and people with no disease. The cutoff (or criterion) point divides screened people into test-positives and test-negatives.

- Healthy people with no disease (solid line) are either correctly classified as TN or misclassified as FP.

- Diseased people (dashed line) are either correctly classified as TP or misclassified as FN.

The diagram is a useful model of the real world, where values of screening test measures (such as blood pressure) are generally different for diseased (hypertensive) and nondiseased (normotensive) people, but the distributions overlap.

The measures of screening test performance can be displayed on the diagram by identifying the appropriate areas under the curves. For example, the numerator for sensitivity is TP, whereas the denominator is everyone under the curve labeled "disease."

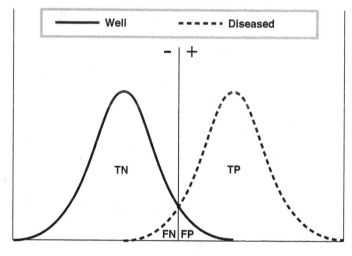

Screening Test Diagram

Summarized 2 × 2 Tables

Measure		Disease		Predictive Values	
		Present	Absent	Equation	Notes
	Positive	TP	FP	$PPV = \dfrac{TP}{TP + FP}$	Each value looks at a 'positive'
	Negative	FN	TN	$NPV = \dfrac{TN}{TN + FN}$	Each value looks at a 'negative'
Screening Test Measures	Equation	$Sensitivity = \dfrac{TP}{TP + FN}$			$Specificity = \dfrac{TN}{TN + FP}$
	Notes	Want to identify all possible causes. Use everything in 'diseased' column = TP + FN.			Want to more specifically identify those that do not have disease. Use everything in 'no diseased,' column.

REVIEW QUESTIONS

Screening Tests

A new screening test is applied to a representative sample of 1,000 people in the population. Based on the data presented in the following table, calculate the requested screening test measures.

	Diseased	Well	
Positive	90	60	150
Negative	10	840	850
	100	900	1,000

Response options for **Questions 20–25**:

A. 90/150

B. 90/100

C. 90/1,000

D. 90

E. 60

F. 10

G. 840/850

H. 840/900

I. 930/1,000

J. 900/1,000

K. 100/1,000

L. Cannot be calculated

20. What is the sensitivity of the screening test?

21. What is the specificity of the screening test?

22. What is the positive predictive value of the screening test?

23. What is the accuracy of the screening test?

24. What is the number of false positive test results?

25. What is the prevalence of disease, assuming screening of a representative sample?

Questions 26–31

The Centers for Disease Control and Prevention is concerned about optimizing the detection of a disease that poses a serious public health threat. CDC health officials are considering lowering the usual screening test cutoff point from X to Y.

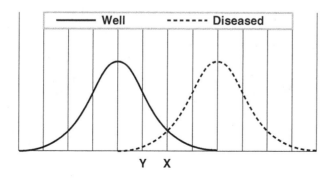

26. Moving cutoff in the manner being considered by the CDC causes the number of false positives to

    A. increase

    B. decrease

    C. remain unchanged

    D. cannot be determined

27. Moving the cutoff in the manner being considered by the CDC causes the positive predictive value to

    A. increase

    B. decrease

    C. remain unchanged

    D. cannot be determined

28. Moving the cutoff in the manner being considered by the CDC causes the accuracy to

    A. increase

    B. decrease

    C. remain unchanged

    D. cannot be determined

29. Moving the cutoff in the manner being considered by the CDC causes the sensitivity to

    A. increase

    B. decrease

    C. remain unchanged

    D. cannot be determined

30. Assuming that everyone who receives a positive test result is referred for medical follow-up, moving the cutoff in the manner being considered by the CDC will cause the numbers of screened people who are referred for follow-up to

    A. increase

    B. decrease

    C. remain unchanged

    D. Cannot be determined

31. At Cutoff Point X, sensitivity is

    A. 100%

    B. 85%

    C. 50%

    D. 25%

    E. 0%

32. A physician interviews an 18-year-old woman who mentions that she just received a negative syphilis test result from the county health department, and she feels relieved. She explains that she has been a sex worker for about a year, working several nights a week. Typically, she has oral or vaginal sex with several customers per night, sometimes without a condom. On the basis of these findings, the physician is likely to be most concerning with which of the following screening test measures?

   A. Sensitivity

   B. Specificity

   C. Positive predictive value

   D. Negative predictive value

   E. Accuracy

33. A 55-year-old man visits his primary care physician with a complaint of urinary infrequency. Examination finds a 1-cm nodule on his prostate gland. The physician orders a prostate-specific antigen (PSA) serum test. By common standards, a PSA level >4 ng/mL is considered abnormal. Using this standard, this test has a sensitivity of 80% and a specificity of 90%. A recently published epidemiologic article found that in a cross-sectional study, 10% of men of this age have prostate cancer. The result on the patient's PSA is 7 ng/mL. What is your best estimate of the likelihood that this man actually has prostate cancer?

   A. 13%

   B. 25%

   C. 36%

   D. 47%

   E. 58%

   F. 69%

   G. 72%

   H. 81%

20. **Answer: B.** Sensitivity = TP/All diseased people = 90/100

21. **Answer: H.** Specificity = TN/All well people = 840/900

22. **Answer: A.** PPV = TP/All test positives = 90/150

23. **Answer: I.** Accuracy = (TP + TN)/All screened people = 930/1,000

24. **Answer: E.** False positives = Well people who are misclassified by the test = 60

25. **Answer: K.** Prevalence = All diseased people/All screened people = 100/1,000

26. **Answer: A.** At Y, FP will increase as more well people are misclassified.

27. **Answer: B.** Although there will be more TP at Cutoff Y, there will be a large increase in numbers of FP. The ratio, TP/(TP + FP), will decrease. A positive test result will be less predictive of actual disease.

28. **Answer: B.** X is the point of overlap and the point of maximal accuracy. Moving to Y will decrease accuracy.

29. **Answer: A.** At Y, more diseased people will receive a (correct) positive test result. They will be TP. TP, the numerator for sensitivity, will increase while the denominator (total people with disease) will be unchanged.

30. **Answer: A.** Larger numbers of people would be screened positive at Cutoff Y and referred for follow-up.

31. **Answer: B.** Notice that Cutoff Point X separates the curve of diseased people into two areas; above the cutoff point, approximately 85% of diseased people receive a (correct) positive test result. They are true positives. Sensitivity = TP /All people with disease.

32. **Answer: D.**

33. **Answer: D.**

STUDY DESIGNS

The following form is used for displaying the relationship of exposure to disease status:

2 × 2 Table Format

	Disease	No Disease	
Exposed	a	b	a + b
Nonexposed	c	d	c + d
	a + c	b + d	a + b + c + d

When epidemiologists observe the relationships between exposures and disease outcomes in free-living populations, they are conducting observational studies. When epidemiologists or clinicians test interventions aimed at minimizing the disease-producing exposures and optimizing health-promoting exposures or factors, they are performing experimental studies.

In **observational studies**, nature is allowed to take its course; no intervention.

In **experimental studies**, there is an intervention and the results of the study assess the effects of the intervention.

Observational Studies

Case report: Brief, objective report of a *clinical characteristic or outcome from a single clinical subject or event*, n = 1. For example, a 23-year-old man with treatment-resistant TB. No control group.

Case series report: Objective report of a *clinical characteristic or outcome from a group of clinical subjects*, n >1, i.e., patients at local hospital with treatment-resistant TB. No control group.

Cross-sectional study: The *presence or absence of disease and other variables* are determined in each member of the study population or in a representative sample *at a particular time*. The co-occurrence of a variable and the disease can be examined.

- Disease prevalence rather than incidence is recorded.
- The temporal sequence of cause and effect cannot usually be determined in a cross-sectional study, e.g., who in the community now has treatment-resistant TB.

Case-control study: Identifies *a group of people with the disease and compares them with a suitable comparison group without the disease.* It is almost always retrospective, e.g., comparing cases of treatment-resistant TB with cases of nonresistant TB.

- Cannot assess incidence or prevalence of disease
- Can help determine causal relationships
- Very useful for studying conditions with very low incidence or prevalence

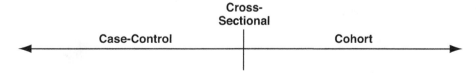

Differentiating Study Types by Time

Cohort study: *Population group identifies who has been exposed to risk factor and is followed over time and compared with a group not exposed to the risk factor.* Outcome is disease incidence in each group, e.g., following a prison inmate population and marking the development of treatment-resistant TB.

- Allows you to evaluate whether potential risk factors are related to subsequent outcomes

- Prospective; subjects tracked forward in time

- Can determine incidence and causal relationships

- Must follow population long enough for incidence to appear

- Historical examples: Framingham study

Analyzing Observational Studies (measure of effect)

For cross-sectional studies, use Chi-square (χ^2); for cohort studies, use relative risk and/or attributable risk.

Relative risk (RR): Comparative probability asking, "How much more likely is the exposed person going to get the disease compared to the nonexposed?"

- Incidence rate of exposed group *divided by* the incidence rate of the unexposed group. How much greater chance does one group have of contracting the disease compared with the other group?

- For example, if infant mortality rate in whites is 8.9 per 1,000 live births and 18.0 in blacks per 1,000 live births, then the relative risk of blacks versus whites is 18.0 divided by 8.9 = 2.02. Compared with whites, black infants are twice as likely to die in the first year of life.

- For statistical analysis, it yields a *p* value.

Attributable risk (AR) (Also called absolute risk reduction): Comparative probability asking, "How many more cases in one group?"

- Incidence rate of exposed group *minus* the incidence rate of the unexposed group

- Using the same example, attributable risk is equal to 18.0 − 8.9 = 9.1. Of every 1,000 black infants, there were 9.1 more deaths than were observed in 1,000 white infants. In this case, attributable risk gives the excess mortality.

- Note that both relative risk and attributable risk tell us if there are differences but do not tell us why those differences exist.

For case-control studies: Use odds ratio (OR).

Odds ratio (OR): Looks at the increased odds of getting a disease with exposure to a risk factor versus nonexposure to that factor.

- Odds of exposure for cases divided by odds of exposure for controls

- The odds that a person with lung cancer was a smoker versus the odds that a person without lung cancer was a smoker

Odds Ratio

	Lung Cancer	No Lung Cancer
Smokers	659 (A)	984 (B)
Nonsmokers	25 (C)	348 (D)

$$OR = \frac{A/C}{B/D} = \frac{AD}{BC}$$

Use OR = AD/BC as the working formula.

For the above example:

$$OR = \frac{AD}{BC} = \frac{659 \cdot 348}{984 \cdot 25} = 9.32$$

- The odds of having been a smoker are more than 9 times greater for someone with lung cancer compared with someone without lung cancer.

- OR approaching 1 = increased risk of outcome with exposure

REVIEW QUESTIONS

Study Design

34. How would you analyze the data from this case-control study?

	No Colorectal Cancer	Colorectal Cancer	TOTALS
Family history of colorectal cancer	120	60	180
No family history of colorectal cancer	200	20	220
TOTALS	320	80	400
ANSWER:	$\dfrac{AD}{BC}$	$\dfrac{(60)(200)}{(120)/(20)}$	OR = 5.0

34. **Answer: A.** This means that the odds of having a family history of colorectal cancer are 5 times greater for those who have the disease than for those who do not.

Differentiating Observational Studies

Characteristic	Cross-Sectional Studies	Case-Control Studies	Cohort Studies
Time	One time point	Retrospective	Prospective
Incidence	No	No	Yes
Prevalence	Yes	No	No
Causality	No	Yes	Yes
Role of disease	Measure disease	Begin with disease	End with disease
Assesses	Association of risk factor and disease	Many risk factors for single disease	Single risk factor affecting many diseases
Data analysis	Chi-square to assess association	Odds ratio to estimate risk	Relative risk to estimate risk

Computational Measures by Type of Observational Study

Measure	Cross-Sectional Study	Case-Control Study	Cohort Study
Prevalence of disease	Yes	No	No
Prevalence of exposure	Yes	No	No
Odds ratio	No	Yes	No
Incidence rate in the exposed	No	No	Yes
Incidence rate in the nonexposed	No	No	Yes
Relative risk	No	No	Yes
Attributable risk	No	No	Yes

Experimental Studies: Clinical Trials

Clinical trials (intervention studies): Research that involves the administration of a test regimen to evaluate its safety and efficacy.

- **Control group:** Subjects who do not receive the intervention under study; used as a source of comparison to be certain that the experiment group is being affected by the intervention and not by other factors. In clinical trials, this is most often a placebo group. Note that control group subjects must be *as similar as possible to intervention group* subjects.

- For Food and Drug Administration (FDA) approval, 3 phases of clinical trials must be passed.

    Phase 1: Testing safety in healthy volunteers
    Phase 2: Testing *protocol and dose levels* in small group of patient volunteers
    Phase 3: Testing *efficacy and occurrence of side effects* in larger group of patient volunteers. Phase 3 is considered the definitive test.

- **Randomized controlled clinical trial (RCT):**

    1. Subjects in study are *randomly allocated* into "intervention" and "control" groups to receive or not receive an experimental preventive or therapeutic procedure or intervention.

    2. Generally regarded as *the most scientifically rigorous* studies available in epidemiology.

    3. **Double-blind RCT** is the type of study *least subject to bias*, but also the *most expensive* to conduct. Double-blind means that neither subjects nor researchers who have contact with them know whether the subjects are in the treatment or comparison group.

- **Community trial:** Experiment in which the unit of allocation to receive a preventive or therapeutic regimen is an *entire community or political subdivision*. Does the treatment work in real world circumstances?

- **Crossover study:** For ethical reasons, no group involved can remain untreated. *All subjects receive intervention* but at different times (e.g., AZT trials). Assume double-blind design. For example, Group A receives AZT for 3 months; Group B is control. For the second 3 months, Group B receives AZT and Group A is control.

Comparison of Case-Control and Cohort Studies

Case-Control Study	Cohort Study
Small number of subjects	Large number of subjects
Lower cost	Higher cost
Short time period	Longer time period
One disease: multiple past exposures	**One exposure: multiple future diseases**
Low prevalence or high prevalence diseases	High incidence diseases only
Major source of bias: recall	Major source of bias: selection

STUDY DESIGNS: BIAS IN RESEARCH

Bias in research is deviation from the truth of inferred results.

Reliability: Ability of a test to *measure something consistently*, either across testing situations (test–retest reliability), within a test (split half reliability), or across judges (inter-rater reliability). Think of the clustering of rifle shots at a target (*precision*).

Validity: Degree to which a test measures that which was intended. Think of a marksman hitting the bulls-eye. Reliability is a necessary, but insufficient, condition for validity (*accuracy*).

Types of bias

Selection bias (sampling bias): The *sample selected is not representative* of the population. Examples:

- Predicting rates of heart disease by gathering subjects from a local health club

- Using only hospital records to estimate population prevalence (Berkson's bias)

- People included in study are different from those who are not (nonrespondent bias)

Measurement bias: Information is gathered in a manner that distorts the information. Examples:

- Measuring patients' satisfaction with their respective physicians by using leading questions, e.g., "You don't like your doctor, do you?"

- Subjects' behavior is altered because they are being studied (Hawthorne effect). This is a factor only when there is no control group in a prospective study.

Experimenter expectancy (Pygmalion effect): *Experimenter's expectations inadvertently communicated to subjects*, who then produce the desired effects. Can be avoided by **double-blind** design, where neither the subject nor the investigators who have contact with them know which group receives the intervention under study and which group is the control.

Lead-time bias: Gives a *false estimate of survival rates*. For example, patients seem to live longer with the disease after it is uncovered by a screening test. Actually, there is no increased survival, but because the disease is discovered sooner, patients who are diagnosed seem to live longer.

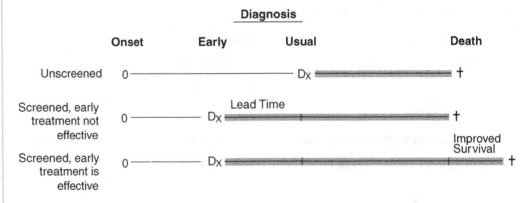

Diagnosis, Time, and Survival

Recall bias: Subjects *fail to accurately recall events* in the past. For example, "How many times last year did you kiss your mother?" This is a likely problem in retrospective studies.

Late-look bias: *Individuals with severe disease are less likely to be uncovered in a survey because they die first.* For example, a recent survey found that persons with AIDS reported only mild symptoms.

Confounding bias: *The factor being examined is related to other factors of less interest.* Unanticipated factors obscure a relationship or make it seem like there is one when there is not. More than one explanation can be found for the presented results. An example would be comparing the relationship between exercise and heart disease in two populations when one population is younger and the other is older. Are differences in heart disease due to exercise or to age?

Type of Bias in Research and Important Associations

Type of Bias	Definition	Important Associations	Solutions
Selection	Sample not representative	Berkson's bias, nonrespondent bias	Random, independent sample
Measurement	Gathering the information distorts it	Hawthorne effect	Control group/placebo group
Experimenter expectancy	Researcher's beliefs affect outcome	Pygmalion effect	Double-blind design
Lead-time	Early detection confused with increased survival	Benefits of screening	Measure "back-end" survival
Recall	Subjects cannot remember accurately	Retrospective studies	Confirm information with other sources
Late-look	Severely diseased individuals are not uncovered	Early mortality	Stratify by severity
Confounding obscure results	Unanticipated factors	Hidden factors affect results	Multiple studies, good research design

REVIEW QUESTIONS

Response options for **Questions 35–40:**

   A. 520/695

   B. 600/1,000

   C. 520/600

   D. 695/1,000

   E. 80/305

   F. (520/695)/(80/305)

   G. (520 × 225)/(175 × 80)

   H. (520/695) − (80/305)

   I. Cannot be determined for this type of study

	Disease	Well	
Exposed	520	175	695
Nonexposed	80	225	305
	600	400	1,000

35. Assume the table represents a cohort study: What is the incidence rate in the exposed?

36. Assume the table represents a cross-sectional study: What is the relative risk?

37. Assume the table represents a case-control study: What is the odds ratio?

38. Assume the table represents a cross-sectional study: What is the prevalence of disease?

39. Assume the table represents a disease outbreak investigation: What is the attack rate for people who did not eat the food?

40. Assume the table represents a cohort study: What is the attributable risk?

41. A study compares the effectiveness of a new medication for treatment of latent tuberculosis infection with the standard medication, isoniazid. Subjects with latent TB infection are sorted with equal likelihood of selection to receive the new medication or isoniazid. Neither the subjects themselves nor the clinicians know the treatment condition for each patient. This study is best described as a

   A. double-blind randomized cohort study

   B. randomized controlled trial with crossover design

   C. double-blind randomized clinical trial

   D. double-blind randomized clinical trial with crossover design

   E. double-blind quasi-experimental trial

42. A group of 200 hypertensive subjects and a comparable group of 200 normotensive subjects are recruited and enrolled into a longitudinal study to examine the effect of a diagnosis of hypertension on subsequent occurrence of coronary heart disease. Study subjects are followed for 5 years. Final data are presented in the table below. What is the attributable risk for hypertension?

	CHD	No CHD	Total
Hypertension	25	175	200
No hypertension	10	190	200
Total	35	365	400

A. 0.075

B. 2.5

C. 2.7

D. 0.125

E. Cannot be computed for this type of study

43. A study is conducted relating percentage of calories from fat in the habitual diet to subsequent incidence of clinical diabetes mellitus. Four groups of initially well persons are selected from the community to represent persons within each of four categories of fat intake. The percentages of daily calories from fat are: <20%, 20–40%, 35–49%, >50%. The groups are followed longitudinally for 5 years and assessed annually for diabetes. The type of study design is best described as a

A. case-series trial

B. case-control study

C. cross-sectional study

D. cohort study

E. community trial

44. Alcohol consumption and cigarette smoking both contribute causally to the occurrence of esophageal cancer. These risk factors are not independent; in fact, they operate synergistically. A study of cigarette smoking in relation to esophageal cancer that fails to stratify or otherwise control for level of alcohol consumption would be guilty of which of the following threats to validity?

    A. Ascertainment bias

    B. Confounding bias

    C. Design bias

    D. Lead time bias

    E. Observer bias

    F. Recall bias

    G. Response bias

    H. Selection bias

35. **Answer A.**

36. **Answer I.**

37. **Answer G.**

38. **Answer B.**

39. **Answer E.**

40. **Answer H.**

41. **Answer C.**

42. **Answer A.**

43. **Answer D.**

44. **Answer B.**

6

Biostatistics

PROBABILITY BASICS

Combine probabilities for independent events by multiplication.

- Events are independent if the occurrence of one tells you nothing about the occurrence of another.

- If the chance of having blond hair is 0.3 and the chance of having a cold is 0.2, the chance of meeting a blond-haired person with a cold is $0.3 \times 0.2 = 0.06$ (or 6%).

- If events are nonindependent, then multiply the probability of one times the probability of the second, given that the first has occurred. For example, if one has a box with 5 white and 5 black balls in it, the chance of picking two black balls is $(5/10) \times (4/9) = 0.5 \times 0.44 = 0.22$ (or 22%).

Combine probabilities for mutually exclusive events by addition.

- Mutually exclusive means that the occurrence of one event precludes the occurrence of the other (i.e., cannot both happen). If a coin lands heads, it cannot be tails; the two are mutually exclusive. For example, if a coin is flipped, the chance that it will be either heads or tails is $0.5 + 0.5 = 1.0$ (or 100%).

- If two events are not mutually exclusive, the combination of probabilities is accomplished by adding the two together and subtracting out the multiplied probabilities. For example, if the chance of having diabetes is 10%, and the chance of someone being obese is 30%, the chance of meeting someone who is obese or has diabetes is $0.1 + 0.30 - (0.1 \times 0.30) = 0.37$ (or 37%).

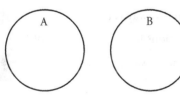 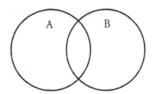

Mutually Exclusive   Nonmutually Exclusive

Venn Diagram Representations of Mutually Exclusive and Nonmutually Exclusive Events

Suppose survival rates after surgery are as follows:

N: 183
1 Year: 90%
2 Year: 75%
3 Year: 50%
4 Year: 40%

The life expectancy after surgery would be 3 years. If a patient survives for 2 years, the chance of surviving for 3 years would be 50/75.

Now suppose a study is conducted to see how many pediatric patients have parents who exercise regularly. After research, it is concluded that 40% of pediatric patients have parents who exercise regularly. Assuming the events are independent, what is the probability that 2 pediatric patients with parents who exercise regularly will come into the office on the same day?

(A) 0.16

(B) 0.4

(C) 0.8

(D) 0.96

(E) 0.08

(F) 0.04

(choice A; this requires the multiplication rule)

DESCRIPTIVE STATISTICS

Measures (Indices) of Central Tendency

Measures of central tendency is a general term for several characteristics of the distribution of a set of values or measurements around a value at or near the middle of the set.

Mean (synonym: "average"): The sum of the values of the observations divided by the numbers of observations.

$$\text{Mean: } \frac{\text{Sum of the observed measurements}}{\text{Number of observations}}$$

Median:

- Simplest division of a set of measurements is into two parts—the upper and lower half

- Point on the scale that divides the group in this way is the median

- Measurement below which half the observations fall: the 50th percentile

Mode: The most frequently occurring value in a set of observations.

Normal Distribution

Normal distribution is continuous frequency distribution of infinite range defined by a specific mathematical function with the following properties:

- A continuous, symmetrical distribution; both tails extend to infinity.

- The arithmetic mean, mode, and median are identical.

- The shape is completely determined by the mean and standard deviation.

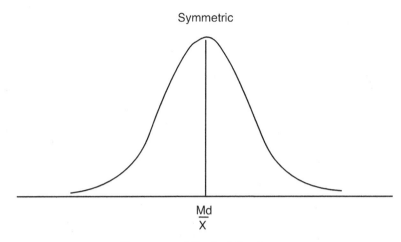

Measures of Central Tendency

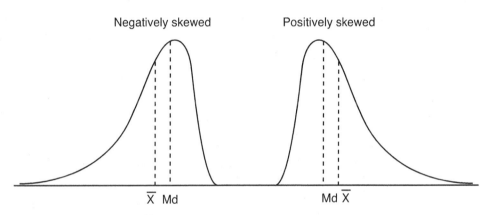

Skewed Distribution Curves

Dispersion of Data

The dispersion of data helps us identify the spread, or the variation, of the data.

Deviation score: The distance from the mean. Found by subtracting the distribution mean from the distribution values you are evaluating. For example, the mean of the distribution is 120 and you want to know the deviation score of the value 150.

$$x = 150 - 120$$
$$= 30$$

This is used to obtain the variance of a distribution.

Range: The difference between the largest and smallest values in a distribution.

Variance: A measure of the variation shown by a set of observations, defined by the sum of the squares of deviation scores of each value divided by the number of degrees of freedom in the set of observations or $n - 1$.

Standard deviation

- The most widely used measure of dispersion of a frequency distribution

- It is equal to the positive square root of the variance.

- Whereas the mean tells where the group of values are centered, the standard deviation is a summary of how widely dispersed the values are around the center.

$$s = \sqrt{\frac{\sum(X - \overline{X})^2}{n - 1}}$$

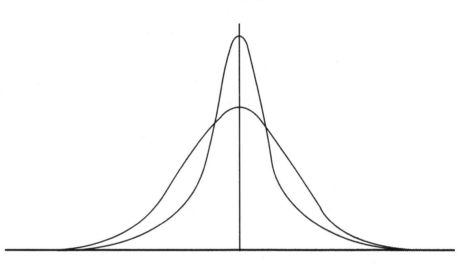

**Comparison of Two Normal Curves with the Same Means,
but Different Standard Deviations**

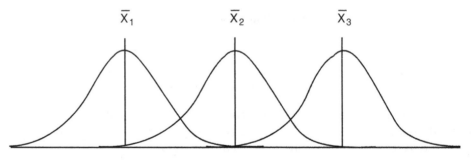

**Comparison of Three Normal Curves with the Same
Standard Deviations, but Different Means**

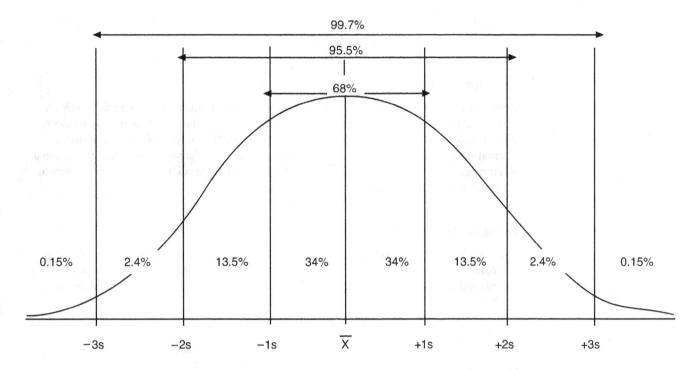

Note: Percentages are rounded so they are easier to memorize. Total area under the curve is 100%.

Percentage of Cases Within One, Two, and Three Standard Deviations of the Mean in a Normal Distribution

The standard deviation (s or sd) is stated in score units. The normal curve has the property that within one standard deviation a certain proportion of the cases is included. The property is as follows: Between the mean and the value of one standard deviation from the mean in either direction there will be 34% of the cases; there will be 68% of the cases between the score at 1s above and 1s below the mean. Within two standard deviations of the mean are 95.5% of the cases. Between 1s and 2s from the mean in either direction, there will be 13.5% of the cases, or 27% for both. Within 3s of the mean are 99.7% of the cases. And between 2s and 3s from the mean there will be almost 2.5% of the cases, 4.7% for the two extremes together. There will be a few cases, of course, 0.3%, beyond 3s from the mean both above and the mean. You must know these figures. For example: What percentage of the cases are 2s below the mean? (2.5%)

Students will *not* be asked to calculate a standard deviation or a variance on the exam, but students need to know what they are and how they relate to the normal curve.

INFERENTIAL STATISTICS

Generalizations from a Sample to the Population as a Whole

The purpose of inferential statistics is to designate *how likely it is that a given finding is simply the result of chance*. Inferential statistics would not be necessary if investigators studied all members of a population. However, because we can rarely observe and study entire populations, we try to select samples that are representative of the entire population so that we can *generalize the results from the sample to the population*.

Inferential statistics focuses on drawing conclusions about an entire population (i.e., parameter) based on information in a sample.

Confidence Intervals

Confidence intervals are a way of admitting that any measurement from a sample is only an *estimate* of the population. Although the estimate given from the sample is likely to be close, the true values for the population may be above or below the sample values. A confidence interval *specifies how far above or below a sample-based value the population value lies* within a given range, from a possible high to a possible low. The true mean, therefore, is most likely to be somewhere within the specified range.

Confidence Interval of the Mean

The confidence interval contains two parts: *1*) An estimate of the quality of the sample for the estimate, known as the *standard error of the mean*; and *2*) the degree of confidence provided by the interval specified, known as the standard or Z-score. The confidence interval of the mean can be calculated by:

Mean $\pm$ appropriate Z-score $\times$ standard error of the mean $= \overline{X} \pm Z\,(S/\sqrt{N})$

- Increasing sample size will narrow the confidence interval.

Standard error of the mean is the standard deviation divided by the square root of the sample size. It demonstrates the sample mean deviation from the true population mean.

- If the standard deviation is larger, the chance of error in the estimate is greater.

- If the sample size is larger, the chance of error in the estimate is less.

The Z-score or standard score is a score from a normal distribution with a mean of 0 and a standard deviation of 1. Any distribution can be converted into a Z-score distribution using the formula:

$$Z = (\overline{X} - \overline{X})\,/\,S \text{ or}$$

$$Z = \text{Sample mean} - \text{population mean/Standard deviation}$$

- The Z-score distribution is easy to use for calculations because it has simple values. All points in a Z-score distribution are *represented in standard deviation units*.

- Positive scores are above the mean; negative scores are below the mean. Therefore, a Z-score of $+2.0$ is exactly two standard deviations above the mean; a Z-score of -1.5 is exactly 1.5 standard deviations below the mean.

Z-scores are used in computing confidence intervals to set the level of confidence. Recall that in a normal distribution, 95.5% of the cases are within two standard deviations (2s) of the mean. To get 95% confidence and 99% confidence, all we need to know is what symmetric Z-score to use to contain exactly 95% and 99% of the cases.

- For 95% confidence $= 1.96$; for calculation purposes, use Z-score of 2.0.

- For 99% confidence $= 2.58$; for calculation purposes, use Z-score of 2.5.

- Note that a 99% confidence interval will be wider than a 95% interval.

Confidence Intervals for Relative Risk and Odds Ratios

If the given confidence interval contains 1.0, then there is no statistically significant effect of exposure. Example:

Relative Risk	95% Confidence Interval	Interpretation
1.57	(1.12–2.25)	Statistically significant (increased risk)
1.65	(0.89–2.34)	Not statistically significant (risk is the same)
0.76	(0.56–0.93)	Statistically significant (decreased risk)

Hypothesis Testing

A hypothesis is a statement that postulates a difference between 2 groups. Statistics are used to evaluate the possibility that this difference occurred by chance.

- **Null hypothesis** says that the *findings are the result of chance or random factors.* If you want to show that a drug works, the null hypothesis will be that the drug does *not* work.
  - One-tailed, i.e., directional or "one-sided," such that one group is either greater than, or less than, the other. For example, Group A is not $<$ Group B, or Group A is not $>$ Group B.
  - Two-tailed, i.e., nondirectional or "two-sided," such that two groups are not the same. For example, Group A $=$ Group B
- **Alternative hypothesis** says what is left after defining the null hypothesis. In this example, the drug actually *does* work.

Significance Testing

To test your hypothesis, you would draw a random sample from a population (e.g., men with hypertension) and make an inference. But before you sample, you set a significance level, alpha, which is the risk of error you are willing to tolerate. Customarily, the level of significance is set at 0.05 and the risk is associated with the rejection of the null hypothesis, even though it is true (e.g., type I error).

Interpretation

p-Value

The p-value and alpha level are very similar, usually set at 0.05, and both symbolize significance. They are only slightly different in that the alpha level represents risk and is independent of data, whereas p-value measures the strength (i.e., significance) of the data against the null hypothesis.

A p-value is for interpreting output from a statistical test; focus on the p-value. The term refers to two things. In its first sense, the p-value is a standard against which we compare our results. In the second sense, the p-value is a result of computation.

The computed p-value is compared with the p-value criterion to test statistical significance. If the computed value is less than the criterion, we have achieved statistical significance. In general, the smaller the p the better.

The p-value criterion is traditionally set at $p \leq 0.05$. (Assume that these are the criteria if no other value is explicitly specified.) Using this standard:

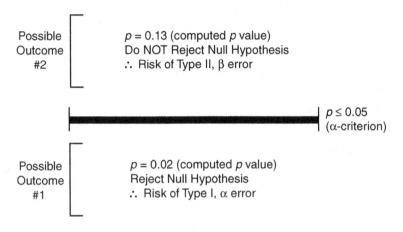

Making Decisions Using *p*-Values

- If $p \leq 0.05$, reject the null hypothesis (reached statistical significance).
- If $p > 0.05$, do not reject the null hypothesis (has not reached statistical significance).

Therefore:

- If $p = 0.13$, fail to reject the null hypothesis, i.e., decide that the drug does not work.
- If $p = 0.02$, reject the null hypothesis, i.e., decide that the drug works.

Types of errors

Just because we reject the null hypothesis, we are not certain that we are correct. For some reason, the results given by the sample may be inconsistent with the full population. If this is true, any decision we make on the basis of the sample could be in error. There are two possible types of errors that we could make:

Type I error (α error): *rejecting the null hypothesis when it is really true*, i.e., assuming a statistically significant effect on the basis of the sample when there is none in the population or asserting that the drug works when it doesn't. The chance of a Type I error is given by the p-value. If p (or α) $= 0.05$, then the chance of a Type I error is 5 in 100, or 1 in 20.

Type II error (β error): *failing to reject the null hypothesis when it is really false*, i.e., declaring no significant effect on the basis of the sample when there really is one in the population or asserting the drug does not work when it really does. The chance of a Type II error cannot be directly estimated from the p-value.

β **Error** can be calculated by subtracting power from 1: $1 - \text{Power} = \beta$.

- Power is the capacity to detect a difference if there is one.
- Increasing sample size (n) increases power.

Meaning of the *p*-value

- Provides criterion for making decisions about the null hypothesis.
- Quantifies the chances that a decision to reject the null hypothesis will be wrong.
- Tells statistical significance, not clinical significance or likelihood of benefit.
- Generally, *p*-value is considered statistically significant if it is equal to or less than 0.05.

Limits to the *p*-value

The *p*-value does not tell us *1*) the chance that an individual patient will benefit, *2*) the percentage of patients who will benefit, and *3*) the degree of benefit expected for a given patient.

Types of Scales

To convert the world into numbers, we use 4 types of scales: nominal, ordinal, interval, and ratio scales.

Types of Scales in Statistics

Type of Scale	Description	Key Words	Examples
Nominal (Categorical)	Different groups	This or that or that	Gender, comparing among treatment interventions
Ordinal	Groups in sequence	Comparative quality, rank order	Olympic medals, class rank in medical school
Interval	Exact differences among groups	Quantity, mean, and standard deviation	Height, weight, blood pressure, drug dosage
Ratio	Interval + true zero point	Zero means zero	Temperature measured in degrees Kelvin

Nominal or categorical scale

A nominal scale puts people into boxes, without specifying the relationship between the boxes. Sex is a common example of a nominal scale with two groups, male and female. Anytime you can say, "It's either this or that," you are dealing with a nominal scale. Other examples: cities, drug versus control group.

Ordinal scale

Numbers can also be used to express ordinal or rank-order relations. For example, we say Ben is taller than Fred. Now we know more than just the category in which to place someone. We know something about the relationship between the categories (quality). What we do not know is how different the two categories are (quantity). Class rank in medical school and medals at the Olympics are examples of ordinal scales.

Interval scale

An interval scale uses a scale graded in equal increments. In the scale of length, we know that one inch is equal to any other inch. Interval scales allow us to say not only that two things are different, but by how much. If a measurement has a mean and a standard deviation, treat it as an interval scale. It is sometimes called a "numeric scale."

Ratio scale

The best measure is the ratio scale. This scale orders things and contains equal intervals, like the previous two scales, but it also has one additional quality: *a true zero point*. In a ratio scale, zero is a floor—you can't go any lower. Measuring temperature using the Kelvin scale yields a ratio scale measurement.

SELECTING A STATISTICAL TEST

Types of Scales and Basic Statistical Tests

Name of Statistical Test	Variables		Comment
	Interval	**Nominal**	
Pearson Correlation	2	0	Is there a linear relationship?
Chi-square	0	2	Any # of groups
t-test	1	1	2 groups only
One-way ANOVA	1	1	2 or more groups
Matched pairs *t*-test	1	1	2 groups, linked data pairs, before and after
Repeated measures ANOVA	1	1	More than 2 groups, linked data

Meta-Analysis

- A statistical way of *combining the results of many studies* to produce one overall conclusion
- A mathematic literature review

Correlation Analysis (*r*, Ranges from —1 to +1)

- A *positive value* means that *two variables go together in the same direction*, e.g., MCAT scores have a positive correlation with medical school grades.
- A *negative value* means that the *presence of one variable is associated with the absence of another variable*, e.g., there is a negative correlation between age and quickness of reflexes.
- The further from zero, the stronger the relationship ($r = 0$).
- A zero correlation means that two variables have no linear relation to one another, e.g., height and success in medical school.

Graphing correlations using scatterplots

A scatterplot will show points that approximate a line. For the exam, know how to interpret scatter plots of data: positive slope, negative slope, and which of a set of scatterplots indicates a stronger correlation.

There are 2 types of correlation: the **Pearson correlation** compares two interval level variables, and the **Spearman correlation** compares two ordinal level variables.

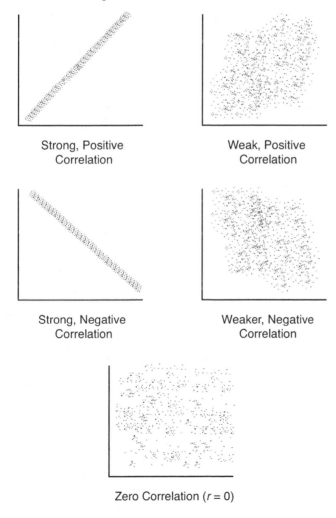

Scatter Plots and Correlations

t-Tests

The output of a *t*-test is a "*t*" statistic.

- *Comparing the means of two groups* from a single nominal variable, using means from an interval variable to see whether the groups are different

- Used for two groups only, i.e., compares two means. For example, do patients with MI who are in psychotherapy have a reduced length of convalescence compared with those who are not in therapy?

- Pooled *t*-test: regular *t*-test, assuming the variances of the two groups are the same

- Matched pairs *t*-test: if each person in one group is matched with a person in the second. Applies to before and after measures and linked data.

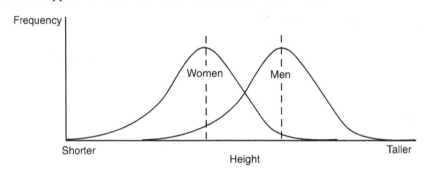

Comparison of the Distributions of Two Groups

Analysis of Variance (ANOVA)

Output from an ANOVA is one or more "F" statistics.

- **One-way:** *Compares means of many groups* (two or more) *of a single nominal variable* using an interval variable. Significant *p*-value means that at least two of the tested groups are different.

- **Two-way:** *Compares means of groups generated by two nominal variables* using an interval variable. Can test effects of several variables at the same time.

- Repeated measures ANOVA: multiple measurements of same people over time.

Chi-Square

- Nominal data only

- Any number of groups

- Tests to see whether two nominal variables are independent, e.g., testing the efficacy of a new drug by comparing the number of recovered patients given the drug with those who are not

Chi-Square Analysis for Nominal Data

	New Drug	Placebo	Totals
Recovered	45	35	80
Not Recovered	15	25	40
Totals	60	60	120

REVIEW QUESTIONS

1. The American Medical Association commissions a health study of a representative sample of U.S. physicians. Enrolled physicians complete detailed surveys and undergo an extensive battery of medical tests. For a number of analyses, physicians are classified by subspecialty. Although numerous physiologic measures are assessed, the following questions describe analyses of just one of these, mean fasting plasma glucose. Select the appropriate statistical test for a comparison of mean fasting plasma glucose values for representative samples of surgeons and cardiologists.

    A. *t*-test
    B. Matched pairs *t*-test
    C. One-way ANOVA
    D. Two-way ANOVA
    E. Chi-square

2. An experimenter tests a new medication as compared to a current one. Alpha is selected to be 0.05. At the end of the trial, the patients receiving the new medication show more improvement than those on the standard medication. The *p*-value is 0.002. What will the experimenter conclude?

    A. Do not reject the null hypothesis.
    B. The new medication has more clinical benefits than the standard medication.
    C. The likelihood that a type I error has actually been committed is less than the maximum risk the experimenter was willing to accept.
    D. The result is not significant.
    E. A type II error has been committed.

3. BMI is found to correlate to the following physiologic measures. Which has the strongest correlation?

    A. Physical activity ($r = -0.56$)
    B. Percentage of calories from complex carbohydrates ($r = -0.32$)
    C. Systolic blood pressure ($r = +0.43$)
    D. Triglycerides ($r = +0.37$)
    E. LDL cholesterol ($r = +0.49$)

4. A new medication for high cholesterol is piloted on a group of 100 men, age 45–59, with total serum cholesterol ranging 260–299 mg/dL. After 3 months on the medication, the mean cholesterol for the treatment group is 250 mg/dL with a standard deviation 20 mg/dL. What is the 95% confidence interval on the mean for this study?

    A. 210–290 mg/dL

    B. 230–270 mg/dL

    C. 246–254 mg/dL

    D. 248–252 mg/dL

    E. 249–251 mg/dL

5. The Wechsler Adult Intelligence Scale–Revised (WAIS-R) is a standardized IQ test with a mean of 100 and a standard deviation of 15. A person with an IQ of 115 is at what percentile of IQ?

    A. 50th

    B. 68th

    C. 84th

    D. 95th

    E. 99th

6. From a published article describing the results of the study presented above, the following data table is abstracted. This table presents the relative risks (RR) of clinical diabetes for each of the categories of fat intake relative to the baseline category of <20%. Interpret the study findings from the tabular data.

	% of Calories from Fat	RR for Diabetes	95% Confidence Interval
Baseline	<20	1	—
Level 2	20–34	1.3	0.8–1.8
Level 3	35–49	2	1.6–2.6
Level 4	>50	3	2.7–3.3

    A. Levels 2, 3, and 4 have significantly elevated risks for diabetes relative to baseline.

    B. Levels 2 and 3 are significantly different from each other.

    C. Levels 3 and 4 are significantly different from baseline and risk elevating.

    D. Levels 3 and 4 are not significantly different from each other.

    E. RR for levels 2, 3, and 4 are numerically different but not significantly different from baseline.

1. **Answer: A.**

2. **Answer: C.**

3. **Answer: A.**

4. **Answer: C.**

5. **Answer: C.**

6. **Answer: C.**

Interpretation of Medical Literature

7

INTRODUCTION

The purpose of this chapter is to provide you with an approach to reading and understanding research articles and pharmaceutical advertisements. It is based on principles of epidemiology.

An understanding of these concepts is fundamental to the comprehension of medical literature. We have sacrificed depth for the sake of brevity since our goal was to provide a few fundamental tools and avoid complexity.

RESEARCH ABSTRACT 1

Wedge resection or lobectomy: comparison of tumor recurrence rates and overall survival in NSCLC patients receiving preoperative chemotherapy

Wedge resection for non-small-cell lung cancer (NSCLC) stage I patients still remains controversial with many physicians. The primary outcomes of tumor recurrence and overall survival (OS) remain unclear when compared with complete lobectomy, which has traditionally been considered a far more effective procedure. However, a recent compilation of case reports and case series reports have validated impressive tumor recurrence and OS rates that were previously only believed to be seen in patients receiving lobectomy. Our primary objective was to compare and analyze the tumor recurrence rates and OS for both wedge resection and lobectomy in patients with stage I NSCLC following preoperative chemotherapy.

Methods

We systematically reviewed individual case reports and case series reports from 152 institutions in the United States for patients who first received preoperative chemotherapy and then underwent either wedge resection (248 patients) or lobectomy (329 patients). A propensity score algorithm was used to reduce the confounding that can occur when examining the effects and variables related to both treatment measures. Following the procedures, tumor recurrence and OS were assessed at 3 and 5 years in all patients.

Results

Preoperative mortality related to chemotherapy complications for patients scheduled to have wedge resection or lobectomy was 0.8% and 1.5%, respectively ($p = 0.22$). Perioperative mortality in patients undergoing lobectomy was 3.8% versus 0.8% in those receiving wedge resection ($p = 0.02$). During the predetermined follow-up times at 3 and 5 years, overall tumor recurrence (both locoregional and metastases) was assessed:

- At the 3 year follow-up, overall tumor recurrence was 5.9% for wedge resection and 4.2% for lobectomy ($p = 0.41$).

- At the 5-year follow-up, overall tumor recurrence was 6.3% for wedge resection and 6.1% for lobectomy ($p = 0.29$).

When comparing the OS for wedge resection with lobectomy the 3-year OS rates were 82% vs 71%, respectively; $p = .09$) and 5-year OS rates were 69% v 68%, respectively; ($p = .29$). Wedge resection was not found to be an independent predictor of tumor recurrence (hazard ratio, 1.23; 99% CI, 0.96 to 1.15) or OS (hazard ratio, 1.43; 99% CI, 0.92 to 1.23).

Conclusion

Wedge resection and lobectomy are associated with similar overall tumor recurrence and overall survival rates when performed after preoperative chemotherapy. However, perioperative complications and mortality are significantly lower in patients receiving wedge resection compared with lobectomy. Since patients generally maintain superior overall lung function with wedge resection, we recommended that wedge resection be performed in all eligible patients with Stage I NSCLC unless there is a compelling reason to perform a lobectomy.

PRACTICE QUESTIONS

1. Information from the abstract most strongly supports which of the following conclusions?

   A. Both wedge resection and lobectomy have lower mortality and tumor recurrence rates when patients first receive preoperative chemotherapy.

   B. Perioperative mortality was lower in patients undergoing wedge resection.

   C. Postoperative complications were lower in patients undergoing wedge resection.

   D. Pulmonary function tests at 1 year were significantly higher in patients receiving wedge resection.

   E. The overall survival for wedge resection at 3 years was proven to be higher than that of lobectomy.

The correct answer is choice B. You are asked to determine which answer choice is most strongly supported by the information provided in the abstract. In this type of question, the correct answer is found in the abstract itself and the reader needs only to interpret the information. Of the answer choices, choice B is most supported by the information provided in the drug abstract. The statement, "Perioperative mortality was lower in patients undergoing wedge resection" is supported by the data provided in the Results section. We are told that perioperative mortality in those receiving lobectomy was 3.8% versus 0.8% for those receiving wedge resection (P = 0.02). This data shows that mortality in those receiving a lobectomy was almost 5x higher than seen in those receiving wedge resection. Furthermore, the p value is 0.02, which shows statistical significance.

The stated objective of the researchers was to "compare and analyze the tumor recurrence rates and OS for both wedge resection and lobectomy in patients with stage I NSCLC following preoperative chemotherapy." In other words, researchers assessed tumor recurrence and OS in patients receiving 2 different surgical procedures. Since all patients received preoperative chemotherapy, one cannot draw a conclusion about the impact of preoperative chemotherapy based on the information presented (**choice A**). Remember, there would have to be a subset of patients who did not receive preoperative chemotherapy in order for a comparative analysis to be performed.

Postoperative complications (**choice C**) were not discussed in the abstract.

A clinician could reasonably conclude that pulmonary function tests would be higher at 1 year in patients receiving wedge resection when compared with lobectomy (**choice D**). However, this "reasonable assumption" is not supported, as data regarding lung function at 1 year was not presented in the abstract.

Choice E states "The overall survival for wedge resection at 3 years was proven to be higher than that of lobectomy." In the Results section of the abstract, it says, "When comparing the OS for wedge resection with lobectomy, the 3-year OS rates were 82% vs 71%, respectively; ($p = .09$)." At first glance it may appear to be a correct statement; however, the p value is 0.09. Therefore, the 2 percentages are not statistically different.

2. Which of the following best describes the type of study performed?

A. Case-control study

B. Crossover study

C. Meta-analysis

D. Propensity-matched analysis

E. Randomized, controlled clinical trial

The correct answer is choice D. You are asked to determine what type of study/analysis the researchers performed. The researchers reviewed individual case reports and case series reports from a number of institutions. After reviewing and compiling the data, they used an algorithm to reduce confounding variables and subsequently analyze the data. Based on this information, we can conclude that the researchers performed a **propensity-matched analysis**. Propensity score matching (PSM) is used in the statistical analysis of observational data. PSM is a statistical matching technique which attempts to approximate the effect of a treatment by accounting for the covariates that predict receiving a given treatment. This type of statistical analysis is used to reduce bias caused by confounding variables. Propensity scores (obtained from a propensity-matched analysis) are valuable when attempting to draw causal conclusions from observational studies (such as case reports) where the "treatment" or "independent variable" was not originally randomly assigned.

Case-control studies (**choice A**) are retrospective observational studies used to identify risk factors that are believed to be associated with a particular disease or condition. Subjects are initially classified as having or not having the disease in question and then their histories are explored to identify the presence or absence of any risk factors. Data are usually analyzed by means of an odds-ratio, and interpreted such that if something occurs in the history of the diseased group, but not in the non-diseased group, then it will be identified as a risk factor.

Cross-over studies (**choice B**) are clinical trials in which 2 comparison groups (for example) both receive the drug being tested and the comparative intervention (often a placebo) at different times. This interventional study will generally begin with one group (group A) receiving the investigational drug while a comparison group (group B) receives a placebo. Then, at some predetermined time, there will be a washout period and then Group A is switched to the placebo, while the Group B is given the investigational drug. This study design allows comparison of those on and off the drug, but also satisfies the ethical requirement that everyone in the study is exposed to whatever benefit the experimental drug may provide.

A meta-analysis (**choice C**) will meticulously examine several interventional clinical studies on a particular disease state (or treatment measure) and then combine the results using an acceptable statistical methodology. The results will be presented as if they were from 1 large study. The classical meta-analysis compares 2 types of treatment measures while multiple treatment meta-analysis (or network meta-analysis) can provide estimates of treatment efficacy of multiple treatment regimens, even when direct comparisons are unavailable. One of the key differences between a meta-analysis and a propensity matched analysis is that a meta-analysis is used with interventional studies, and a propensity-matched analysis is used with observational reports or studies.

A randomized, controlled clinical trial (**choice E**) is a type of interventional study where a researcher will administer a medication or treatment measure to one group of participants and evaluate its effects against a control group who receives another treatment measure or placebo. Subjects in the study are randomly allocated into "intervention" and "control" groups to receive or not receive an experimental preventive or therapeutic procedure or intervention. In the "wedge resection" analysis, researchers compiled the results from several observational studies. The data evaluated was derived from case reports where patients were NOT originally assigned to receive either a wedge resection or lobectomy.

3. The next step in follow-up of these research results would be to conduct which type of study?

    A. Case-control study

    B. Cohort study

    C. Cross sectional study

    D. Randomized, controlled clinical trial

    E. Replication in a different biological model

The correct answer is D. In the current study, researchers reviewed and compiled the data from numerous case reports and case series reports. They then attempted to draw causal conclusions from these observational studies where the treatment was not originally randomly assigned. Using this approach, researchers are able to determine if further investigation is warranted. In this particular analysis, researchers identified a higher than expected overall survival rate and lower than expected tumor recurrence rate associated with a procedure (wedge resection) that is believed to be associated better postoperative lung function as compared to lobectomy. Since the results of their analysis essentially showed no real difference in overall tumor recurrence rates and overall survival rates, the next step would be to further validate these results with an interventional study, such as a prospective, randomized controlled trial (RCT). In an RCT, researchers will likely randomly assign patients to receive either wedge resection or lobectomy following preoperative chemotherapy. Researchers will then be able to determine if there is a statistical difference between the two treatment options.

Case-control studies (**choice A**) are retrospective observational studies used to identify risk factors that are believed to be associated with a particular disease or condition. Subjects are initially classified as having or not having the disease in question and then their histories are explored to identify the presence or absence of any risk factors.

Cohort studies (**choice B**) are observational studies in which subjects are classified as having or not having a risk factor and then followed forward in time so incidence rates for the two groups can be compared. Although cohort studies are a type of prospective study, the next step would be to use an "interventional" prospective study, such as a randomized controlled clinical trial.

Cross-sectional studies (**choice C**) are observational studies used to assess the prevalence of a disease in a given population and the factors which co-occur with that disease at a particular time.

Replication in a different model (**choice E**) is a type of study generally used in early animal testing of experimental medications. For example, early animal testing for a new compound may involve a small number of rats. Once data is obtained from a single animal test, there is still a lot of information that needs to be obtained and questions that need to be answered before this new compound (experimental drug) can be considered for human trials. Therefore, researchers often perform several different types of animal tests using a variety of rat species followed by testing in other animal models.

RESEARCH ABSTRACT 2

Mekanib improved overall survival and decreased vemurafenib resistance in BRAF-mutated metastatic melanoma

BRAF mutations have been observed in approximately 50% of all malignant melanomas. The most predominant BRAF mutations found in melanoma are those that introduce an amino acid substitution at valine 600. Approximately 80–90% of these mutations are classified as BRAF V600E. Other predominant BRAF mutations include V600K, V600R and V600D. All of these mutations result in heightened BRAF kinase activity and amplified phosphorylation of downstream targets, which in particular includes MEK. BRAF inhibitor therapy (with vemurafenib or dabrafenib) is associated with well-documented clinical benefit in most patients with BRAF V600E-mutated melanoma (and other subtypes). However, resistance to these drugs and tumor progression generally occurs in patients within the first year. It is believed that BRAF mutations stimulate melanoma cell proliferation and survival predominantly through activation of MEK. The purpose of this study was to determine if the addition of the allosteric MEK1/MEK2 inhibitor mekanib (KAP071714) to vemurafenib delayed expected vemurafenib resistance, as well as improved progression free survival (PFS) and overall survival (OS) in comparison with dacarbazine.

Methods

This was a phase 3, multicenter, double-blinded, randomized clinical trial comparing the effectiveness of mekanib (KAP071714) in 447 total participants with previously untreated, metastatic melanoma with the BRAF V600E mutation. Patients were randomly assigned into 2 cohorts. Cohort A (222 participants) received dacarbazine (1000 mg per square meter of body-surface area intravenously every 3 weeks); Cohort B (225 participants) received vemurafenib (960 mg orally twice daily) + mekanib (150 mg orally daily). PFS was the primary end point and OS was a secondary end point.

Results

Median PFS was 11.6 months in the mekanib group and 2.3 months in the dacarbazine group (hazard ratio for disease progression or death in the mekanib group, 0.23; 95% confidence interval [CI], 0.30 to 0.58; $p<0.007$). At 15 months, the rate of overall survival was 78% in the mekanib group and 42% in the dacarbazine group (hazard ratio for death, 0.43; 95% CI, 0.52 to 0.88; $p = 0.02$). Elevated hepatic enzymes, rash, diarrhea, and hypertension were the most common toxic effects in the mekanib group. Nausea, vomiting alopecia, facial flushing, myalgia, leukopenia and hepatotoxicity were the most common toxic effects in the dacarbazine group. There were 8 patients in the mekanib group and 15 patients in the dacarbazine group who withdrew from the study due to severe side effects. Secondary skin neoplasms were not observed in either group.

Conclusions

Mekanib, as compared with traditional dacarbazine chemotherapy, improved rates of PFS and OS among patients with the BRAF-mutated metastatic melanoma, as well as delayed vemurafenib drug resistance. Mekanib should be considered for use in conjunction with vemurafenib for the treatment of BRAF-mutated metastatic melanoma.

(Funded by SMILE Pharmaceuticals, ClinicalTrials.gov number NCT0123456789101112)

1. Information from the abstract above most strongly supports which of the following conclusions about mekanib?

    A. In the treatment of select cases of metastatic melanoma, mekanib alone provides higher rates of PFS and OS than dacarbazine alone.

    B. Mekanib does not produce severe side effects.

    C. Mekanib produces fewer side effects than dacarbazine.

    D. Metastatic melanoma patients with BRAF V600K mutations have improved PFS and OS rates when taking vemurafenib + mekanib versus dacarbazine.

    E. Most metastatic melanoma patients appropriately prescribed vemurafenib and mekanib are likely to complete their treatment regimen.

The correct answer is choice E. You are being asked to determine which answer choice is most supported by the information provided in the abstract. While several answer choices might "look good," you will be able to eliminate the incorrect answer choices once you examine the meaning of each statement. Of the answer choices, choice E is most supported by the information provided in the drug abstract. The Results section indicates that "Eight patients in the mekanib group and 15 patients in the dacarbazine group withdrew from the study due to severe side effects." Of the 225 patients originally enrolled in the mekanib + vemurafenib arm of the study, 217 persons or 96% of the original study group completed the study. Hence, you can reasonably conclude that most metastatic melanoma patients appropriately prescribed vemurafenib and mekanib are likely to complete their treatment regimen.

The statement, "In the treatment of select cases of metastatic melanoma, mekanib alone provides higher rates of PFS and OS than dacarbazine alone" can be eliminated (**choice A**) since the study was not designed to evaluate mekanib versus dacarbazine. This study evaluated mekanib PLUS vemurafenib versus dacarbazine.

"Mekanib does not produce severe side effects" (**choice B**) is an incorrect statement because the abstract only lists a few of the most common side effects. It does not mention the severe (and less common) side effects. These findings are likely to be found in the body of the published study. Remember, this is an abstract and only provides limited information.

"Mekanib produces fewer side effects than dacarbazine" (**choice C**) is incorrect because the abstract only lists a few of the most common side effects for both drugs. It does not outline the number and frequency of occurrence of side effects. These findings are likely to be found in the complete study.

The statement "Metastatic melanoma patients with BRAF V600K mutations have improved PFS and OS rates when taking vemurafenib + mekanib versus dacarbazine" can be eliminated (**choice D**), because the study was only performed in metastatic melanoma patients with BRAF V600E mutations. Hence, the reader cannot draw conclusions about the effect of vemurafenib plus mekanib in this patient population.

2. In the conclusion section of the abstract, the authors indicate that when mekanib was added to vemurafenib the drug delayed vemurafenib drug resistance. Which of the following is the most likely reason that the reader should question the validity of this claim?

   A. Insufficient follow-up of study participants

   B. Insufficient information on adverse effects and drug-drug interactions

   C. Lack of an appropriate control group

   D. Subject attrition

   E. Use of hazard ratio instead of relative risk

The correct answer is choice C. You are asked to determine the most likely reason why one should question the validity of the claim that mekanib delays vemurafenib-resistance. The correct answer is lack of an appropriate control group. In order for researchers to conclude that mekanib decreases vemurafenib resistance, the control group must be vemurafenib alone and the study group must be vemurafenib PLUS mekanib. In this study, the control group was dacarbazine and study group was vemurafenib plus mekanib; hence, there is not an appropriate control group to answer the question "Does mekanib delay vemurafenib resistance?" In other words, there is no data available to support the claim that the addition of mekanib did in fact decrease vemurafenib resistance. Furthermore, the background states that "resistance to these drugs (vemurafenib and dabrafenib) and tumor progression generally occurs in patients within the first year" and the Results section states that the median PFS was 11.6 months in the mekanib group. The median PFS is a little less than a year; hence, the reader should actually question if mekanib actually provided any benefit at all.

The Results section provides information about median PFS and survival rates at 15 months. The length of the study was sufficient to assess the effects it was designed to assess (**choice A**).

The Results section provides information on adverse effects but does not provide any information on drug-drug interactions (**choice B**). Although a drug interaction could potentially decrease the effectiveness of mekanib, the most likely reason to question the validity of the claim (in the question stem) is because of a lack of an appropriate control group.

The Results section states that "Eight patients in the mekanib group and 15 patients in the dacarbazine group withdrew from the study due to severe side effects." Out of an original 447 patients, only 23 patients withdrew from the study. Hence, the subject attrition rate is low for this study (**choice D**).

By definition, the hazard ratio is a measure of relative risk over time in situations where the researchers are interested not only in the total number of events, but also in the timing of these events. For example, the event of interest may be subject death or it could be a non-fatal event such as readmission or symptom change. The use of a hazard ratio in this particular study is appropriate (**choice E**).

3. In the background section of the abstract, researchers state that the purpose of the study was to determine whether the addition of the allosteric MEK1/MEK2 inhibitor mekanib (KAP071714) to vemurafenib treatment would delay drug resistance, as well as improve progression-free survival (PFS) and overall survival (OS) in comparison to dacarbazine. Which of the following study design changes could have been made to appropriately evaluate all the specified outcomes?

   A. Add a vemurafenib-only cohort to the study

   B. Prescribe all 3 medications to each participant but at different dosage ranges

   C. Replace the dacarbazine cohort with a vemurafenib-only cohort

   D. Use a crossover study instead of a randomized clinical trial

   E. No changes were needed since the study was properly designed to meet the specified outcomes

The correct answer is choice A. You are asked to determine what changes could have been made to the original study design so that the 3 initial study outcomes could be appropriately evaluated. Based on the purpose outlined in the question stem, the 3 outcomes being evaluated are as follows:

1. Decreased vemurafenib resistance when mekanib is added

2. Improved PFS for vemurafenib + mekanib compared to dacarbazine

3. Improved OS for vemurafenib + mekanib compared to dacarbazine

The current study design appropriately evaluates PFS and OS between vemurafenib + mekanib AND dacarbazine because participants were administered either vemurafenib + mekanib OR dacarbazine. However, the only way to assess whether mekanib decreases vemurafenib-resistance is to evaluate this regimen against a vemurafenib-only cohort. Hence, in order to appropriately evaluate all 3 outcomes described in the question stem, there would need to be 3 cohorts:

1. Dacarbazine only

2. Vemurafenib only

3. Vemurafenib + mekanib

If researchers prescribed all 3 medications to each participant but at different dosage ranges (**choice B**), then none of the initial 3 outcomes could have been measured because there is no comparison against either dacarbazine only or vemurafenib only.

If researchers replaced the dacarbazine cohort with a vemurafenib-only cohort (**choice C**), then they would be able to assess the "resistance outcome." However, they would not be able to assess the effects of mekanib + vemurafenib against dacarbazine.

In cross-over studies, all subjects receive both interventions unless it is a placebo-controlled study (then all participants receive treatment and placebo). If a crossover study design were used with the existing study, then group A (for example) would receive dacarbazine only, and group B would receive vemurafenib + mekanib. Then, at some predetermined point there would be a washout period, and group B would receive dacarbazine only and group A would receive vemurafenib + mekanib. This type of study design (**choice D**) would not be able to assess the "vemurafenib resistance outcome" as outlined above.

PHARMACEUTICAL AD 1

Tazofect

(tanzopanib 10 and 20 mg capsules)

For newly diagnosed and treatment-resistant EGFR-mutated NSCLC, an effective treatment is now available to improve progression-free survival (PFS)!

- Tazofect is indicated for treatment of EGFR-mutated NSCLC
- Tazofect has shown efficacy in PIK3CA, PTEN, and KRAS-mutated NSCLC

Tazofect is like extra time in a capsule...

...so your patients have more time to do what they want to do!

Tazofect has been proven to:

- Increase PFS by an average of 9 months in all NSCLC study participants (first-line and erlotinib resistant)
- Increase PFS by an average of 10 months in first line NSCLC study participants over those receiving Tarceva® (erlotinib)
- Almost double the PFS in carboplatin resistant NSCLC study participants over those receiving Tarceva® (erlotinib)

The side effect profiles for both Tazofect and erlotinib were similar.

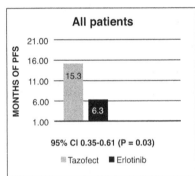

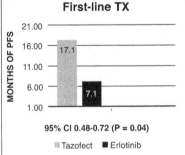

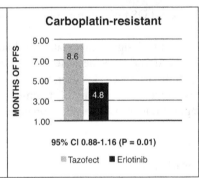

- The effects of Tazofect (10-20 mg qd) and erlotinib (150-200 mg qd) in subjects with EGFR exon 19 deletions or exon 21 (L858R) substitution mutations are presented above. The results were taken from a phase 3, randomized, double blinded multicenter clinical trial. Per protocol, each of these agents was continued until clinically significant disease progression occurred plus an additional 2 months unless mortality occurred. The average follow-up time for patients who completed the study in both Tazofect groups was 17.3 months and 8.3 months in both erlotinib groups.

- Of the 800 initial participants enrolled in the phase 3, randomized, double blinded multicenter trial, 225 (of 398) participants completed the study in the Tazofect group and 388 (of 402) participants completed the study in the erlotinib group.

- Of the original number of study participants, 103 Tazofect patients and 102 erlotinib patients were classified as carboplatin-resistant.

Increased progression-free survival!

Additional product information provided below

SMILE Pharmaceuticals

Smile for life with SMILE Pharmaceuticals

Improved patient outcomes!

HIGHLIGHTS OF PRESCRIBING INFORMATION

Please see Tazofect (tanzopanib) drug package insert for complete prescribing information

Indications and Usage: Tazofect (tanzopanib) is a kinase inhibitor indicated for first-line treatment of NSCLC with EGFR exon 19 deletions and EGFR exon 21 (L858R) substitution mutations in patients age 18 years and older.

Mechanism of Action: Tanzopanib is a kinase inhibitor that acts by inhibiting intracellular tyrosine kinase domain of epidermal growth factor receptor (EGFR) thus resulting in cell cycle arrest and angiogenesis inhibition. Tanzopanib has an elimination half-life of approximately 28 hours in patients with normal hepatic and renal function.

Dosage and Administration: Treatment of NSCLC with EGFR exon 19 deletions and EGFR exon 21 (L858R) substitution mutations in patients aged 18 years and older with normal hepatic and renal function: 10–20 mg daily until clinically significant disease progression.

Contraindications: Hypersensitivity to tanzopanib; use in patients with severe hepatic impairment, active infection and thrombocytopenia.

Warnings and Precautions: May cause reactivation of tuberculosis and hepatitis B. Use caution in patients receiving other chemotherapeutic agents, thyroid disorders, dehydration, mild to moderate renal and hepatic dysfunction

Adverse Reactions:

Common (≥5%): elevated AST & ALT (15%), diarrhea (15%), fatigue (13%), elevated bilirubin (12%), infection (10%), cough (8%), thrombocytopenia (7%)

Less Common (<5%): hepatorenal syndrome (2%), hepatotoxicity (2%), toxic epidermal necrolysis (1%), Stevens-Johnson syndrome (1%), acute renal failure (1%), hypothyroidism (1%), hemolytic anemia (<1%)

1. The data provided in the drug advertisement most strongly supports which of the following conclusions?

   A. In the treatment of cancer, Tazofect and erlotinib can be used interchangeably.

   B. Tazofect is not indicated for treatment of EGFR exon 19 insertion in non-small cell lung cancer.

   C. Tazofect should be considered for use in patients with PIK3CA mutated NSCLC.

   D. The combination of Tazofect and erlotinib will improve the PFS to a greater extent than either agent alone.

   E. The dose of Tazofect should be adjusted in patients with hepatic dysfunction.

The correct answer is B. In the Indications section of the prescribing information, the following is stated. "Tazofect (tanzopanib) is a kinase inhibitor indicated for first-line treatment of NSCLC with EGFR exon 19 deletions and EGFR exon 21 (L858R) substitution mutations in patients aged 18 years and older." There is no mention of "EGFR exon 19 insertions." That is not to say that the drug cannot be used in NSCLC patients with EGFR exon 19 insertions. However, Tazofect is not indicated (FDA approved) for use in these patients by the FDA. Hence this is a true statement and the correct answer.

Both Tazofect and erlotinib are indicated for EGFR exon 19 deletions or exon 21 (L858R) substitution mutations. Also both drugs are noted to have similar side effect profiles (as indicated in the primary drug ad). However, erlotinib is also indicated for the treatment of pancreatic cancer. Since erlotinib has a broader range of clinical indications and **choice A** states "in the treatment of cancer," these agents are not interchangeable. It should also be pointed out that almost half of the Tazofect patients dropped out of the trial. Without knowing the reasons why, it would not be advisable to interchange Tazofect with erlotinib. Choice A is a false statement.

Choice C states that "Tazofect should be considered for use in patients with PIK3CA mutated NSCLC." Although the main drug ad states that "Tazofect has shown efficacy in PIK3CA, PTEN and KRAS Mutated NSCLC," there is no data in the prescribing information or drug ad itself to support this claim. Also what exactly does "shown efficacy" mean? The drug may be marginally effective in a small percentage of PIK3CA patients, for example. In other words, there is no data to support this claim in the drug ad. Choice C is an incorrect statement.

Choice D states that "The combination of Tazofect and erlotinib will improve the PFS to a greater extent than either agent alone." There is no information indicating whether the combination of the 2 agents will provide more benefit, less benefit or the same benefit as either agent used alone. Choice D is an incorrect statement.

Choice E refers to making a dosing adjustment in patients with hepatic dysfunction. In the prescribing information section, there is a contraindication for use in severe hepatic impairment as well as a precaution about use in patients with mild-moderate hepatic dysfunction. However, there is no information provided in the drug ad related to a dosing adjustment in patients with hepatic dysfunction. Choice E is an incorrect statement.

2. Consider the following statement: "Tazofect was proven to provide approximately double the PFS in carboplatin resistant NSCLC study participants over those receiving Tarceva® (erlotinib)." When evaluating the drug ad and highlights of prescribing information, which of the following provides the best evidence that this statement is inaccurate?

    A. Number of patients treated in the carboplatin resistant group for both drugs

    B. The calculation of months of PFS for the carboplatin resistant graph

    C. The confidence interval for the carboplatin resistant graph

    D. The p value for the carboplatin resistant graph

    E. The y axis data points for the carboplatin resistant graph

The correct answer is C. You are asked to evaluate a statement found on the main drug ad and then indicate what information invalidates this statement. Of all the answer choices, the data provided on the confidence interval for the carboplatin resistant graph provides the best evidence that the statement is inaccurate. A confidence interval gives an estimated range of values which is likely to include an unknown parameter (such as actual PFS), the estimated range being calculated from a given set of sample data. In the original statement, the drug company claimed that their drug (Tazofect) was proven to provide approximately double the PFS in carboplatin resistant NSCLC study participants over those receiving Tarceva® (erlotinib). However, the confidence interval provided with the carboplatin resistant graph contains the number 1. If the 95% confidence interval for a study includes 1.0, then there is >1 in 20 chance that random variation in outcome incidence among the study groups (Tazofect-study and erlotinib-control) is what produced the observed correlation between treatment and outcome. In the instance the p value is also likely to be >0.05. In summary if the confidence interval contains the relative risk of 1.00, the result is not significant. As discussed, this should also lead the reader to believe that the p-value (provided on the same graph, choice D) is also inaccurate. However, without the data seen with the confidence interval, the reader would have no way of suspecting that the provided p-value is also likely inaccurate. Therefore, choice C is the best answer

In the key under the 3 graphs, it is stated that 103 Tazofect patients and 102 erlotinib patients were classified as carboplatin resistant. This is a sufficient number of patients in each group (**choice A**).

The statement makes reference to the number of months of PFS in the Tazofect group being "almost double" the erlotinib group in carboplatin resistant patients. The PFS for Tazofect is 8.6 months and the PFS for erlotinib is 4.8 months. This statement could have been phrased differently, but is not completely inaccurate (**choice B**).

When comparing the data points on the y-axes of the 3 graphs, the y-axis on the carboplatin resistant group was clearly manipulated so that a more "profound graphical representation" of the actual results is evident. Although this should cause the reader to question the integrity of the authors, choice C is still the best answer.

3. Shortly after Tazofect is released for use in the general population, the FDA and drug manufacturer begin to receive numerous reports of complete treatment failure in both carboplatin resistant patients and first line therapy patients as well as higher than expected percentages of adverse events in all patients. Which of the following is the most likely reason for these reports on Tazofect?

   A. Insufficient follow-up of study participants

   B. Insufficient information on adverse effects

   C. Insufficient information on drug indications

   D. Subject attrition

   E. Type II error was committed

The correct answer is choice D. In the question stem we are told that shortly after the drug is used in the general population there are reports of treatment failure in both carboplatin resistant patients and first line treatment patients. We are also told that higher-than-expected percentages of adverse events are occurring. The question is asking for the most likely cause of this occurrence. The most likely reason based on the data provided in the drug ad and highlights of prescribing information is subject attrition. Under the 3 graphs it is stated that "Of the 800 initial participants enrolled in the phase 3, randomized, double blinded multicenter trial, 225 (of 398) participants completed the study in the Tazofect group and 388 (of 402) participants completed the study in the erlotinib group." Approximately half (225/398 participants) of the original Tazofect study participants never completed the trial. Furthermore, the authors did not provide an explanation as to why they did not complete the study. Is it likely that they did not complete the trial because of severe adverse effects and/or death?

Without knowing the reasons why the participants never completed the trial, it is difficult to evaluate the safety and efficacy of Tazofect in both first line therapy and carboplatin resistant patients. Also, it is quite possible that only a small percentage of the 103 participants in the carboplatin resistant arm of the study never completed the study. Without more information, it is hard for the reader to make a valid conclusion. In summary, the authors should have indicated why almost half of the study participants never completed the study; hence, the primary reason why these reports are occurring (due to treatment failures and increased adverse effect occurrence) is directly related to the circumstances surrounding the high level of subject attrition in this trial.

The phase 3 trial for Tazofect lasted in each patient until clinically significant disease progression occurred plus an additional 2 months unless mortality occurred. Furthermore, the average follow-up time for patients who completed the study was listed. The length of the study was sufficient to assess the effects it was designed to assess. Choice A is an incorrect response.

At the bottom of the highlights of prescribing information page of the drug ad, there is an extensive list of adverse effects and percentage of occurrence of each of these side effects. Hence, sufficient information on these adverse effects was provided. Choice B is an incorrect response. However, this information was based on the number of patients who completed the clinical trial. Since almost half of the study participants (in the Tazofect arm) never completed the trial, an accurate accounting of side effect appearance was not available. This is directly related to subject attrition.

At the top of the highlights of prescribing information page of the drug ad, it clearly states that "Tazofect (tanzopanib) is a kinase inhibitor indicated for first-line treatment of NSCLC with EGFR exon 19 deletions and EGFR exon 21 (L858R) substitution mutations in patients aged 18 years and older." The drug is NOT indicated for use in carboplatin resistant patients. Although there is a graph on the first page of the drug ad and comments about proven effects, the drug ad never claimed that the drug was "indicated" for use in carboplatin patients. Choice C is an incorrect response.

A type II or beta error is where the researcher fails to reject the null hypothesis when it is really false. In other words, the researcher declared that there was no significant effect on the basis of the sample when there really is one in the population. The likely impact of this type of error is that the drug (Tazofect) would NOT obtain FDA approval and the general population would not receive this medication. Choice E is an incorrect response.

PHARMACEUTICAL AD 2

GluSense™ ... because it makes sense!

(Glugliflozin 75 mg, 150 mg and 300 mg tablets)

Diabetes is a complex disease ...

GluSense is a simple treatment measure with proven therapeutic outcomes!

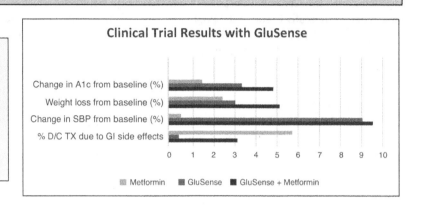

Clinical Trial Results with GluSense

Change in A1c from baseline (%)
Weight loss from baseline (%)
Change in SBP from baseline (%)
% D/C TX due to GI side effects

0　1　2　3　4　5　6　7　8　9　10

☐ Metformin　■ GluSense　■ GluSense + Metformin

- The clinical effects of GluSense (150-mg qd), metformin (1000 mg bid) and combination therapy (GluSense 150 mg qd + metformin 1000 mg bid) in patients with newly diagnosed type 2 diabetes who failed to meet glycemic goals with diet and exercise alone are presented above. The results were taken from a phase 3, randomized, double-blinded multicenter clinical trial.

- Each therapy was administered in conjunction with a structured diet and exercise program.

- A baseline A1c, body weight and systolic blood pressure reading were obtained at the onset of the trial and every 8 weeks during the trial. All participants were enrolled in the study for 12 months.

- Of the 1600 initial participants enrolled in the trial, 462 (of 510) participants in the metformin-only group completed the study, 358 (of 533) of the GluSense-only group completed the study, and 313 (of 577) in the GluSense + metformin group completed the study.

- The primary reason (as stated by the patient) for withdrawing from the study was unwanted side effects.

GluSense demonstrated <u>greater reductions</u> in A1c, weight loss & blood pressure than metformin alone at 52 weeks!

- GluSense is indicated for treatment of T2DM as monotherapy & in combination with metformin.

- GluSense has shown efficacy when used in conjunction with other oral hypoglycemic agents.

The treatment your T2DM patients have always needed is finally here!!

SMILE Pharmaceuticals

Smile for life with SMILE Pharmaceuticals

GluSense has been proven to:

- Reduce A1c in T2DM patients by an average of 3.4% as monotherapy (P<0.001) & in combination with metformin an average of 4.9% (P<0.002) – mean baseline A1c = 8.05%

- Reduce baseline weight in T2DM patients by an average of 3.1% as monotherapy (P<0.02) & in combination with metformin an average of 5.2% (P<0.03) – mean baseline weight = 182 lbs (87.3 kg)

- Reduce baseline systolic blood pressure in T2DM patients by an average of 9.1% as monotherapy (P<0.006) & in combination with metformin an average of 9.6% (P<0.001) – mean baseline SBP = 177 mm Hg.

Additional product information provided below

HIGHLIGHTS OF PRESCRIBING INFORMATION

Please see GluSense (glugliflozin) drug package insert for complete prescribing information.

Indications and Usage: GluSense (glugliflozin) is an SGLT2 inhibitor with insulin-sensitizing properties, indicated for the treatment of type 2 diabetes in conjunction with diet and exercise as monotherapy, and in combination with metformin in patients aged 18 years and older.

Mechanism of Action: Glugliflozin is an SGLT2 inhibitor with insulin-sensitizing properties. This agent has a dual mechanism of action. It acts by:

- Inhibiting the sodium-glucose cotransporter 2 (SGLT2), thereby reducing glucose reabsorption and increasing urinary glucose excretion

- Decreasing insulin in the periphery and liver, resulting in increased insulin-dependent glucose disposal and decreased hepatic glucose output. Glugliflozin is an agonist for peroxisome proliferator-activated receptor-gamma (PPARγ). Activation of PPARγ nuclear receptors in the liver, skeletal muscle, and adipose tissue modulates the transcription of a number of insulin responsive genes involved in the control of glucose and lipid metabolism.

- Other: antagonizes peripheral alpha-1 adrenergic receptors

Pharmacokinetics

- Glugliflozin has an elimination half-life of approximately 16 hours in patients with normal hepatic and renal function.

- Following oral administration of glugliflozin, Tmax occurs within 3 hours.

- Glugliflozin is extensively metabolized by hydroxylation and oxidation; the metabolites also partly convert to glucuronide or sulfate conjugates.

- Following oral administration of glugliflozin, approximately 15–20% of the drug dose is recovered in the urine.

Dosage and Administration: Treatment of type 2 diabetes in patients aged 18 years or older who have failed to meet glycemic goals with diet and exercise alone:

- Monotherapy: 150–300 mg PO qd; start at 75 mg PO qd and increase by 75 mg qwk; max dose 450 mg/day

- Combination with metformin: same as monotherapy and standard metformin dose of 2000 mg daily (in divided doses)

Contraindications: Type 1 diabetes mellitus, hypersensitivity to glugliflozin and/or sulfonamides; NYHA class III or IV heart failure, severe hepatic impairment, hyperkalemia, use with medications causing hyperkalemia and diabetic ketoacidosis

Warnings and Precautions: May cause hypoglycemia, hypotension, and AST/ALT elevation. Caution use in elderly patients with poorly controlled diabetes and patients with past history of cardiovascular disease.

Adverse Reactions (for a complete list, see drug package insert)

Common (5%):	Less Common (<5%):
Hyperkalemia	Fatigue
Hypoglycemia	Hepatic dysfunction
Orthostatic hypotension	Thirst
Dizziness	Fainting
Tachycardia	Mental impairment
Hyperhidrosis	Pancreatitis

Drug Interactions (see drug package insert)

1. The data provided in the drug advertisement most strongly supports which of the following conclusions?

    A. GluSense is a substitute for diet and exercise in type 2 diabetes due to its weight loss properties.

    B. GluSense is recommended for use in patients with a history of myocardial infarction.

    C. GluSense is safer to use in patients with type 2 diabetes than metformin.

    D. The antihypertensive effects of GluSense are comparable to some currently available antihypertensive medications.

    E. The combination use of GluSense and a sulfonylurea is recommended for those who initially fail sulfonylurea monotherapy.

The correct answer is D. This type of question generally requires a process of elimination. The statement "The antihypertensive effects of GluSense are comparable to some currently available antihypertensive medications" is most strongly supported by the drug ad. Relevant information to support this statement can be found in several places: First in the table, GluSense is associated with 9.1% decrease in average systolic blood pressure. This percentage decrease is comparable to the diuretics, low-moderate doses of ACE inhibitors, alpha antagonists as well as varying doses of other drugs from different drug classes. Second, the mechanism of action section of the highlights of prescribing information states that this drug antagonizes peripheral alpha-1 adrenergic receptors. This is the same mechanism of action as drugs like terazosin and doxazosin. Finally, the side effects of the drug (orthostatic hypotension, dizziness, and tachycardia) also support its antihypertensive properties since these are side effects commonly seen in alpha antagonists. Hence, out of all of the answer choices, this statement is most strongly supported by the drug ad.

There are several places which indicate GluSense is used in conjunction with diet and exercise, such as the key under the chart on the main ad page and in the Indications and Usage section in the highlights of prescribing information. Although the drug promotes weight loss, GluSense is not a substitute for diet and exercise (**choice A**).

The Warnings and Precautions section states that GluSense should be used cautiously in patients with past history of cardiovascular disease. Furthermore, in Contraindications, it is stated that GluSense is contraindicated for use in patients with NYHA Class III or IV heart failure. Since myocardial infarction (**choice B**) is a form of cardiovascular disease and a common precipitating cause of heart failure, GluSense would not be recommended for use in these cases. GluSense may potentially be used "cautiously" in patients with a mild form of cardiovascular disease but is not "recommended."

The drug ad does not have a safety profile comparison between GluSense and metformin (**choice C**). The only related comparison between the drugs is the appearance of severe GI side effects leading to withdrawal from the study.

The only statement relating to the use of GluSense and another drug is found in the main area of the drug ad: "GluSense has shown efficacy when used in conjunction with other oral hypoglycemic agents." It does not specify the names or drug classes of the other agents (**choice E**). Furthermore, it does not provide any data to support this claim.

2. Of the initial trial participants, 175 persons from the GluSense-only group and an even large number from the GluSense and metformin group withdrew from the study. Which of the following is the most likely reason for participant withdrawal?

    A. Appearance of drug interactions

    B. Hypersensitivity to sulfonamides

    C. Severe hypoglycemia

    D. Severe hypotension

    E. Severe GI side effects

The correct answer is C. You are asked to determine the most likely reason why participants withdrew from the study. In the key under the graph on page 1, it states "The primary reason (as stated by the patient) for withdrawing from the study was unwanted side effects." However, it is not stated what side effect caused them to withdraw. Therefore, you must determine the most likely reason based on information provided in the drug ad. The Adverse Reactions section of the highlights of prescribing information provides only a "partial" list of side effects with a percent occurrence above and below 5% so this section alone cannot be used to answer the question. The correct answer can be derived from the section on the bottom right of the main drug ad. It states that GluSense has been proven to reduce A1c in type 2 diabetes (T2DM) patients by an average of 3.4% as monotherapy ($p < 0.001$) and in combination with metformin an average of 4.9% ($p < 0.002$). The mean baseline A1c was 8.05% for study participants. If the mean baseline A1c was 8.05%, that means that some patients likely started with an A1c around 7%. Remember that an A1c 6% is an average daily glucose level of 126 mg/dL. If you lower this A1c by 3.4% (GluSense only) or 4.9% (Glusense + metformin), the resulting A1c levels are 3.6% and 2.1%, respectively. Since the A1c is a long-term average of the daily blood glucose levels, it is likely that this agent caused severe hypoglycemia in participants; hence, the likely reason for withdrawal from the study. Furthermore, it is stated that hypoglycemia is one of the most common adverse effects. Choice C is the best answer choice.

The drug ad does not specifically mention any problems with drug-drug interactions (**choice A**) in the clinical trial and there is a comment indicating that the reader should please see GluSense (glugliflozin) drug package insert for complete prescribing information. Based on this information, it is unlikely that drug-drug interactions are the primary reason for patient withdrawal.

The Contraindications section states that GluSense is contraindicated for use in patients with sulfonamide hypersensitivity (**choice B**). However, there is nothing which would lead the reader to believe this is the primary reason for withdrawal from the study.

The bottom right of the ad states that GluSense has been proven to reduce baseline SBP (systolic blood pressure) in T2DM patients by an average of 9.1% as monotherapy ($p < 0.006$) and in combination with metformin an average of 9.6% ($p < 0.001$). The mean participant baseline SBP was 177 mm Hg. Even if the starting blood pressure was 100 mm Hg, the patient would still not be hypotensive with a 9.6% drop in blood pressure. Note, too that orthostatic hypotension is listed as a common side effect, but with the information presented it is unlikely that was the primary reason for patient withdrawal (**choice D**).

It is unlikely that severe GI side effects (**choice E**) were the primary reason for participant withdrawal since the table shows that the GluSense-alone arm had almost no withdrawals from study. GluSense also improved the GI side effect withdrawal rate for patients receiving metformin when the 2 medications were combined.

3. A 64-year-old man comes to the physician with complaints of increasing polyuria and polydipsia. His past medical history is significant for type 2 diabetes, hypertension, hyperlipidemia, and a myocardial infarction 4 years ago. Allergy history includes an anaphylactic reaction to levofloxacin. He is currently receiving metformin 1000 mg 2× daily, enalapril 10 mg daily, pravastatin 20 mg daily, and spironolactone 25 mg twice daily. Physical examination shows blood pressure of 126/82 mm Hg, heart rate 62/min, height 172.7 cm (5 feet, 8 inches), weight 88.6 kg (195 lbs), and BMI 29.6.

    Laboratory studies show:

    - Blood glucose: 215 mg/dL

    - A1c: 10.5%

    - Albumin: 3.8 g/dL

    - Creatinine: 1.3 mg/dL

    - AST: 20 IU/L

    - ALT: 22 IU/L

    - Sodium: 138 mEq/L

    - Potassium: 4.9 mEq/L

    - Calcium: 9.6 mg/dL

    - Ejection fraction: 66%

    If the attending physician is considering the addition of GluSense to this patient's medication regimen, which of the following is a contraindication for prescribing this medication?

    A. Allergy contraindication

    B. Cardiovascular contraindication

    C. Drug interaction contraindication

    D. Hepatic contraindication

    E. Renal contraindication

    F. There is no contraindication in this patient and the medication can be prescribed

The correct answer is C. You are being asked for the most likely reason to not prescribe this medication to a given patient. Therefore, you need to look for either an absolute or relative contraindication for prescribing this medication in the drug ad. The Contraindications section states that GluSense is contraindicated for "use with medications causing hyperkalemia." The patient is currently receiving enalapril and spironolactone. Both of these medications are associated with the development of hyperkalemia. Furthermore, the patient's potassium level is 4.9 mEq/L, which is at the high level of normal. The patient is likely to become hyperkalemic once starting this medication. Based on this information, a drug-drug interaction (**choice C**) between GluSense and both enalapril and spironolactone is the most likely contraindication for use of this medication in this patient. Choice C is correct and (**choice F**) is incorrect.

The patient has a history of anaphylaxis to the fluoroquinolone levofloxacin. Although GluSense is contraindicated for use in patients with a sulfonamide allergy, there is no allergy contraindication for using this medication in patients with a fluoroquinolone allergy (**choice A**).

The only cardiovascular contraindication (**choice B**) listed for GluSense is NYHA Class III or IV heart failure. This patient has a normal ejection fraction of 66% (normal 55–70%) so does not meet the cardiovascular contraindication criteria for this drug. Although the patient's past history of myocardial infarction predisposes him to heart failure, the patient currently does not have heart failure so there is no contraindication. However, there is a warning for use of GluSense in patients with cardiovascular disease. As indicated, this patient has a past history of a myocardial infarction as well as hyperlipidemia and hypertension. Therefore, this medication should be used cautiously in this patient. If GluSense is prescribed, the patient should be monitored closely but there is no cardiovascular contraindication for the use of this drug in this patient.

The patient has normal hepatic function (AST: 20 IU/L (normal <35 IU/L) and ALT 22 IU/L (normal <35 IU/L)); hence, there is no hepatic contraindication for using GluSense in this patient (**choice D**).

The patient has normal renal function (creatinine: 1.3 mg/dL (normal 0.5–1.4 mg/dL)); hence, there is no renal contraindication for using GluSense in this patient (**choice E**).

PART V

PATIENT SAFETY AND QUALITY IMPROVEMENT

Clinical Applications of Patient Safety and Quality Improvement

8

Case: Within the past 2 years, a major tertiary care referral hospital experiences separate cases of a blood transfusion reaction due to incompatibility, 2 inpatient falls leading to significant injury, a wrong-site surgery, and a medication-dosing error causing a patient death.

- What is the most probable single underlying cause behind these medical errors? **Systems failures due to the complexity of health care delivery**

Health care is not a single system, but rather multiple systems which all interact. These clinical microsystems are defined as a group of clinicians and staff working together with a shared clinical purpose to provide health care for a population of patients. Individual health care organizations contain multiple microsystems which evolve over time. It is the complexity of these systems that predispose patients to harm from medical error.

Health care in the United States is capable of achieving incredible results for even the most severely ill patients. However, it does not do so reliably and consistently. Medical errors plague our health delivery systems. The Institute of Medicine (IOM) estimates that 44,000–98,000 patients die each year in the United States from preventable medical errors. This translates to more annual deaths than motor vehicles accidents, HIV, and breast cancer. In addition to the toll that this takes in the form of human suffering, medical errors also represent a significant source of inefficiency and increased cost in the health care system.

The causes of these adverse events are not usually from people intentionally seeking to harm patients, but rather from the complexity of the health care system together with the inherent capability for human error. The causes of these errors are varied, and can include failures made in administering medication, performing surgery, reporting lab results and making a diagnosis, to name a few. The most severe of these medical errors are referred to as **sentinel events.** A sentinel event is an adverse event in which death or serious harm to a patient has occurred; it usually refers to an event that is not at all expected or acceptable (e.g., operating on the wrong patient or body part, abduction of an infant from the hospital, patient suicide while admitted to the hospital). The choice of the word *sentinel* reflects the egregiousness of the injury (e.g., amputation of the wrong leg) and the likelihood that investigation of such an event will reveal serious problems in current policies or procedures.

It is unacceptable for patients to suffer preventable harm caused by a health care system whose purpose is to provide healing and comfort. Improving patient safety is the responsibility of every health care professional and requires a comprehensive team effort. Collectively, health care needs to learn from past errors and develop systems of care which prevent future errors from harming patients (e.g., process of root cause analysis).

Systems in health care delivery can be redesigned to **make it difficult for health care personnel to do the wrong thing** and **easier to consistently do the right thing**.

UNDERSTANDING MEDICAL ERROR

Classifications of Medical Errors

Medical errors can be classified as **errors of commission** (doing something wrong) or **errors of omission** (failing to do the right thing). Errors of omission are more difficult to recognize than errors of commission, but are thought to represent a larger percentage of medical errors.

Examples are ordering a medication for a patient with a documented allergy to that medication (**error of commission**), and failing to prescribe low-dose unfractionated heparin as venous thromboembolism prophylaxis for a patient undergoing hip replacement surgery (**error of omission**).

> Case: A 47-year-old man presents to the outpatient clinic with complaints of shoulder pain and is diagnosed with arthritis. The clinician treating him administers a shoulder corticosteroid injection without reviewing the patient's medication list prior to the procedure. The patient has been taking Coumadin for atrial fibrillation and develops hemarthrosis.
>
> • Error classified as a lapse or omission

Lapses are missed actions or omissions (e.g., forgetting to monitor serum sodium in a patient undergoing diuresis for congestive heart failure). Lapses are not directly observable (i.e., you cannot directly 'see' a lack of memory). **Slips** are observed actions that are not carried out as intended (e.g., accidentally injecting a medication intravenously when it was meant to be given subcutaneously). **Mistakes** are a specific type of error brought about by a faulty plan or incorrect intentions; the intended action is wrong (e.g., barium swallow on a patient with suspected esophageal perforation or giving steroids to a patient with acute glaucoma).

The figure below clarifies the relationship further.

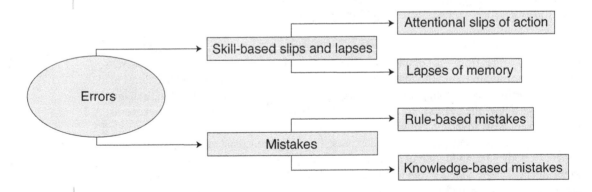

> Case: After an unexpected 3-hour delay in the operating room due to a problem in the electrical system, an operating room team rushes to get started in order to complete the scheduled elective procedures. The team elects not to perform the mandatory sponge count at the end of the first surgery in order to get the next case started sooner. The patient returns 2 weeks later with abdominal pain and is found on x-ray to have a retained foreign object (a sponge) in the abdominal cavity.
>
> • Error due to **'violation' in policy**

Violations are conscious failures to adhere to procedures or regulation. Violations differ from slips, lapses and mistakes because they are deliberate actions, i.e., intentionally doing something against the rules. Reasons for violations may include time constraints, unfamiliarity with policy, or motivation by personal gain. A health care professional may consider that a violation is well-intentioned; however, if it results in an adverse event it would still technically constitute a 'violation' rather than an error.

> Case: A 65-year-old man presents to the emergency department with sudden epigastric pain. He has a history of alcoholism, and the treating physician suspects a diagnosis of pancreatitis. Despite the fact that the patient denies alcohol use for several years, has normal blood levels of pancreatic enzymes, and has an abnormal EKG, he is treated for pancreatitis and the actual diagnosis of myocardial infarction is delayed.

- Error due to **'anchoring bias'**

Anchoring bias describes when a clinician relies on and clings steadfastly to the initial diagnostic impression, despite subsequent information to the contrary. In many cases the features of a patient's presentation allow the clinician to make a correct initial diagnostic impression; however, in certain cases subsequent developments in the patient's course will prove inconsistent with the first impression. Anchoring bias refers to the tendency to hold on to the initial diagnosis, even in the face of disconfirming evidence.

> Case: A 33-year-old woman with a breast lump is asked if it is tender. When she says that it is tender, the clinician confirms the suspected diagnosis of a cyst. No further history is obtained and the clinician fails to realize there has been an increase in size, associated adenopathy and fixation to the chest wall (hence the tenderness), all suggesting breast cancer.

- Error due to **'confirmation bias'**

Confirmation bias may accompany anchoring, and refers to the tendency to focus on evidence that supports an initial diagnosis, rather than to look for evidence that refutes it or provides greater support to an alternative diagnosis.

> Case: A 24-year-old sexually active woman is seen by her ob/gyn physician for complaints of abdominal pain. She is evaluated briefly and treated for a UTI without any other tests being performed. The next day, the patient presents to the emergency department and is diagnosed with a ruptured appendicitis.

- Error defined as **'premature closure'**

Premature closure is acceptance of a diagnosis before it has been fully vetted by considering alternative diagnoses or searching for data that contradict the initial diagnosis. In this case the physician finds a cause that fits the clinical picture and ceases to search for other diagnostic possibilities.

> Case: A 4-week-old infant is brought to the emergency department by his parents after he develops an episode of emesis with an observed period of apnea. Three other infants were seen in the emergency department earlier this week with the flu. The infant is discharged home with instructions for flu management, but the parents return with him later, reporting that the child had another episode of apnea. The patient is further evaluated and subsequently transferred to the children's hospital with the clinical diagnosis of apnea from gastroesophageal reflux.

- Cognitive error classified as **'availability bias/heuristic'**

Availability bias/heuristic is the tendency to make the diagnosis of a current patient biased by recent or vividly recalled cases or events, rather than on prevalence or probability.

> Case: During her third visit to an outpatient clinic for shortness of breath, a 57-year-old woman with documented pneumonia is treated with antibiotics and sent home. She later presents to the emergency department with exacerbation of dyspnea and is admitted to the medical service, where she is found to have hypoxia from heart failure.
>
> • Error due to **'diagnosis momentum'**

Diagnosis momentum is a bias that occurs when the diagnosis considered by one clinician becomes a definitive diagnosis as it is passed from one clinician to the next; it then becomes accepted without question by clinicians down the line. It is the medical equivalent of "following the crowd."

> Case: A patient with a known heroin addiction presents with abdominal pain. The treating physician assumes the pain to be a sign of opiate withdrawal and manages the patient accordingly with admission to the inpatient med-psychiatry ward. Later during the hospital stay the patient's pain increases and he develops peritonitis from a missed bowel perforation.
>
> • Error related to **'framing effects'**

Framing effects: Diagnostic decision-making unduly biased by subtle cues and collateral information. This can lead to diagnostic error by allowing the way the story is framed to influence the diagnosis.

Human Factors that Cause/Influence Medical Errors

An understanding of medical error requires comprehension of the personal situations and factors associated with the risk of error. Human beings have limited memory and attention capacity. People can make errors when distracted or overtasked. The risk of error is exacerbated by conditions of fatigue, stress, and illness.

> Case: A 9-year-old-boy is admitted to the pediatric oncology service for the treatment of a hemolytic malignancy, and is started on chemotherapy ordered from the pharmacy. The hospital pharmacist is working a double shift because 2 other pharmacists called in sick. The hospital is particularly busy and the pharmacist has not had a break all day. He accidentally sends the wrong dose of chemotherapy to the floor, after which the patient develops a hypotensive reaction. The patient is successfully resuscitated with fluids and supportive care.
>
> • What contributed to this adverse patient event?

The risk of medical error is increased when health care professionals work under less than ideal circumstances, especially when well-designed safety systems are not in place. Poor working conditions include:

- Inexperience (especially when combined with lack of supervision)
- Time pressures
- Poor safety procedures (e.g., lack of staffing, lack of safety policies)
- Poorly designed human-equipment interfaces (e.g., difficult to program infusion pumps)
- Inadequate information (e.g., missing or outdated labs, illegible written orders, failure to communicate change in status, language barriers)

A helpful acronym which can be used by health care providers to assess their suitability to provide patient care is **IM SAFE**.

Illness

Medication

Stress

Alcohol

Fatigue

Emotion

The following actions have been demonstrated to limit errors caused by human factors.

- Avoid reliance on memory or vigilance.
- Simplify processes when possible.
- Standardize common procedures and processes.
- Routinely use checklists.

SYSTEMS-BASED PRACTICE

Lessons from high-reliability organizations (e.g., aviation, nuclear power plants) emphasize the importance of approaching errors on a **systems level** rather than a personal level with blame. It is easier to redesign the conditions under which people work than to attempt to change fallible human nature. When a system fails (i.e., medical error occurs), the immediate question should be **why did it fail**, not 'who caused it to fail.'

A classic example of a systems-based approach to patient safety is the removal of concentrated potassium from general hospital wards. This action was intended to prevent the inadvertent preparation of IV solutions with concentrated potassium, an error that had produced small but consistent numbers of deaths for many years. This particular approach is called a 'forcing function,' where the system is redesigned in a way that forces an individual to avoid making the error due to process design, rather than relying on individual memory. Think of a car that won't allow you to start the engine unless your foot is on the brake.

The "Swiss-cheese model of error" (James Reason, 1991) helps to identify the multiple factors that can often contribute to an error resulting in patient harm.

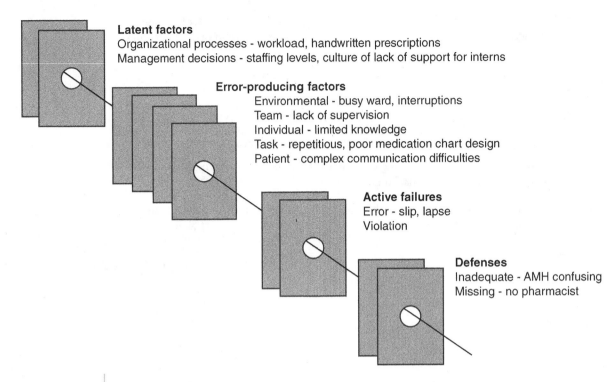

Latent factors
Organizational processes - workload, handwritten prescriptions
Management decisions - staffing levels, culture of lack of support for interns

Error-producing factors
Environmental - busy ward, interruptions
Team - lack of supervision
Individual - limited knowledge
Task - repetitious, poor medication chart design
Patient - complex communication difficulties

Active failures
Error - slip, lapse
Violation

Defenses
Inadequate - AMH confusing
Missing - no pharmacist

Source: James Reason, 1991

The layers represent barriers that prevent human error from causing patient harm. In a perfect world, these defenses would be impenetrable and patients would always be safe. In reality, these defenses have holes (hence, 'Swiss cheese'), which represent latent hazards (e.g., poor system design, lack of supervision, equipment defects). Occasionally the holes line up and a patient is injured.

Patient harm can be avoided by building systems with successive layers of protection (e.g., awareness, alarms, policies) and removal of latent errors (i.e., plug the holes).

Case: A 45-year-old man presents for treatment of acute sinusitis. He is prescribed antibiotics, after which he suffers a severe allergic reaction requiring hospitalization. Despite attempts of resuscitation, the patient sustains a cardiac arrest and dies. Later review of his medical record reveals a documented allergy to the antibiotic that was prescribed.

- How do we learn from this event to prevent a similar occurrence in the future?

An example of the "Swiss cheese model" follows below.

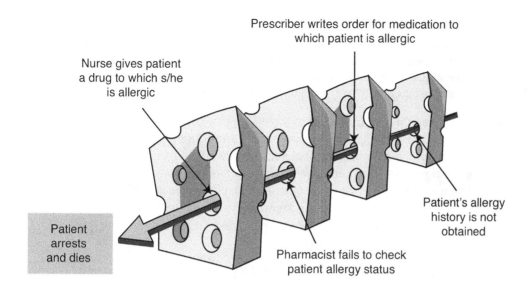

This example details a **medication error**. The patient's medication allergy is not obtained in the initial history, thus leading to the wrong medication being prescribed by the clinician, filled by the pharmacist, and administered by the nurse. The final result is the patient's death.

Applying 'systems-thinking' here, the question to be addressed is, "How can the system be redesigned so it is able to absorb the error before it reaches the patient?"

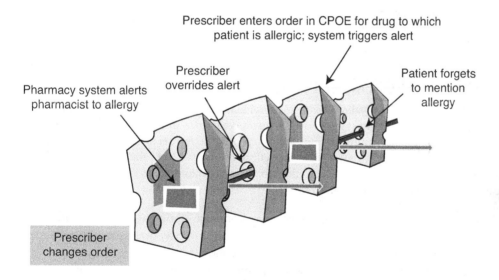

A systems-based redesign seeks not to *remove* the possibility of error, but rather to **create/ reinforce barriers to harm**. For this case, one example would have been to implement a computer physician order entry (CPOE) based on the patient's electronic health record, which could have alerted the prescriber and pharmacist to the allergy.

Disclosure of Medical Errors

Known medical errors should be openly disclosed to the affected patient or, in certain circumstances, their families. During error disclosure, it is crucial to prepare the appropriate environment for disclosure. Be sure to arrange to have the proper time, place, and people involved, including arrangement of follow-up care and psychosocial support.

> Case: A 29-year-old man is brought to the emergency department after falling from a ladder. He is evaluated in the trauma bay and subsequently admitted to the hospital with a bilateral calcaneal fracture and stable L4/L5 compression fracture of the spine. The nurse notices that the blood pressure cuff used on the patient had blood stains on it from a prior patient treated for a motor vehicle collision. The prior patient was known to have hepatitis C. Somehow the cuff was not changed or cleaned before being used on the new patient, thus potentially exposing him to hepatitis C.
>
> • What information should be conveyed to the patient who was exposed?

An error disclosure should include the following 3 elements:

1. Accurate description of the events and their impact on the patient
2. Sincere apology showing care and compassion
3. Assurance that steps are being taken to prevent the event from happening in the future

Often the most senior physicians responsible for the patient and most familiar with the case will make the official disclosure.

QUALITY IMPROVEMENT PRINCIPLES

Only 5% of patient harm is directly due to individual incompetence or poor intentions. People need to be accountable, but system-based changes are needed to truly transform care. Blaming individuals and taking punitive actions for honest mistakes/errors do little to improve the overall safety of the health system. The most effective approach is to **find out how the error happened**, rather than who did it, and then **fix the system** to prevent a similar error from causing harm to patients in the future.

> Case: Two days after undergoing a hysterectomy for uterine fibroids, a woman is restarted on her outpatient dose of rivaroxaban (a new oral anticoagulant). The patient has a known history of deep venous thrombosis, for which she receives pain control via an epidural catheter. Before removal of the epidural catheter, the anesthesia intern on the pain service reviews the medication list for anticoagulants, yet does not realize that rivaroxaban is an anticoagulation agent. Five days after removal of the catheter, the patient develops an epidural hematoma and sustains paraplegia.
>
> • What should be done with the intern to improve safety in the future? **Find out *how* the intern made this error (i.e., how the system allowed the error to occur and result in harm to the patient) and then fix the system to prevent a similar error from causing injury to patients in the future.**

Error Reporting

Collecting data on medical errors is essential for improving patient care. Reporting errors provides this data and allows opportunities to improve care by learning from failures of the healthcare system. Error reporting is facilitated by

- Anonymous reporting
- A simple and easy-to-use system
- Timely feedback
- Absence of punitive actions

Note that while 'near misses' do not necessarily need to be disclosed to patients, they should be reported to the system so they can be studied and used to inform system changes.

Root Cause Analysis

"Root cause analysis" (RCA) is a retrospective approach to studying errors. It allows a team to identify problems in the system or process of care. It should be conducted by a knowledgeable team (consisting of representatives from all the specialties/professions involved in the event), focus on systems/process analysis rather than individual performance, and identify potential improvements that can be made to reduce the chance of similar errors in the future.

> Case: A 16-year-old patient comes to deliver her baby. During the process of her care, an infusion intended exclusively for the epidural route is connected instead to the peripheral IV line and infused by pump. Within minutes, the patient experiences cardiovascular collapse. A cesarean section results in the delivery of a healthy infant, but the medical team is unable to resuscitate the mother.

- Describe an effective approach to studying this error so that future cases of patient harm are prevented.

The fishbone diagram (also known as a 'Cause and Effect' or Ishikawa diagram) is used to explore all the potential causes that result in a poor outcome. An example is as follows:

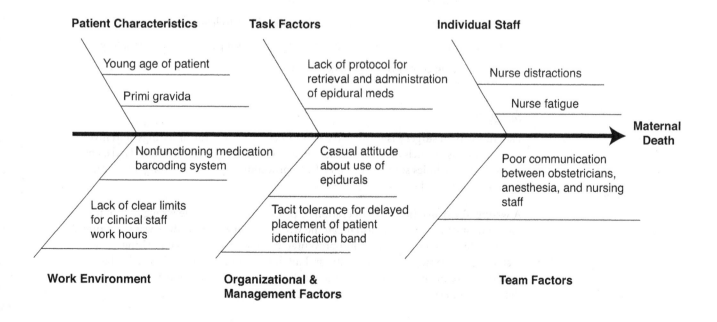

CLINICAL PEARL

Be aware of the second victim of medical error: the health care professionals involved in the adverse event. Without proper support, their shame and fear can lead to depression, anxiety, and even suicide. Colleagues who have been involved in medical error must feel supported; as much as possible, the goal is to learn from the error and move on.

In the case presented here, systemic problems identified by the RCA would include medications being kept in the room, communication problems, inexperienced staff, and technology failures. Many solutions were then generated, including the removal of barriers to barcode scanning and changing the current medication ordering and dispensing policy. Another consideration would be to add a 'forcing function,' by redesigning the Luer lock on the epidural bag to be unable to connect to an IV line.

Failure Mode and Effects Analysis

The Failure Mode and Effects Analysis (FMEA) is a systematic tool that allows practitioners to anticipate what might go wrong with a device, product or process; determine the impact of that failure; and determine the likelihood of failure being detected before it occurs. Unlike the retrospective nature of RCA, the FMEA is a proactive approach to patient safety. It produces a risk priority number (RPN) based on the probability and relative impact of a failure.

$$RPN = \textbf{severity of the effect} = \textbf{probability of occurrence of the cause} \times \textbf{probability of the detection}$$

For example: inadvertent esophageal intubation during elective surgery can severely affect patient outcome (rating of 10), but it has a low level of occurrence (2) and can be detected fairly easily (3).

Therefore, RPN for this failure mode = $\textbf{10} \times \textbf{2} \times \textbf{3} = \textbf{60}$.

BUILDING A SAFER HEALTH SYSTEM

In 2001 the IOM provided 6 aims to improve patient safety and quality; health care should be **S**afe, **T**imely, **E**quitable, **E**fficient, **E**ffective, and **P**atient-centered (STEEEP). Basic concepts for building a health care system which achieves these aims include:

- Standardizing care whenever possible, reducing reliance on memory (e.g., using checklists for important steps)
- Using systems-based approaches to build safety nets into the health care delivery process to compensate for human error
- Openly report and study errors (e.g., using RCA to learn from error)
- Engaging with patients (i.e., patient education is a powerful tool for safety)
- Improving communication and teamwork

Surgery

Patient safety in surgery is similar to patient safety in non-surgical settings, and involves many of the same issues including medication error, hospital-acquired infection (HAI), and readmissions. It also includes some errors specific to procedures including wrong-site surgery, retained foreign objects, and surgical site infections.

A **wrong-site procedure** is an operation or procedure done on the wrong part of the body or on the wrong person. It can also mean the wrong surgery or procedure was performed. Wrong-site procedures are rare and preventable, but they do still occur. Using a standard system of confirming the patient, site, and intended procedure with the medical team and patient before the procedure starts is a widely employed method of reducing or eliminating these types of errors.

Case: A 59-year-old man with unresectable lung cancer presents to the emergency department with acute shortness of breath. A chest radiograph demonstrates a right sided malignant pleural effusion. The thoracic surgeon intending to drain the pleural effusion mistakenly places the chest tube on the left side after reading an x-ray of another patient. Post-procedure chest x-ray shows a persistent pleural effusion on the right lung. A second chest tube is then placed, this time in the patient's right chest. The patient remains stable and his breathing improves. The left chest tube is removed after confirmation that there is no air leak. There are no further sequelae.

- How could this adverse event be prevented?

A team supported by the World Health Organization's "**Safe Surgery Saves Lives**" program designed a surgical safety checklist designed to improve team communication and consistency of care with the intent of reducing complications and deaths associated with surgery. The premise of the safe surgical checklist is that many common surgical complications are preventable. Implementation of the checklist was associated with significant reductions in the rates of death and complications including wrong-site surgery.

Among other benefits, the surgery checklist helps ensure appropriately administered antibiotic prophylaxis which reduces the incidence of surgical wound infection. The timing of antibiotic administration is critical to efficacy.

- The first dose should be given preferably within 30 minutes before incision.

- Re-dosing at 1 to 2 half-lives of the antibiotic is recommended for the duration of the procedure.

- In general, postoperative administration is not recommended.

Antibiotic selection is influenced by the organism most likely to cause a wound infection in the specific procedure.

Common Elements of Safe Surgery Checklist

- Confirm patient identity, planned procedure and marking of site

- Review patient allergies

- Ensure necessary equipment is present (e.g., pulse-oximetry)

- Introduce team members to each other

- Review critical steps of the procedure

- Address need for preoperative antibiotics

- Determine airway risk

- Determine estimated blood loss

Medications

Medication errors occur when a patient receives the wrong medication or when the patient receives the right medication but in the wrong dosage or manner (e.g., medication given orally instead of IV, or correct medication given at the wrong time). These errors represent one of the most common causes of preventable patient harm.

Case: A 54-year-old woman (Susan Jones) is admitted to the hospital and diagnosed with metastatic breast cancer for which chemotherapy is administered. During her hospitalization she mistakenly receives an anticoagulation medication intended for the woman next to her in the room who has a similar name (Suzanne Jonas). The mistake is recognized after the first dose and the medication is discontinued without any complications. Later during the same admission, she is inadvertently given an overdose of Dilaudid when the verbal order of 2 mg is administered intravenously instead of orally. She experiences lethargy and hypotension which resolve with supportive care during a brief stay in the ICU.

- What are the risk factors contributing to the occurrence of these medication errors?

Several factors can increase the risk of medication errors:

- Inadequate confirmation of patient identity prior to medication administration
- Look-alike and sound-alike (rifampin/rifaximin) medications

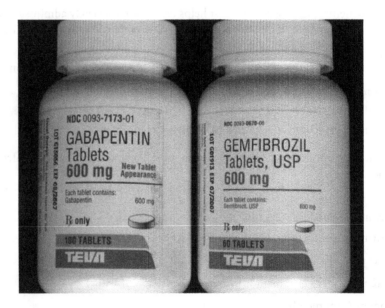

Look-alike Medications

- Illegible hand-written prescriptions/orders can result in a pharmacist or nurse administering the wrong drug or wrong dose of medication
- Use of certain abbreviations can result in misinterpretation of the order

The Joint Commission recently created a **"Do Not Use"** list of abbreviations for health professionals.

Official "Do Not Use" List[1]

Do Not Use	Potential Problem	Use Instead
U, u (unit)	Mistaken for "O" (zero), the number "4" (four) or "cc"	Write "unit"
IU (International Unit)	Mistaken for IV (intravenous) or the number 10 (ten)	Write "International Unit"
Q.D., QD, q.d., qd (daily)	Mistaken for each other	Write "daily"
Q.O.D., QOD, q.o.d, qod (every other day)	Period after the Q mistaken for "I" and the "O" mistaken for "I"	Write "every other day"
Trailing zero (X.0 mg)* Lack of leading zero (.X mg)	Decimal point is missed	Write X mg Write 0.X mg
MS	Can mean morphine sulfate or magnesium sulfate	Write "morphine sulfate" Write "magnesium sulfate"
MSO_4 and $MgSO_4$	Confused for one another	

[1] Applies to all orders and all medication-related documentation that is handwritten (including free-text computer entry) or on pre-printed forms.

Source: jointcommission.org

The "**5R's**" describe a strategy used to help prevent medication error by confirming the following 5 items prior to administering any medication.

- Right drug
- Right patient
- Right dose
- Right route
- Right time

Performing **medication reconciliation** (a review of the patient's complete medication list during any transition of care) is also intended to prevent inadvertent inconsistencies in the medication regimen.

Other systems changes that have saved countless lives:

- Removal of high-risk medications from certain clinical settings
- 'Unit dose administration,' in which medications packaged in ready-to-use units are prepared by the pharmacy and delivered to the clinical floor (this practice has resulted in fewer medication errors compared with having nurses perform mixing and dispensing on the floor)

The **integration of information technology** has also helped to reduce medication errors. Studies have shown that Computerized Physician Order Entry (CPOE) is an effective means of reducing medication error. It involves entering medication orders directly into a computer system rather than on paper or verbally. CPOE can decrease prescribing errors by automatically alerting the prescriber or pharmacist to allergies, potential drug-drug interactions or an incorrect dose.

Other technologies that have been designed to improve medication errors include barcoding to confirm correct patient identity and smart-pumps to prevent inappropriate dosage of IV medications.

Infections

Hospital-acquired infections (HAI) can be avoided. They are preventable, adverse events which may be caused by failing to adhere to evidence-based prevention strategies. Common HAIs include UTI (most common 35–40%), hospital-acquired pneumonia/ventilator-acquired pneumonia (15–20%), surgical site infection (20%), and central line infection (10–15%).

> Case: A 42-year-old man has surgery to repair a right inguinal hernia. His post-operative course is complicated by excessive post-op pain requiring IV narcotics. Ten hours after surgery he develops pubic pain. He has not voided since before surgery. A bedside ultrasound confirms a distended bladder indicating acute urinary retention. A urinary catheter is placed by a new nurse who is not familiar with sterile technique. The catheter immediately yields 800 cc of urine and the patient's pubic pain resolves. The patient requests to have the catheter left in place over the next 2 days. On post-operative day 3 the patient develops a fever to 101°C. A urine analysis and culture reveal an acute urinary infection.
>
> • What steps can be taken to reduce the likelihood of this complication?

There are some common approaches which can help to reduce HAI:

- Hand washing
- Use of sterile technique
- Use of preoperative prophylactic antibiotics (SSI)
- Elevating the head of the bed (ventilation associated pneumonia)
- Limiting use and duration of indwelling urinary catheters (UTI)
- Following evidence-based protocols for central line placement
  - Hand washing prior to procedure
  - Wearing a cap, mask, sterile gown and gloves
  - Preparation of site with chlorhexidine
  - Use of sterile barrier
  - Removal of the line as soon as possible

Pressure Ulcers

Pressure, or decubitus, ulcers are often preventable. Approaches to avoid this complication include performing risk assessments to identify vulnerable patients (e.g., paraplegics, diabetics, malnutrition, immobility, etc.).

> Case: A 65-year-old woman with type 2 diabetes and BMI 44 is being treated in the hospital for diabetic ketoacidosis. She has a urinary catheter in place to monitor urine output and does not get out of bed to go to the bathroom. She has refused ambulation or getting out of bed to a chair due to feeling very fatigued. Later during the hospital stay she develops a fever. Physical exam reveals a stage III infected decubitus ulcer over the sacral prominence.
>
> • How could this complication have been prevented?

Preventive activities for high-risk patients include daily inspection of skin, appropriate skin care and minimizing pressure through frequent repositioning and use of pressure relieving surfaces (e.g., airbeds).

Patient Falls

Patient falls are a common cause of injury, both within and outside of health care settings. More than one-third of adults over 65 fall each year. Injuries can include bone fractures and head injury/intracranial bleeding, which both can lead to death.

> Case: A 70-year-old woman is admitted to the nursing home after being treated in the hospital for a hip fracture sustained during a fall at home. She had an intramedullary nail placed and is currently able to ambulate with a walker. In addition to her hypertension medication, anxiolytic, dementia pills and a beta-blocker, she also takes post-operative pain medication every 4–6 hours. The patient was also placed on warfarin for DVT prophylaxis. On her way to the bathroom at night, she slips and falls, sustaining a head injury and significant intracranial hemorrhage.
>
> • What steps can be taken to reduce the risk of serious injury from a fall?

Performing a fall risk assessment will help to select patients who can benefit from preventative resources (e.g., one-to-one observation, non-slip flooring, lowering the bed height). It is important to identify patients at high risk of sustaining serious injury from a fall. The following are known risk factors for patient fall:

- Advanced age (age >60)
- Muscle weakness
- Use of >4 prescription medications
- Impaired memory
- Difficulty walking (e.g., use of a cane or walker).

Unplanned Readmissions

Unplanned hospital readmissions following discharge are recognized as a serious cause of decreased quality and often result from complications or poor coordination of care. Improving communication, reinforcing patient education, and providing appropriate support to patients at risk for readmissions are all strategies to reduce unplanned readmissions.

Case: A 79-year-old patient is admitted to the cardiology service and treated for acute CHF. He is started on a new medication regimen including a diuretic which relieves his symptoms and improves his cardiac function. He is discharged home, though he returns to the hospital 10 days later with another episode of CHF. During the readmission, the team notices that the patient never filled his new prescriptions and was not taking the prescribed diuretic while at home.

- What actions can be taken to prevent this from happening again?

Recommendations to improve the discharge process and prevent readmissions are as follows:

- Provide timely access to care following a hospitalization
- Communicate and coordinate care plan with patients and other providers
- Improve the discharge planning and transition processes
- Ensure patient education and support to optimize home care

Teamwork

Providing safe health care relies on health care professionals working together as a team. Well-functioning teams deliver higher quality and safer care. The need for improved teamwork has led to the application of teamwork training principles, originally developed in aviation, to a variety of health care settings. Simple changes to behavior and culture have had a profound impact on the culture of teamwork and safety in patient care.

Case: A resident responds to a cardiac code 10 minutes late because he was not aware that he was on code-duty. Upon arrival the patient is actively having chest compressions performed by a physician assistant. A nurse brings in the cardiac arrest cart and a respiratory technician places an oxygen mask on the patient and begins bag-mask ventilation. The resident asks for a blood pressure and heart rate to be checked. The respiratory tech and physician assistant both attempt to find a pulse on the patient's wrist, interrupting chest compressions and ventilation. The nurse simultaneously lowers the bed to place electrodes for an ECG which makes the oxygen mask fall off to the floor. The ECG demonstrates ventricular fibrillation and the resident calls to "shock the patient." No one is certain how to work the defibrillator. The patient expires.

- How can teamwork be improved to achieve a better outcome during the next cardiac code?

Effective teams share the following characteristics:

- Common purpose/shared mental model
- Measurable goals
- Effective leadership
- Effective communication
- Mutual support
- Respect value of all team members

Briefs and **huddles** are effective tools for teamwork. The team *brief* is used for planning, and is a short 'time-out' prior to starting the delivery of care in order to discuss team formation, assign essential roles, establish expectations and climate, and anticipate outcomes and likely contingencies. The *huddle* is used for team problem-solving, and is performed on an ad hoc basis to reestablish situational awareness, reinforce plans already in place, and assess the need to adjust the plan.

Clinical Communication Skills

Communication failures have been identified as a root cause in the majority of serious patient safety events. Patient safety and quality in health care improve when physicians communicate effectively with colleagues, patients, and families. Several techniques have been developed to enhance clinical communication skills.

> Case: A 25-year-old woman is admitted to the ICU following a motor vehicle collision, during which she sustained a significant head injury. She is intubated and monitored for increased ICP. The nurse coming on the night shift notices that the patient's pupils are dilated, and she is uncertain if this is a change in the patient's status. The nurse pages the resident on-call to see the patient. The resident evaluates the patient but does not speak with the nurse and is not aware of the nurse's concern of a change in status. No intervention is taken. The following morning during rounds the neurosurgical team finds the patient brain dead from herniation.

- How could communication be improved to prevent this error?

SBAR is a form of structured communication first developed for use in naval military procedures. It has been adapted for health care as a helpful technique used for communicating critical information that requires immediate attention and action concerning a patient's condition.

The following is an example of SBAR communication:

- **Situation:** What is going on with the patient? "I am calling about Mr. Smith in room 432 who is complaining of shortness of breath."

- **Background:** What is the clinical background or context? "The patient is a 67-year-old man post-operative day one from a left total hip replacement. He has no previous history of pulmonary or cardiac disease."

- **Assessment:** What do I think the problem is? "His breath sounds are decreased bilaterally and his oxygenation is only 87% on room air. He was getting IV Ringer's lactate at a rate of 150 cc/hour, in addition to 5 liters fluid replacement and 4 units of blood in the operating room. I would like to rule out acute pulmonary congestion from fluid overload."

- **Recommendation:** What would I do to correct it or what action is being requested? "I've already started supplemental oxygen and I feel strongly that the patient should be assessed for pulmonary overload, his fluids stopped and potentially given a diuretic. Are you available to come in?"

Case: During resuscitation of a cardiac code, the physician running the code states that she thinks epinephrine should be given intravenously. The nurse is uncertain if this was an order and believes that the doctor may have been just thinking out loud. No epinephrine is given. The doctor mistakenly assumes that the drug was administered and that it was not effective in reviving the patient. Precious time is lost until it is realized that no medication has been given.

- What communication technique can be used to avoid this error?

A **call-out** is a strategy used to communicate important or critical information. The goals of a call-out are to inform all team members simultaneously during team events, help team members anticipate next steps, and help create a shared mental model.

Case: A hospital lab technician phones a nurse to inform him of a critical serum calcium value in one of his patients. The nurse mistakenly hears a different number and believes the calcium to be only mildly elevated. The patient develops a symptomatic arrhythmia and requires transfer to the ICU for further appropriate care.

- How can techniques in effective communication be used to prevent this error?

A **read-back or check-back** is a communication technique commonly used in the military and aviation industry, and is now increasingly employed in health care to guard against miscommunication. Safety organizations encourage health care professionals to make a routine practice of reading back verbal orders or critical labs to ensure accuracy.

Case: During a clinical rotation on the pediatric ICU, you are invited by the chief resident to observe the operative repair of a congenital heart lesion in the pediatric cardiac surgery operating room. When you arrive in the OR the patient is already intubated and anesthetized, and procedures are underway to prep the patient for surgery. During the start of the case you see that an operative team member inserts the urinary catheter with a clear breach in sterile technique. This is neither noticed by the team member inserting the catheter nor mentioned by anyone else in the room. Being new to this setting, you are unaware whether different practices for sterile insertion are used in pediatric patients.

- What would you do to address your concern?

Critical language is a form of assertive structured communication which provides key words that enable members of the team to speak when patient safety concerns arise. These key phrases are uniformly understood by all to mean "stop and listen to me; we have a potential problem."

The acronym **CUS** is used to remember these key words.

- "I'm <u>c</u>oncerned"

- "I'm <u>u</u>ncomfortable"

- "I think this is a <u>s</u>afety issue"

Speaking up for patient safety is the responsibility of every member of the health care team. It is important to speak up for the patient. It may be intimidating to speak up when you are the most junior member of the team and at times uncertain if a safety issue is actually in question; however, as people with the privilege of caring for others, health care workers have to value our responsibility to the patient above all else. **Speak up if you witness an error or the potential for an error**. Make sure to report adverse events so others can study and learn from them—informing system-based approaches to improving patient safety.

Handoffs

Errors during handoffs and sign-outs can be mitigated by ensuring an accurate and effective transfer of pertinent patient information to the receiving health care professional. This has immediate applications to on-call sign-outs and changes of shift, but it also affects other scenarios such as hospital- and unit-floor-transfers.

> Case: A diabetic patient with an ankle fracture is signed-out to the covering intern from a team member in a hurry to leave the hospital. Later that night the patient develops sinus tachycardia thought be related to pain, and the covering intern orders more pain medication. Unknown to the covering intern, the patient was found earlier to have an incidental pulmonary embolism. This information was forgotten during the hurried sign-out. The patient develops chest pain, dyspnea and ultimately dies from progression of the PE.

- How can this adverse event be avoided in the future?

An effective handoff encompasses the following principles:

- Active process

- Prioritize sick patients

- Verbal + written

- Have a set system

- Limit distractions

- Allow sufficient time

- Ensure updated information

Quality Improvement Roadmap

The methods used to approach quality and process improvement are as follows:

1. Identify the problem.
2. Measure the problem.
3. Organize a team.
4. Flowchart the process.
5. Develop a range of interventions to fix the problem.
6. Measure the impact of the interventions.

Case: A hospital is interested in reducing the number of medication errors in the inpatient geriatric unit. The current medication ordering system has been in place for 15 years and consists of written orders on slips of paper being sent to pharmacy by pneumatic tubes, and then receiving the medication in a batched collection system on the unit. Nurses are required to then sort through the batched medications to identify the correct one for their patient(s). Over the past year, the severity of the admitted geriatric patients has increased, along with the number of medications required. There have been reports of possible increased rates of medication errors over the past 6 months.

- How will you approach improving the current process?

The following tools are commonly used in quality improvement:

Flow chart: map of all the steps in the current clinical process being evaluated

- Flow charting a process helps the team clearly see the complexity of the process and the opportunities for improvement.

Pareto analysis: process of rank-ordering quality improvement opportunities to determine which of the various potential opportunities should be approached first

Run chart (time plot): graphical record of a quality characteristic measured over time

- Run charts help the team determine if a change is a true improvement over time or just a random fluctuation.
  - A trend is defined as ≥5 consecutive points constantly increasing or constantly decreasing. If a trend is detected, it might indicate a non-random pattern that should be investigated.
  - A shift is a run containing ≥6 data points all above or all below the median and indicates a non-random pattern that should be investigated.

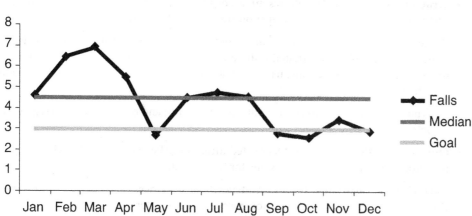

Sample Run Chart Plotting Patient Falls

AHRQ.gov

Control chart: method used to distinguish between variations in a process due to common causes and those due to special causes. It is constructed by obtaining measurements of some characteristic of a process, summarizing with an appropriate statistic, and grouping the data by time period, location, or other process variables.

- Common cause variation is an inherent part of every process. It is random and due to natural or ordinary fluctuations in the system.

- Reducing variation improves the predictability of outcomes and helps reduce the frequency of adverse outcomes for patients.

- Special cause variation is due to irregular or unnatural causes that are neither predictable nor inherent to the process. Special cause variation should be identified and eliminated before making QI changes to a process.

There are many different types of control charts, depending on the statistic analyzed on the chart.

Interventions can take many forms, including automation, standardized process, and checklists. A forcing function is a very effective intervention for patient safety, as it does not rely on human memory or vigilance. A forcing function is an aspect of a design that prevents a target action from being performed. Examples are:

- Computer system that does not allow a drug to be ordered at a dose outside known safety parameters

- Enteral tubing designed to prevent accidental connections with IV ports

Measurements of quality include structure, process, outcomes, and balancing measures.

- **Structure** refers to equipment, resources, or infrastructure (e.g., number of ICU beds, certified infectious disease specialist on staff, ratio of nurses to patients)

- **Process measures** relate to an action involved in the care of patients that is believed to be associated with a particular outcome (e.g., use of preoperative antibiotics to reduce surgical site infections, using 2 means of patient identification prior to blood transfusion).

  - Typically easier to measure than outcome measures, and often serve as surrogates to outcomes

- **Outcome measures** reflect results related directly to the patient (e.g., survival, infection rates, number of admissions for heart failure)

- **Balancing measures** monitor for unintended consequences of a change or intervention made to a process or system. Some well-intended interventions can create unanticipated negative results in quality and safety.

  - For example, alarms have been placed on a number of medical devices and equipment to alert for problems (e.g., oxygen saturation falling below a set level). One negative result has been 'alarm fatigue.' Studies indicate that 85–99% of hospital alarms do not require clinical attention, but failure to respond to the rare critical alarm has resulted in patient death. This is a type of 'boy who cried wolf' phenomenon, where the frequency and prevalence of hospital alarms reduce our attention to them. Strategies are in place to customize alarms to alleviate some of the problem.

Quality models are specific techniques used in improving patient care.

PDSA (plan-do-study-act) refers to a rapid cycle of activities involved in achieving process or system improvement. It is a form of trial and error and consists of planning an intervention, trying it out (i.e., small scale pilot), observing results (e.g., data collection of quality measures), and acting on what is learned (e.g., implement change system-wide or go back to the planning stage with a new intervention).

Six Sigma is a data-driven, patient-centered approach focused on reducing variability. This organized and systematic method for strategic process improvement uses a step-by-step DMAIC method.

- **Define**: define the problem

- **Measure**: measure key quality metric

- **Analyze**: identify root causes

- **Improve**: determine optimal solutions

- **Control**: strive for sustainability of implemented change

Lean process focuses on removing waste from the process or system and adopting a value-added philosophy of patient care. Value-stream maps are created to optimize activities that add value from the patient's point-of-view and remove activities that do not.

The following are steps that any health care practitioner can apply to improve safety and quality for patients.

- Follow safety protocols (e.g., hand washing)
- Speak up when there are safety concerns (e.g., medical errors and near misses)
- Practice good communication skills (e.g., SBAR)
- Educate patients about their care
- Take care of yourself (e.g., get appropriate sleep and control stress)
- Practice patient-centered care/recognize opportunities to enhance value for patients

CARE WELL DONE

The case below describes the incredible potential of the health care system. Applying the principles of patient safety and quality improvement to clinical care will enable health care to move closer to the goal of getting it right for every patient, every time.

A 3-year-old girl falls into an icy fishpond in a small Austrian town in the Alps. She is lost beneath the surface for 30 minutes before her parents find her on the pond bottom and pull her up. CPR is started immediately by the parents on instruction from an emergency physician over the phone, and EMS arrives within 8 minutes. The girl has a body temperature of 36° C and no pulse. Her pupils are dilated and do not react to light. A helicopter takes the patient to a nearby hospital, where she is wheeled directly to an operating room. A surgical team puts her on a heart-lung bypass machine, her body temperature increases almost 10 degrees, and her heart begins to beat. Over the next few days her body temperature continues to rise to normal and her organs start to recover. While she suffered extensive neurologic deficits during this event, by age 5 with the help of extensive outpatient therapy, she recovers completely and is like any other little girl her age.

CHAPTER SUMMARY

- Medical errors result from the complexity of health care combined with the reality of human failure. Although accountability and responsibility are important, simply blaming people for errors they did not intend to commit does not address underlying failures in the system and is an ineffective way of improving safety.
- System-based redesigns in health care delivery are required and hold the greatest potential for advancing patient safety and quality improvement.
- Improving communication, teamwork and the culture of safety are effective methods in improving patient safety.
- Safety is a team effort requiring everyone on the care team to work in partnership with one another and with patients and families.

High Yield Facts

- Systems-based approaches to improving health care are superior to individual-level efforts or blame

- Preoperative checklists can prevent perioperative complications and safety events

- Evidence-based bundles (protocols) prevent central line infection

- Limiting the duration of urinary catheters decreased hospital acquired infections

- Head-of-bed elevation and oral care prevent ventilator associate pneumonia

- Medication reconciliation helps to prevent medication errors during transitions

- Hand hygiene is an important component of infection control

- Avoid the use of hazardous abbreviations

- Computerized physician order entry helps improve medication safety

- Identification of high risk patients is a key step in fall prevention

- Team training and communication can improve quality and safety

PRACTICE QUESTIONS

1. A 36-year-old woman with HIV/AIDS and B-cell lymphoma is hospitalized for *Clostridium difficile*–associated diarrhea. Following treatment, the patient is discharged home with a prescription for a 14-day course of oral vancomycin. She is unable to fill the prescription at her local pharmacy because of a problem with her insurance coverage. While awaiting coverage approval, she receives no treatment. Her symptoms soon return, prompting an emergency department visit where she is diagnosed with toxic megacolon. Which of the following should be addressed in order to bring about changes that improve patient safety?

    A. Prescribing physician

    B. Pharmacist

    C. Insurance company

    D. Patient

    E. Discontinuity of care

The correct answer is choice E. The main failure in this case occurred upon transition of care from the hospital to home. Addressing the discontinuities in care which arise at the time of transition has the greatest potential to improve patient safety.

Rather than dispensing blame to any of the parties involved in the error (**choices A–D**), focus should be given to implementing systems-based transformations to support patients during a transition (e.g., post-discharge telephone follow-up to identify and resolve potential medication issues early).

2. A 23-year-old man with a history of depression is admitted to the inpatient psychiatry ward after his third attempt at suicide with an intentional drug overdose. The patient is stabilized medically; however, he is put under 24-hour monitoring by the nursing staff due to repeated attempts at self-harm. During a change of shift, there is a mistake in communication and no one is assigned to the patient. The mistake is noticed 15 minutes into the new shift, and a member of the nursing team is assigned to watch the patient. Fortunately, during that 15-minute period, the patient made no attempt to harm himself. Which of the following statements is correct about this event?

    A. This is a sentinel event and should be reported to the medical board.

    B. This is a sentinel event and should be reported to the hospital and family.

    C. This is a near-miss and should be reported to the hospital.

    D. This is a near-miss and should be reported to the patient and family.

    E. This is a near-miss and no reporting is required since the patient was not harmed.

The correct answer is choice C. The event described is a near-miss; there was an error which fortunately did not result in patient harm. Most near-misses need not be disclosed to patients or families (**choice D**), but they should be reported to the hospital so that the error can be studied and thus prevented in the future. A sentinel event (**choices A and B**) is an adverse event resulting in serious or permanent injury to a patient.

3. An 85-year-old woman is being transferred to an acute rehabilitation facility following a hospital admission for hip replacement surgery. Postoperatively during her hospital stay, she is started on deep vein thrombosis (DVT) prophylaxis medication with plans to continue the medication upon discharge. The intern and nurse who are discharging the patient fail to convey this new medication to the receiving treatment team at the rehabilitation center. The patient is not continued on her anticoagulation medication and sustains a DVT, leading to a fatal pulmonary embolus 3 weeks after transfer. Which of the following actions will facilitate quality improvement and the prevention of a similar error in the future?

    A. Determine which staff member(s) failed to order the medication

    B. Develop a process to increase the use of medication reconciliation

    C. Send a memo to all staff about the importance of DVT prophylaxis

    D. Educate patients about the dangers of DVT following hip surgery

    E. Conduct monthly audits to monitor medication errors at transitions of care

The correct answer is choice B. The goal of quality improvement (QI) is to achieve improvement by measuring the current status of care and then developing systems-based approaches to making things better. It involves both prospective and retrospective reviews and specifically attempts to avoid attributing blame. QI seeks to create systems to prevent errors from happening. In this case, developing a process to increase the use of medication reconciliation would be following the principles of QI. The other interventions in the answer choices are QA-based and/or simply not as effective in creating and sustaining a positive change. Quality assurance (QA) is an older term describing a process that is reactive and retrospective in nature; it is a form of 'policing' to ensure that quality standards have been followed. It often relies on audits and traditionally has focused on punitive actions for failures in quality, i.e., determining who was at fault after something goes wrong. QA has not proven to be very effective in transforming care.

Population Health Management

9

DEFINING POPULATION HEALTH

What is population health?

> **Case example:** A 65-year-old woman presents to the emergency department at 3:00 AM with the acute onset of an asthma attack. She is treated with steroids and nebulizer treatments to stabilize her respiratory status. This is the third such presentation in the past 9 months. During her course of treatment it becomes evident that the patient is not able to get time off from work to see her primary care physician during clinic hours, did not receive an influenza vaccination this year, and continues to smoke 1 pack of cigarettes per day.
>
> - What day-to-day factors are present that impact this patient's health outcomes with asthma?
>
> - How would you help to optimize her long-term management of asthma?

Health care in the United States has traditionally focused on the management of acute medical problems such as trauma, myocardial infarction, and stroke. Incredible advances have been made in these areas and outcomes from acute presentation of disease have steadily improved over the years, with outcomes among some of the best observed in any health system in the world.

However, the health care system here has lagged significantly in the area of disease prevention and health maintenance. Major disparities in access to preventative care services such as prenatal care, cancer screening, and diabetes management; together with social inequalities with respect to patient education and income; as well as persistent individual behaviors such as poor diet, lack of exercise and cigarette smoking have contributed to the very poor overall health status observed in the United States.

BIG GEMS (mnemonic for determinants of health)

- Behavior

- Income

- Genetics

- Geography

- Environment

- Medical care

- Social-cultural

Problems with patient safety and variations in care that do not follow evidence-based standards further erode the value of patient care. Ironically, the United States spends more on health care than any other nation in the world, yet ranks among the lowest in health measures, compared to other developed nations. Furthermore, the current rate of health care spending in the United States is unsustainable.

Population health is an approach to health care which addresses both individual and public health concerns in order to achieve optimal patient results. It is an approach to patient care which understands that health is influenced by several factors outside of traditional health care delivery models, including (but not limited to) social, economic, and environmental factors.

Population health management is fundamental to the transformation of health care delivery. Its principles recognize the importance of focusing attention not only on improving individual patient care, but also on improving the health of an entire population. In fact, direct health care accounts for only a small proportion of premature deaths in the United States.

- For example, the leading causes of premature death—smoking (435,000 deaths/year), obesity (400,000 deaths/year), and alcohol abuse (85,000 deaths/year)—are all preventable through interventions driven by population health management.

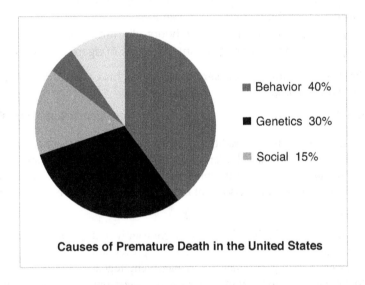

Causes of Premature Death in the United States

Population health management is, in effect, about coordinating care and improving access in order to enhance patient/family engagement and reduce variation in care to achieve better long-term outcomes at a reduced cost. The Institute for Healthcare Improvement (IHI) lists improving the health of the population as one of the 3 dimensions of its Triple Aim approach to optimizing health system performance.

IHI Triple Aim:

- Improve the patient experience of care (including quality and satisfaction)
- **Improve the health of populations**
- Reduce the per capita cost of health care

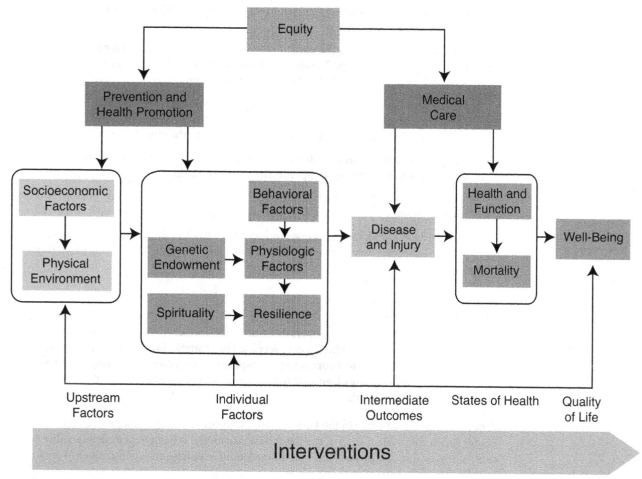

Source: Adapted from Stiefel M. Nolan KA. Guide to Measuring the Triple Aim: Population Health, Experience of Care, and Per Capita Cost. IHI Innovation Series white paper. Cambridge, Massachusetts: Institute for Healthcare Improvement; 2012. (Available on IHI.org)

IHI Population Health Composite Model

Population health management focuses on high-risk patients who are responsible for the majority of health care utilization while simultaneously addressing preventative and chronic care needs of the entire population. One of the first steps in this process is to define the target population (e.g., a hospital or clinic's entire service area or any subset, whether economic, geographic or demographic, or individuals with certain health conditions). Another important step is to identify the specific health status and needs of that group and deploy interventions and prevention strategies to improve the health of the group. The interventions target individuals, but they affect the entire population.

The incorporation of technology (e.g., electronic health records) and innovations in health care (e.g., digital home health monitoring) provide the infrastructure to support efforts in successful population health management. A key factor for the success of population health programs is automation, as managing populations can be highly complex. Technology-enabled solutions are essential to the efficient management of a program.

Let's say a primary care clinic is interested in improving population health for its diabetic patients.

- First, the clinic analyzes the patient registry generated by its electronic health records to identify high-risk type 2 diabetic patients who are not compliant with their medication and who frequently fail to keep their clinic appointments.

- Next, those patients are offered enrollment in a home hemoglobin A1C monitoring program, using a system which digitally records hemoglobin A1C levels taken in the home and then electronically transfers the results to the clinic.

- The system sends an alert to the clinical team when patients' hemoglobin A1C levels are consistently higher than a predetermined threshold.

- A nurse coordinator contacts these patients by phone to help manage medication compliance, answer patient questions, and encourage timely follow-up with clinic visits.

- A nutritionist works with patients to encourage healthy dietary choices, while a social worker addresses any financial constraints to following medical recommendations.

VALUE-BASED CARE

The traditional health care system operates under a **fee-for-service model**, where a fee is collected for each provision of health care service. For example, hospitals and physicians collect a fee each time a patient comes to the hospital for the treatment of congestive heart failure (CHF), including any diagnostic tests or procedures (e.g., chest x-ray, B-type natriuretic peptide, cardiac angiogram).

A new model of health care in the United States, supported by legislation, is accountable care. Under the Accountable Care Act, the fee-for-service model is being replaced with **value-based care**, where health care professionals are rewarded for keeping entire populations of patients healthy.

Using the CHF example, a value-based system would reward health care professionals for encouraging lifestyle changes that prevent hospital admissions for CHF, such as promoting a heart healthy diet, monitoring home fluid intake, and motivating patients to engage in regular exercise. Instead of rewarding exclusively for the treatment of acute medical problems, the new system provides incentives for the health care system to maintain healthy populations, prevent disease, and avoid acute medical problems through the active monitoring and management of chronic disease. **Quality in health care is measured by outcomes achieved**, rather than the *volume* of services delivered.

Note: Value in patient care can be defined as quality of care divided by total cost of care.

Strategies that increase quality and reduce unnecessary costs result in improved value for patients. Unnecessary costs may be generated from the following examples:

- Duplication of services (e.g., a surgeon orders a routine pre-operative ECG for a patient undergoing elective surgery, not realizing the same test was done 1 week ago in the primary care physician's office and was normal)

- Non evidence-based care (e.g., ordering antibiotics for a viral infection)

- Avoidable inefficiencies in care (e.g., a patient returns to the hospital with acute CHF 1 week after being treated for the same condition because he was unaware that a new diuretic had been started in the hospital and was therefore never filled upon discharge)

Failures in preventive health also lead to avoidable health care spending, as in hospitalization for the treatment of acute pneumonia in a patent who did not receive an influenza vaccination. Shifting the focus from volume of care to value of care will improve the overall status of health care in the United States and contain the currently unsustainable costs of care.

It is important **not to confuse value-based care** with **rationing of care**, which seeks to reduce needed services in order to preserve resources. Value-based care seeks to reduce unnecessary or unwanted waste in care which increases cost without increasing quality of care to the patient.

- Studies, for instance, have shown that performing stress cardiac imaging or advanced non-invasive imaging in patients without symptoms on a serial or scheduled pattern (e.g., every 1–2 years or at a heart procedure anniversary) rarely results in any meaningful change in patient management. This practice may, in fact, lead to unnecessary invasive procedures and excess radiation exposure without any proven impact on patients' outcomes.
  - An exception to this rule would be for patients >5 years after a bypass operation.
- Similarly, using antibiotics for a sore throat or runny nose that is due to a viral infection not only provides no immediate benefit to the patient, it may also increase harm from adverse drug reactions or development of antibiotic resistant bacterial strains.

Many health care organizations are developing guidelines and recommendations to promote value-based care. These approaches motivate patients and their clinicians to follow effective care practices and guide them away from unnecessary and ineffective care; the result is greater value and effectiveness of healthcare utilization. For example, Choosing Wisely™ (choosingwisely.org) is a national initiative of the American Board of Internal Medicine Foundation which promotes conversations between patients and physicians about unnecessary medical tests/procedures that increase cost without enhancing patient outcomes.

Population health management employs value-based care principles by promoting preventive care, encouraging care patterns that have been proven effective, and reducing waste and unnecessary care.

Value equation in health care:

$$\uparrow value = \frac{\uparrow quality}{\downarrow cost}$$

IMPLEMENTATION OF POPULATION HEALTH MANAGEMENT

The goal of population health management is to keep a patient population as healthy as possible. The components required to achieve this goal include the following:

- Delivery of patient care through multidisciplinary teams

- Coordination of care across care settings

- Increased access to primary care

- Patient education in disease self-management

- Emphasis on health behaviors and lifestyle choices

- Meaningful use of health information technology for data analysis, clinical communication, and outcome measurement

This requires clinicians to identify target populations of patients who may benefit from additional services, such as patients who require reminders for preventative care appointments or patients not meeting management goals. Continual access to patient data and analysis of outcomes is the key to providing proactive, preventive care.

Steps in Population Health Management

Step 1: Define population

Step 2: Identify care gaps

Step 3: Stratify risks

Step 4: Engage patients

Step 5: Manage care

Step 6: Measure outcomes

Several advances in technology are required to perform effective population health management and accomplish risk stratification; identify gaps in care; achieve patient education, compliance education, disease state monitoring; ensure general wellness; as well as to implement and assess specific interventions targeted to selected populations.

- The electronic health record can produce integrated, accessible population-wide data systems capable of generating reports that drive effective quality and care management processes.

- Web-based tools designed to educate patients about their condition, promote self-care, and encourage preventative behaviors have been used successfully to reduce hospitalization rates by enabling patients to take charge of their health.

- Telemedicine programs have been implemented to establish remote care in order to facilitate patient outreach, allow patient follow-up after discharge from the hospital, and improve health care in rural populations.

- The automation of processes and programs is essential in order to make population health management feasible, scalable, and sustainable, such as a health IT system which targets patients in greatest need of services, generates alerts to those patients seeking appropriate and timely appointments with clinicians, and alerts clinicians in real-time to patient care needs.

However, technology alone will not be sufficient for population health management; effective **teamwork** in patient care is also important. Effective population health involves establishing multidisciplinary care teams to coordinate care throughout the entire continuum of care. High-performance clinical care teams can manage a greater number of patients and more comprehensively respond to patient care needs compared with individual clinicians working in isolation. Care teams can include physicians, nurses, nurse practitioners, physician assistants, pharmacists, patient navigators, medical assistants, dieticians, physical therapists, social workers, and care managers, and others.

The **patient-centered medical home (PCMH)** is one emerging model used to deliver patient-centered, value-based care, and it plays an important role in population health management. The medical home model emphasizes care coordination and communication beyond episodic care in order to transform primary care. It stresses prevention, early intervention and close partnerships with patients to tightly manage chronic conditions and maintain health. The PCMH is not necessarily a physical place, but rather an organizational model that delivers the core functions of primary health care. Key principles in this model include:

- Access to a personal physician who leads the care team within a medical practice
- Adoption of a whole-person orientation to providing patient care
- Integrated and coordinated care
- Focus on quality and safety

The medical home is intended to result in more personalized, coordinated, effective and efficient care. Many of the goals of PCMH directly support efforts in population health.

In 2006, the Massachusetts General Hospital (MGH) worked with the U.S. Centers for Medicare and Medicaid to establish 1 of 6 population health demonstration projects nationwide. During the 3-year demonstration, the MGH implemented strategies to improve health care delivery to its most vulnerable high risk patients—those with multiple health conditions and chronic disease. The hospital system took steps to address the needs of 2,500 of their highest-risk patients.

- Each patient was assigned to a comprehensive care team consisting of a primary care physician, experienced nurse case manager, social worker, and pharmacist.
- A non-clinical community resource specialist was employed to work with the care teams in addressing non-clinical factors influencing health outcomes (for example, if the patient was not able to come to the primary care office for a scheduled visit because of transportation issues, this specialist connected the patient to local transportation resources).

This structure of care allowed clinicians to focus the majority of their time on patients' medical needs. The results revealed a decrease in hospital readmissions by 20% and a decrease in emergency room visits by 13% for the patients enrolled in the program. Satisfaction was extremely high among both patients and caregivers, and the system was associated with significant cost-savings. This is one example of using population health to increase quality while decreasing costs, thereby increasing value in patient care.

CHAPTER SUMMARY

- Population health management is an important strategy for improving the quality of patient outcomes, containing costs, and promoting health maintenance.

- Successful population health management requires data-driven clinical decision-making, transformations in primary care leadership, meaningful use of health technology and patient-family engagement.

- Accountable care involves an integrated, proactive approach to improving the quality of health in identified patient populations.

High Yield Topics

- Understanding and managing population risk (e.g., identifying care gaps)

- Care teams coordinating home health between clinic visits, as well as during clinic encounters

- Informatics: sharing information seamlessly with EHR and patient portals

- Engaging patients in health maintenance: screening, prevention and behavioral health

- Measuring outcomes

- Reducing waste in the system (e.g., duplication, non-value added interventions)

- Improving chronic care: keeping patients out of hospital (optimize home and outpatient care)

KEY DEFINITIONS

- **Care cycle**: array of health services and care settings which address health promotion, disease prevention, and the diagnosis, treatment, management, and rehabilitation of disease, injury, and disability

- **Clinical care pathway**: integrated, multidisciplinary outline of anticipated care placed in an appropriate timeframe to help patients with a specific condition/set of symptoms move progressively through a clinical experience to positive outcomes

- **Clinical outcome**: end result of a medical intervention, such as survival or improved health

- **Clinical variation**: variation in the utilization of health care services that cannot be explained by variation in patient illness or patient preferences (Wennberg JH 2010)

- **Continuum of care**: concept involving an integrated system of care which guides and tracks patients over time through a comprehensive array of health services spanning all levels of intensity of care

- **Cost-effectiveness analysis**: analytic tool in which the costs and effects of at least 1 alternative are calculated and presented, as in a ratio of incremental cost to incremental effect; the effects are health outcomes (e.g., cases of disease prevented, years of life gained, or quality-adjusted life years) rather than monetary measures (e.g., cost-benefit analysis) (Gold et al. 1996)

- **Evidenced-based medicine**: applying the best available research results (evidence) when making decisions about health care

- Health care professionals who perform evidence-based practice use research evidence, along with clinical expertise and patient preferences. Systematic reviews (summaries of health care research results) provide information that aids in the process of evidence-based practice.

  ○ For example, a health care provider recommends acetaminophen to treat arthritis pain in a patient who has recently had stomach bleeding. The health care provider makes this recommendation because research shows that acetaminophen is associated with less risk for stomach bleeds than other common pain relievers. The health care provider's recommendation is an example of evidence-based practice.

- **Health**: a state of complete physical, mental and social well-being, and not merely the absence of disease or infirmity (WHO definition)

- **Health inequity**: those inequalities in health deemed to be unfair or to stem from some form of injustice; the dimensions of being avoidable or unnecessary have often been added to this concept (Kawachi, Subramanian, and Almeida-Filho 2002)

- **Health-related quality of life**: impact of the health aspects of an individual's life on his quality of life or overall well-being (Gold et al. 1996)

- **Intervention**: any type of treatment, preventive care, or test that a person could take or undergo to improve health or to help with a particular problem

  - Health care interventions include drugs (prescription drugs or drugs that can be bought without a prescription), foods, supplements (such as vitamins), vaccinations, screening tests (to rule out a certain disease), exercises (to improve fitness), hospital treatment, and certain kinds of care (such as physical therapy).

- **Life expectancy**: average amount of time a person will live after a certain starting point, such as birth or the diagnosis of a disease

  - The calculation is based on statistical information comparing people with similar characteristics, such as age, gender, ethnicity, and health. In the United States, for example, the life expectancy from birth for men and women combined is 78.1 years. In England, it is 78.7, and in China it is 72.9 years.

- **Patient-centered**: approach to patient care that focuses on the priorities, preferences, and best interests of the patient

  - It is a partnership among practitioners, patients, and their families to ensure that (a) decisions respect patients' wants, needs, and preferences and (b) patients have the education and support needed to make decisions and participate in their own care.

- **Patient centered medical home**: care delivery model whereby patient treatment is coordinated through the primary care physician to ensure that the patient receives the necessary care when and where she needs it, in a manner she can understand

  - The goal is to have a centralized setting that facilitates partnerships between individual patients, their personal physician, and when appropriate, their family. Care is facilitated by registries, information technology, health information exchange, and other means to ensure that patients get optimal care.

- **Population**: any group of individuals for whom consideration of health or health care at the level of the group is likely to advance health

- **Population health**: health of a population as measured by health status indicators, and as influenced by social, economic, and physical environments; personal health practices; individual capacity and coping skills; human biology; early childhood development; and health services (Dunn and Hayes 1999)

- **Public health**: activities that a society undertakes to assure the conditions in which people can be healthy; these include organized community efforts to prevent, identify, and counter threats to the health of the public (Turnock 2004)

- **Quality of life**: a broad construct reflecting a subjective or objective judgment concerning all aspects of an individual's existence, including health, economic, political, cultural, environmental, aesthetic, and spiritual aspects (Gold, Stevenson, and Fryback 2002)

- **Quality measure**: clinical quality measures (CQMs) are a mechanism for assessing observations, treatment, processes, experience, and/or outcomes of patient care

  - In other words, CQMs assess "the degree to which a provider competently and safely delivers clinical services that are appropriate for the patient in an optimal timeframe.

- **Registry**: organized system which uses observational study methods to collect uniform data (clinical and other) to evaluate specified outcomes for a population defined by a particular disease, condition, or exposure, and that serves 1 or more predetermined scientific, clinical, or policy purposes

- **Risk factor**: aspect of personal behavior/lifestyle, environmental exposure, or inborn/ inherited characteristic that, on the basis of epidemiologic evidence, is known to be associated with health-related condition(s) considered important to prevent. (Last 2001)

- **Screening:** using tests or other methods of diagnosis to find out whether a person has a specific disease/condition before it causes any symptoms

  - For many diseases (e.g., cancers), starting treatment earlier leads to better results. The purpose of screening is to find the disease so that treatment can be started as early as possible. For example, a breast exam and mammogram are both screening tests used to find small breast cancers.

- **Social determinant**: proposed or established causal factor in the social environment which affects health outcomes (e.g., income, education, occupation, class, social support)

- **Target population**: entire service area or any subset, whether economic, geographic, or demographic, or individuals with certain health conditions

- **Upstream determinants**: features of the social environment, such as socioeconomic status and discrimination that influence individual behavior, disease, and health status

REVIEW QUESTIONS

1. A 59-year-old man with a history of type 2 diabetes is diagnosed with diabetic retinopathy and referred to ophthalmology for additional management. The patient's primary care physician is interested in reducing the number of patients in the practice who develop similar long-term complications from type 2 diabetes mellitus. Which one of the following is the most important next step?

   A. Develop an intervention to monitor blood glucose levels for all patients in the practice

   B. Utilize the patient registry to identify high-risk patients comprising the target population

   C. Train staff in the clinic to identify early signs of retinopathy

   D. Request to have an ophthalmologist perform fundoscopic exams on all patients in the practice

   E. Place a sign in the office depicting the dangers of diabetes

The correct answer is B. One of the first steps in designing a population health management program is to define the target population and identify common risk factors or gaps in care. Ideally, this should be done prior to implementing any intervention, so that it is clear which patients have the greatest need for the intervention and what risk factor(s) the intervention should address.

- Monitoring blood glucose for all patients, even those without diabetes or not at risk for diabetes, may not be a practical use of resources.

- Training staff to identify retinopathy or having an ophthalmologist perform fundoscopic exams will identify patients who already have long-term complications, rather than adjusting behaviors to prevent complications.

- A sign depicting the dangers of diabetes is not a proactive measure, does not optimally engage patients in self-care, and may only help those who are already in the clinic.

2. An 8-year-old boy is brought to the emergency department by his mother after he develops acute shortness of breath and wheezing. The boy appears anxious but is alert and responsive. He is afebrile and responds well to supplemental oxygen and initial respiratory treatment. He has a history of asthma and has presented with similar symptoms 4 times in the past 12 months. The mother smokes 1–2 packs of cigarettes per day while at home with her son. Which of the following addresses an upstream determinant of health amenable to population health management to improve the patient's long-term outcome?

   A. Rapid use of nebulizer treatments in the emergency department

   B. Administration of weight adjusted dose of steroid treatment

   C. Asking the mom to purchase an inhaler to keep at the home

   D. Parent education on second-hand smoking risk and enrollment in a smoking cessation program

   E. Prophylactic antibiotics

The correct answer is D. Educating parents about the risks of second-hand smoke to children—especially one with a history of asthma—and offering parents enrollment in a smoking-cessation program may have a dramatic benefit to the health of the child and help prevent future asthma attacks. Use of nebulizers or steroids in the emergency department may be necessary to treat the acute episode of care; however, it will not help prevent future attacks. The use of antibiotics without indications of bacterial infection (e.g., no fever) is not warranted.

PART VI

MEDICAL ABBREVIATIONS

Medical Abbreviations 10

4Q	4 quadrants
yo or y/o	year old
m	male
f	female
b	black
w	white
L	left
R	right
Hx	history
h/o	history of
c/o	complaining/complaints of
c	with
NL	normal limits
r/o	rule out
s	without
w/	with
Ø	without or no
+	positive
–	negative
A&0x3	alert & oriented to person, place, and time
AA	Alcoholics Anonymous
AAA	abdominal aortic aneurysm
abd	abdomen

ABG	arterial blood gas
AC	abdominal circumference
ACE	angiotensin-converting enzyme
ACTH	adrenocorticotropic hormone
ADH	antidiuretic hormone
AFB	acid-fast bacilli
AFI	amniotic fluid index
afib	atrial fibrillation
AIDS	acquired immune deficiency syndrome
Alb	albumin
ALP	alkaline phosphatase
ALS	amyotrophic lateral sclerosis
ANS	autonomic nervous system
ant	anterior
A&P	auscultation and percussion
ARDS	acute respiratory distress syndrome
AV	arteriovenous
AP	anteroposterior
ASA	aspirin
AST	aspartate transaminase
ALT	alanine transaminase
ANS	autonomic nervous system
b/l	bilateral
BID	twice a day
BM	bowel movement
BMI	body mass index
BP	blood pressure
BPD	biparietal diameter
BPH	benign prostatic hypertrophy
BPP	biophysical profile

BSA	body surface area
BUN	blood urea nitrogen
Ca	calcium
CA	cancer
CABG	coronary artery bypass grafting
CAD	coronary artery disease
cath	catheterization
CBC	complete blood count
cc	chief complaint
CCB	calcium channel blocker
CCU	cardiac care unit
CEA	carcinoembryonic antigen
CF	cystic fibrosis
chemo	chemotherapy
CHF	congestive heart failure
chol	cholesterol
Cl	chloride
CLL	chronic lymphocytic leukemia
CML	chronic myelogenous leukemia
CMV	cytomegalovirus
CN	cranial nerve
CNS	central nervous system
COPD	chronic obstructive pulmonary disease
CPAP	continuous positive airway pressure
CPK	creatine phosphokinase
CPR	cardiopulmonary resuscitation
Cr	creatinine
C&S, C/S	culture and sensitivity
CSF	cerebrospinal fluid
CST	contraction stress test

CT	computed tomography
CTA	clear to auscultation
CVA	cerebrovascular accident
CVP	central venous pressure
Cx	cervix
CXR	chest x-ray
D&C	dilatation and curettage
DI	diabetes insipidus
DM	diabetes mellitus
DSRP	daily record of severity of problems
DTR	deep tendon reflexes
DVT	deep vein thrombosis
dx	diagnosis
ECC	endocervical curettage
EKG/ECG	electrocardiogram
EEG	electroencephalogram
ED	emergency department
EGD	esophagogastroduodenoscopy
EMG	electromyogram
ENT	ears, nose, and throat
EOMI	extraocular muscles intact
ERCP	endoscopic retrograde cholangiopancreatography
ESR	erythrocyte sedimentation rate
EtOH	alcohol
ext	extremities
FBS	fasting blood sugar
Fe	iron
fFN	fetal fibronectin

FSH	follicle stimulating hormone
FH	family history
FUO	fever of unknown origin
Fx	fracture

GA	general appearance
GERD	gastroesophageal reflux disorder
GI	gastrointestinal
Glu	glucose
GnRH	gonadotropin-releasing hormone
GTT	glucose tolerance test
GU	genitourinary

HA	headache
HBsAg	hepatitis B surface antigen
HC	head circumference
Hct	hematocrit
HDN	hemolytic disease of the newborn
HEENT	head, eyes, ears, nose, and throat
Hgb	hemoglobin
HIV	human immunodeficiency virus
HOCM	hypertrophic cardiomyopathy
HRT	hormone replacement therapy
HPI	history of present illness
HR	heart rate
HSM	hepatosplenomegaly
HTN	hypertension

IBD	inflammatory bowel disease
IBS	irritable bowel syndrome
ICU	intensive care unit

IDDM	insulin-dependent diabetes mellitus
IM	intramuscularly
INR	international ratio
IUD	intrauterine device
IV	intravenously
JVD	jugular venous distension
JVP	jugular venous pressure
K	potassium
KUB	kidney, ureter, and bladder
LAD	lymphadenopathy or left anterior descending
LDH	lactate dehydrogenase
LE	lower extremity
LH	luteinizing hormone
LLL	left lower lobe
LLQ	left lower quadrant
LMP	last menstrual period
loc	loss of consciousness
LP	lumbar puncture
LUL	left upper lobe
LUQ	left upper quadrant
M, R, G	murmurs, rubs, or gallops
mets	metastases
MI	myocardial infarction
MRI	magnetic resonance imaging
MRSA	methicillin-resistant *Staphylococcus aureus*
MS	multiple sclerosis
MVP	mitral valve prolapse (cardiology) or maximum vertical pocket (obstetrics)

Na	sodium
NC/AT	normocephalic atraumatic
neuro	neurologic
NIDDM	non–insulin-dependent diabetes mellitus
NKA	no known allergies
NKDA	no known drug allergy
NPH	normal pressure hydrocephalus
NSR	normal sinus rhythm
NST	non-stress test
NSVD	normal spontaneous vaginal delivery
N/V	nausea and vomiting

occ	occasional
OCP	oral contraceptive pills
OD	right eye
OS	left eye
OTC	over-the-counter

PA	posteroanterior
PAN	polyarteritis nodosa
PCP	primary care provider
PCP	*Pneumocystis carinii* pneumonia
PE	physical examination
PE	pulmonary embolus
PEEP	positive end-expiratory pressure
PERRLA	pupils are equal, round, and reactive to light and accommodation
PET	positron emission tomography
PFTs	pulmonary function tests
PID	pelvic inflammatory disease
PMI	point of maximum impulse

po	orally
POC	products of conception
pos	positive
PPD	packs per day
PPD	purified protein derivative
PRN	as needed
PSA	prostatic specific antigen
PT	prothrombin time
PTSD	post-traumatic stress disorder
PTT	partial prothrombin time
PUD	peptic ulcer disease
PVD	peripheral vascular disease
RA	rheumatoid arthritis
RBC	red blood cells
RDS	respiratory distress syndrome
RLL	right lower lobe
RLQ	right lower quadrant
RMG	rubs, murmurs, or gallops
ROM	range of motion
RR	respiratory rate
RRR	regular rate and rhythm
RUL	right upper lobe
RUQ	right upper quadrant
SBO	small bowel obstruction
SCFE	slipped capital femoral epiphysis
SERM	selective estrogen receptor modulator
SH	social history
SLE	systemic lupus erythematosus
SLR	straight leg raising

sob	shortness of breath
SQ	subcutaneous
Staph	staphylococcus
STD	sexually transmitted disease
Strep	streptococcus
SAB	subarachnoid bleed
T	temperature
T1DM	type 1 diabetes mellitus
T2DM	type 2 diabetes mellitus
TB	tuberculosis
TIA	transient ischemic attack
TSH	thyroid stimulating hormone
TURP	transurethral prostatectomy
TVF	tactile vocal fremitus
U/A	urinalysis
UE	upper extremity
UGI	upper gastrointestinal
URI	upper respiratory tract infection
U/S	ultrasound
UTI	urinary tract infection
vag	vaginal
VAS	vibroacoustic stimulation (vibration and sound)
VCUG	voiding cystourethrogram
VDRL	Venereal Disease Research Laboratory
vs	vital signs
WBC	white blood cells
wks	weeks
WNL	within normal limits
wt	weight